1571

REVIEWS OF UNITED KINGDOM STATISTICAL SOURCES

Volume IX

HEALTH SURVEYS
AND
RELATED STUDIES

REVIEWS OF UNITED KINGDOM STATISTICAL SOURCES

Editor W. F. Maunder

Volume I
1. *Personal Social Services*, B. P. Davies
2. *Voluntary Organizations in the Personal Social Service Field*, G. J. Murray

Volume II
3. *Central Government Routine Health Statistics*, Michael Alderson
4. *Social Security Statistics*, Frank Whitehead

Volume III
5. *Housing in Great Britain*, Stuart Farthing
6. *Housing in Northern Ireland*, Michael Fleming

Volume IV
7. *Leisure*, F. M. M. Lewes and S. R. Parker
8. *Tourism*, L. J. Lickorish

Volume V
9. *General Sources of Statistics*, G. F. Lock

Volume VI
10. *Wealth*, A. B. Atkinson and A. J. Harrison
11. *Personal Income*, T. Stark

Volume VII
12. *Road Passenger Transport*, D. Munby
13. *Road Goods Transport*, A. H. Watson

Volume VIII
14. *Land Use*, J. T. Coppock
15. *Town and Country Planning*, L. F. Gebbett

REVIEWS OF UNITED KINGDOM STATISTICAL SOURCES

Edited by W. F. MAUNDER

Professor of Economic and Social Statistics
University of Exeter

VOLUME IX

HEALTH SURVEYS AND RELATED STUDIES

by

MICHAEL ALDERSON

Professor of Epidemiology
Institute of Cancer Research
London University

and

ROBIN DOWIE

Research Fellow
Health Services Research Unit
University of Kent

Published for

The Royal Statistical Society and
the Social Science Research Council

by

PERGAMON PRESS

OXFORD · NEW YORK · TORONTO · SYDNEY · PARIS · FRANKFURT

U.K.	Pergamon Press Ltd., Headington Hill Hall, Oxford OX3 0BW, England
U.S.A.	Pergamon Press Inc., Maxwell House, Fairview Park, Elmsford, New York 10523, U.S.A.
CANADA	Pergamon of Canada, Suite 104, 150 Consumers Road, Willowdale, Ontario M2 J1P9, Canada
AUSTRALIA	Pergamon Press (Aust.) Pty. Ltd., P.O. Box 544, Potts Point, N.S.W. 2011, Australia
FRANCE	Pergamon Press SARL, 24 rue des Ecoles, 75240 Paris, Cedex 05, France
FEDERAL REPUBLIC OF GERMANY	Pergamon Press GmbH, 6242 Kronberg-Taunus, Pferdstrasse 1, Federal Republic of Germany

First published 1979

British Library Cataloguing in Publication Data

Reviews of United Kingdom statistical sources. Vol. 9.
Health surveys and related studies.
1. Great Britain—Statistical services
I. Maunder, Wynne Frederick   II. Alderson, Michael
III. Dowie, Robin   IV. Royal Statistical Society
V. Social Science Research Council. Great Britain
314.1   HA37.G7   78–40963
ISBN 0–08–022459–8

For bibliographical purposes this volume should be cited as:
Alderson, M. R. and Dowie, R., *Health Surveys and Related Studies*, Pergamon Press Ltd. on behalf of the Royal Statistical Society
and the Social Science Research Council, 1979

Set, printed and bound in Great Britain by Cox & Wyman Ltd., London, Fakenham and Reading

VOLUME CONTENTS

Foreword　　　vii

Introduction to Volume IX　　　ix

Review No. 16: Health Surveys and Related Studies　　　1

Subject Index to Health Surveys and Related Studies　　　349

FOREWORD

The Sources and Nature of the Statistics of the United Kingdom, produced under the auspices of the Royal Statistical Society and edited by Maurice Kendall, filled a notable gap on the library shelves when it made its appearance in the early post-war years. Through a series of critical reviews by many of the foremost national experts, it constituted a valuable contemporary guide to statisticians working in many fields as well as a benchmark to which historians of the development of Statistics in this country are likely to return again and again. The Social Science Research Council and the Society were both delighted when Professor Maunder came forward with the proposal that a revised version should be produced, indicating as well his willingness to take on the onerous task of editor. The two bodies were more than happy to act as co-sponsors of the project and to help in its planning through a joint steering committee. The result, we are confident, will be adjudged a worthy successor to the previous volumes by the very much larger 'statistics public' that has come into being in the intervening years.

<table>
<tr><td>

Dr C. S. Smith

Secretary
Social Science Research Council

March 1978

</td><td>

R. F. A. Hopes

Honorary Secretary
Royal Statistical Society

March 1978

</td></tr>
</table>

INTRODUCTION

At the seminar which considered Professor Alderson's first review on Central Government Routine Health Statistics, and in later discussions among those interested, the idea was bruited that there was a certain amount of material which ought properly to be covered by the series but did not fall within the precise limits of the initial brief. Indeed, the suggestion began to emerge that there was likely to be enough additional material to justify a further separate, if perhaps brief, review. Although Professor Alderson was aware that, by contrast with his first assignment, the gap to be filled had somewhat vague boundaries, he began by thinking of it as a 'supplement' and certainly nobody else with whom I was in contact warned me of the formidably vast extent of the material that might be covered. That this was the case became apparent no doubt to the authors as soon as serious work started, but the ultimately gargantuan proportions of the undertaking were somewhat slower in dawning on me.

The boundary of the commitment was particularly ill-defined with regard to the 'soft data' area of medical care delivery, making this aspect especially sensitive to nice judgement; it was by a happy turn of circumstances that Professor Alderson was able to recruit Mrs Robin Dowie as co-author with a special interest on this side. The end result can hardly fail to meet the expectations of those who advanced and approved the suggestion at the first seminar; the statistical sources on the social aspects of health and health care would seem now to be reasonably completely documented. A basic problem throughout, of course, has been to determine the proper boundary of the latter with general medical literature and it is to be hoped that the decisions made will turn out to be satisfactory to users.

The primary aim of this series is to act as a work of reference to the sources of statistical material of all kinds, both official and unofficial. It seeks to enable the user to discover what data are available on the subject in which he is interested, from where they may be obtained, and what the limitations are to their use. Data are regarded as available not only if published in the normal printed format but also if they are likely to be released to a *bona fide* enquirer in any other form, such as duplicated documents, computer print-out or even magnetic tape. On the other hand, no reference is made to material which, even if it is known to exist, is not accessible to the general run of potential users. The distinction, of course, is not clear-cut and mention of a source is not to be regarded as a guarantee that data will be released; in particular cases it may very well be a matter for negotiation. The latter caution applies with particular force to the question of obtaining computer print-outs of custom-specified tabulations. Where original records are held on magnetic tape it might appear that there should be no insuperable problem, apart from confidentiality, in obtaining any feasible analysis at a cost; in practice, it may well turn out that there are capacity restraints which override any simple cost calculation. Thus, what is requested might make demands on computer and programming resources to the extent that the routine work of the agency concerned would be intolerably affected.

The intention is that the sources for each topic should be reviewed in detail, and the brief supplied to authors has called for comprehensive coverage at the level of 'national interest'. This term does not denote any necessary restriction to statistics collected on a national basis (still less, of course, to national aggregates) but it means that sources of a purely local character, without wider interest in either content or methodology, are excluded. Indeed, the mere task of identifying all material of this latter kind is an impossibility. The interpretation of the brief has obviously involved discretion and it is up to the users of these reviews to say what unreasonable gaps become apparent to them. They are cordially invited to do so by communicating with me.

To facilitate the use of the series as a work of reference, certain features have been incorporated which are worth a word or two of explanation.

First, the text of each review is designed, in so far as varying subject matter permits, to follow a standard form of arrangement so that users may expect a similar pattern to be followed throughout the series. The starting-point is a brief summary of the activity concerned and its organization, in order to give a clear background understanding of how data are collected, what is being measured, the stage at which measurements are made, what the reporting units are, the channels through which returns are routed and where they are processed. As a further part of this introductory material, there is a discussion of the specific problems of definition and measurement to which the topic gives rise. The core sections on available sources which follow are arranged at the author's discretion—by origin, by subject subdivision, or by type of data; there is too much heterogeneity between topics to permit any imposition of complete uniformity on all authors. The final section is devoted to a discussion of general shortcomings and possibly desirable improvements. In case a contrary expectation should be aroused, it should be said that authors have not been asked to produce a comprehensive plan for the reform of statistical reporting in the whole of their field. However, a review of existing sources is a natural opportunity to make some suggestions for future policy on the collection and publication of statistics within the scope concerned.

Secondly, detailed factual information about statistical series and other data are given in a Quick Reference List (QRL). The exact nature of the entries is best seen by glancing at the list and accordingly they are not described here. Again, the ordering is not prescribed except that entries are not classified by publication source since it is presumed that it is this which is unknown to the reader. In general, the routine type of information which is given in the QRL is not repeated verbally in the text; the former, however, serves as a search route to the latter in that a reference (by section number) is shown against a QRL entry when there is a related discussion in the text.

Third, a subject index to each review acts as a more or less conventional line of inquiry on textual references; however, it is a computerized system and, for an individual review, the only peculiarity which it introduces is the possibility of easily permuting entries. Thus an entry in the index to the review in this volume is:

Clearing house of health indexes

which is shown also as

Health indexes, clearing house of

as well as

Indexes, clearing house of health

The object at this level is merely to facilitate search by giving as many variants as possible. In addition, individual review subject indexes are merged into a cumulative index which is held on magnetic tape and may possibly be used to produce a printed version from time to time if that seems desirable. Computer print-outs of the cumulative index to date are available on application to me at the Department of Economics, University of Exeter. In addition, selective searches of this index may be made by the input of key-words; the result is a print-out of all entries in which the key-word appears in the initial position in the subject index of any review. Like the cumulative index itself, this is a facility which may be of increasing help as the number of reviews in print grows.

Fourth, each review contains two listings of publications. The QRL Key gives full details of the publications shown as sources and text references to them are made in the form [QRL serial number]; this list is confined essentially to data publications. The other listing is a general bibliography of works discussing wider aspects; text references in this case are made in the form [B serial number].

Finally, usually an attempt is made to reproduce the more important returns or forms used in data collection so that it may be seen what tabulations it is possible to make as well as helping to clarify the basis of those actually available. Unfortunately, there are severe practical limitations on the number of such forms that it is possible to append to a review and authors always perforce have to be highly selective. In the case of this volume any attempt at selection would have been inappropriate and clearly to have reproduced all forms was a task quite impossible to entertain.

If all or any of these features succeed in their intention of increasing the value of the series in its basic function as a work of reference it will be gratifying; the extent to which the purpose is achieved, however, will be difficult to assess without 'feedback' from the readership. Users, therefore, will be rendering an essential service if they will send me a note of specific instances where, in consulting a review, they have failed to find the information sought.

As editor, I must express my very grateful thanks to all the members of the Joint Steering Committee of the Royal Statistical Society and the Social Science Research Council. It would be unfair to saddle them with any responsibility for shortcomings in execution but they have directed the overall strategy with as admirable a mixture of guidance and forbearance as any editor of such a series could desire. Especial thanks are due to the Secretary of the Committee who is an unfailing source of help even when sorely pressed by the more urgent demands of his other offices.

Very sincere thanks are due to all those who gave up their time to attend the seminar held to discuss the first draft of this review which contributed materially to improving the final version. Both the authors and I are most grateful to Mr Thomas Dalby of Pergamon Press Limited for his always attentive help during the vital production stages. The Subject Index entries were compiled by Mrs Juliet Horwood who has also been responsible for many other aspects of the work. Our thanks go also to Mrs Gill Skinner, of the Social Studies Data Processing Unit at the University of Exeter, who has written the computer programs for the production of the Subject Indexes.

University of Exeter
September 1977   W. F. MAUNDER

16: HEALTH SURVEYS
AND
RELATED STUDIES

Michael Alderson
London University

Robin Dowie
University of Kent

LIST OF ABBREVIATIONS USED IN THE TEXT

A & E	Accident and Emergency
AHA	Area Health Authority
AMO	Area Medical Officer
BG	Board of Governors
BMA	British Medical Association
BNF	British National Formulary
CGP	College of General Practitioners
CGRHS	Central Government Routine Health Statistics
CMI	Cornell Medical Index
CMO	Chief Medical Officer
CSM	Committee on Safety of Medicines
CSO	Central Statistical Office
DCP	District Community Physician
DES	Department of Education and Science
DGH	District General Hospital
DHSS	Department of Health and Social Security
DNA	Did not attend
EBS	Emergency Bed Service
EC	Executive Council
ECG	Electrocardiogram
ESN	Educationally subnormal
FES	Family Expenditure Survey
FPC	Family Practitioner Committee
GHS	General Household Survey
GLC	Greater London Council
GMC	General Medical Council
GP	General Practitioner
GPA	Group Practice Allowance
GRO	General Register Office
HAA	Hospital Activity Analysis
HAS	Hospital Advisory Service
HES	Health Examination Survey
HIPE	Hospital In-patient Enquiry
H Inf S	Health Information System
HIS	Health Interview Survey
HMC	Hospital Management Committee
HMSO	Her Majesty's Stationery Office
ICD	International Classification of Disease

IMTA	Institute of Municipal Treasurers and Accountants
IQ	Intelligence Quotient
LCC	London County Council
LEA	Local Education Authority
LHA	Local Health Authority
LMC	Local Medical Committee
MHE	Mental Health Enquiry
MMR	Mass Miniature Radiography
MoH	Ministry of Health
MOH	Medical Officer of Health
MRC	Medical Research Council
NHS	National Health Service
NMS	National Morbidity Study
NPHT	Nuffield Provincial Hospitals Trust
OM	Organization and Method
OPCS	Office of Population Censuses and Surveys
PEP	Political and Economic Planning
QRL	Quick Reference List
RCGP	Royal College of General Practitioners
RCN	Royal College of Nursing
RG	Registrar General
RHA	Regional Health Authority
RHB	Regional Hospital Board
RMO	Regional Medical Officer
RRL	Road Research Laboratory
SAMO	Senior Administrative Medical Officer
SCM	Specialist in Community Medicine
SCPR	Social and Community Planning Research
SCT	Society of County Treasurers
SEN	State Enrolled Nurses
SHHD	Scottish Home and Health Department
SRN	State Registered Nurses
SSRC	Social Science Research Council
UK	United Kingdom
USA	United States of America
WHO	World Health Organization

ACKNOWLEDGEMENTS

In the preparation of this review the authors have had a series of stimulating and useful discussions with a wide range of people concerned with the collection, processing and interpretation of health statistics. The following have contributed to these discussions: Dr A. M. Adelstein, Mr D. E. Allen, Dr J. S. A. Ashley, Dr D. Bainton, Dr D. J. P. Barker, Professor H. Campbell, Dr D. L. Crombie, Dr G. Cust, Dr P. N. Dixon, Dr R. D. T. Farmer, Dr J. Fry, Dr P. Gentle, Dr D. J. Hall, Dr M. A. Heasman, Professor W. W. Holland, Professor M. Jefferys, Professor E. G. Knox, Mr A. Rowntree, Dr A. L. Walby, Professor M. D. Warren, Professor W. E. Waters, Dr B. Williams. This breadth of advice has been most helpful; in addition, a number of the views expressed in this review are a distillation of other conversations and contacts with a wide range of colleagues, to whom the authors are equally grateful.

Mrs J. Causer, Mrs L. Harvey and Mrs C. Thorpe helped check some of the abstracts of published statistics and entries into the QRL, and the authors are most grateful to them for their assistance. Professor W. F. Maunder, the editor of the series, has provided continual support and encouragement during an overlengthy period of drafting; the authors thank him for his continued assistance. The production of this review has involved a considerable load of typing, which has been particularly shouldered by Mrs E. A. Layzell, Mrs B. Lloyd and Mrs C. Phillips; we are most grateful for this help.

The early work on this review was carried out whilst Professor Alderson was Honorary Director of the Wessex Medical Information Unit; the general activity of this unit which was jointly funded by the Wessex Regional Health Authority and the Department of Health and Social Security provided the basic stimulus to become involved in this review. Throughout this period, Mrs Robin Dowie was a Research Fellow in the Health Services Research Unit at the University of Kent, supported by the DHSS. Both authors thank the DHSS and their colleagues in these Units for their support, understanding, and help.

REFERENCE DATE OF SOURCES REVIEWED

This review is believed to represent the position, broadly speaking, as it obtained at 31 December 1976. The following comments have been inserted at the proof-reading stage (1 October 1978), taking account, as far as possible, of any major changes in the situation.

The preparation of this review has involved the consideration of material from a very wide range of conceptual areas, and a high proportion of references that stem from once-off surveys (whether at national, regional or local level). This poses two problems: first, the material is more likely to date than the previous review of Central Government Routine Health Statistics; secondly, the span of the review makes it impossible to do justice to the steady flow of relevant publications that have appeared in the rather distressingly long interval between the preparation of the text and the appearance of the proofs. A highly pragmatic approach has therefore had to be taken in the preparation of this short addendum with no attempt being made to mention any local studies unless they fill a major gap which has been identified in the main review.

The first issue that warrants attention is whether there have been any publications that contribute a significant advance to method for obtaining data relevant to the ground covered in this review. It does not seem that there has been publication of any major step forward; on reflection it seems that there is a perceptible move away from mounting fairly large-scale surveys collecting data to give a broad brush picture of a problem, towards the initiation of studies frequently based upon a small number of 'cases' that probe a particular issue in some depth. Such studies often collect pertinent subjective comments rather than spuriously precise factual data.

Chapter 4 mentioned the report of the Resource Allocation Working Party for England; since the text was finalized both the Scottish Home and Health Department [B 501] and the Welsh Office [B 502] have adopted similar formulae for sharing resources amongst their constituent health authorities. Subsequently there has been a lengthy argument about the method used for these reports; this particularly hinges upon the use of regional Standardized Mortality Ratios as an index of 'outcome' and an indirect measure of need in the regions. The publications to date have not provided definitive guidance to the fresh use of statistics in the management of the health service, but this point is mentioned here because the various resource allocation reports indicate a major step forward in attempting to apply the best data that are available to a crucial issue, i.e. adjusting the balance of health facilities across the country. Some of the issues involved have been critically reviewed by Forster [B 495], Knox [B 498], Snaith [B 503], and Senn and Shaw [B 502].

Turning now to publication of statistics that are relevant to the spectrum of need/ unmet demand/resources/workload/outcome there is only limited material that demands mention. The General Household Survey has produced two further reports for

for 1974 and 1975 [B 499, 500]. The questions on sickness and use of services are unchanged, but those dealing with smoking have been modified. No further questions have been asked about drug consumption since 1972. In 1975 the sampling design was altered; it has a two-stage sample (with stratification for Region) using wards as the primary stage. The technique to get quarterly data has also been modified. It seems a pity that there are no tables of trends in the latest publication now that data are available for a five-year span; however, the statistics are being published with minimum commentary and shorter delay. The introduction to the 1975 reports warns that the health section was radically revised for the following year's survey.

The other study which complements some aspects of the GHS is the National Morbidity Survey; there has been no further major publication from this work, which leaves a great deficit in the overall picture of the health care of the population. Chapter 7 (see Subsections 7.3.2.1 and 7.3.2.3) drew attention to the present deficiency of data from Primary Medical Care; the plea is reiterated here for further action on this topic.

Apart from the statistics from the GHS, there has been no major national publication that spans a wide range of medical problems and provides data that are relevant to the chapters or QRL sections on Need, Unmet Demand, or Outcome.

Likewise, with regard to the chapters on Resources and Use of Services, it appears that most recently there has been very little published from relevant surveys of national or regional samples. One Scottish manpower study is *Women In Nursing* directed by Hockey [B 496] and it is the initial report of this study from the Nursing Research Unit at the University of Edinburgh. In the report by Hunt [B 497] on the elderly living in the community in England in 1976 there are statistics on accessibility to health services and contacts made with various agencies. This enquiry was conducted by the Office of Population Censuses and Surveys: 11,849 addresses were contacted and at 3167 addresses one or more of the residents was aged 65 or over. Eventually, 2622 persons were interviewed.

The final chapter in this review discussed information systems in the future; this is an important topic but one that only evolves slowly. Barr [B 494] has provided a provocative and thoughtful paper, giving leads to a fresh approach in this field. Reference has already been made to the trend to perform case-studies rather than collect volumes of superficial statistics. Another change (though more relevant to the review on Central Government Health Statistics [B 14]) is the radical change that has occurred in the publishing programme of the OPCS—perhaps the most marked change in this since 1839. The statistics are now being presented in a series of topic specific 'booklets', with considerable effort going into the detailed probing of all available data upon one specific topic at a time; more extensive interpretation is provided than used to appear in the routine reports of the RG's Statistical Reviews.

References

[B 494] Barr, A. 'Information for management and planning in the NHS.' *Hospital and Health Services Review*, **73**, 387 (1977).

[B 495] Forster, D. P. 'Mortality, morbidity, and resource allocation.' *Lancet*, **1**, 997 (1977).

[B 496] Hockey, L. *Women in Nursing*. London, Hodder & Stoughton, 1976.

[B 497] Hunt, A. *The Elderly at Home*. London, HMSO, 1978.

[B 498] Knox, G. 'Principles of allocation of health care resources.' *Journal of Epidemiology and Community Health*, **32**, 3 (1978).

[B 499] Office of Population Censuses and Surveys. *The General Household Survey, 1974*. London, HMSO, 1977.

[B 500] Office of Population Censuses and Surveys. *The General Household Survey, 1975*. London, HMSO, 1978.

[B 501] Scottish Home and Health Department. *Scottish Health Authorities Revenue Equalisation (SHARE). Report of the Working Party on Revenue Resource Allocation*. Edinburgh, HMSO, 1977.

[B 502] Senn, S. J. and Shaw, H. 'Resource allocation: Some problems in applying the national formula to area and district revenue allocations.' *Journal of Epidemiology and Community Health*, **32**, 22 (1978).

[B 503] Snaith, A. H. 'Subregional resource allocations in the National Health Service.' *Journal of Epidemiology and Community Health*, **32**, 16 (1978).

[B 504] Welsh Office. *The Distribution of Resources to Health Authorities in Wales*. Second report of the Steering Committee, December, 1977. Cardiff, Welsh Office, 1978.

CONTENTS OF REVIEW 16

1	**Introduction**	15
1.1	*Aim*	15
1.2	*Potential readership*	15
1.3	*Boundaries to coverage*	16
1.4	*Organization of the National Health Service*	16
1.5	*Layout of the review*	19
1.6	*Material covered in the text*	20
1.7	*The application of published statistics*	20
	1.7.1 *Study design*	21
	1.7.2 *Accuracy of data—general considerations*	21
	1.7.3 *Accuracy of subjects' responses*	22
	1.7.4 *Accuracy of examination findings*	24
	1.7.5 *Accuracy of investigation results*	24
	1.7.6 *Bias introduced by non-response*	25
	1.7.7 *Items required in a report*	26
	1.7.8 *The problems of routine data*	27
	1.7.9 *Interpretation and application of published statistics*	27
1.8	*Contents of QRL*	28
1.9	*Data-collection forms*	28
1.10	*Guides to available statistics*	29
	1.10.1 *Abstracts*	29
	1.10.2 *Bibliographies*	29
	1.10.3 *Indexes to publications*	30
	1.10.4 *Indexes to research in progress*	31
	1.10.5 *Archived statistics*	32
2	**Need**	34
2.1	*Introduction*	34
	2.1.1 *The value of data from population studies*	37
	2.1.2 *The value of mortality and morbidity data*	39
2.2	*Population studies*	41
	2.2.1 *National population studies*	41
	2.2.1.1 *The survey of sickness*	41
	2.2.1.2 *The General Household Survey*	42
	2.2.2 *Local population studies*	45
	2.2.2.1 *An early study*	45
	2.2.2.2 *South Wales studies*	46
	2.2.2.3 *Bermondsey and Southwark*	50

	2.2.2.4 Lambeth	50
	2.2.2.5 Miscellaneous epidemiological surveys	51
2.3	Morbidity statistics from the NHS	51
	2.3.1 Screening	52
	2.3.2 Morbidity statistics from general practice	52
	2.3.2.1 The first National Morbidity Study	55
	2.3.2.2 The second National Morbidity Study	56
	2.3.2.3 Other studies from general practice	58
	2.3.3 Morbidity statistics from hospitals	59
2.4	Morbidity statistics from industry	60
2.5	Problem specific studies	61
	2.5.1 Abortion	62
	2.5.2 Accidents	62
	2.5.3 Addiction	63
	2.5.4 Adverse drug reactions	63
	2.5.5 Alimentary disease	63
	2.5.6 Arthritis	64
	2.5.7 Blood diseases	64
	2.5.8 Cancer	64
	2.5.9 Cardiovascular disease	65
	2.5.10 Children	65
	2.5.10.1 Cohort studies of children	65
	2.5.10.2 Congenital abnormality	71
	2.5.10.3 Infancy	71
	2.5.10.4 Children: non-accidental injury	73
	2.5.10.5 School children	73
	2.5.11 Deafness	74
	2.5.12 Dental health	75
	2.5.13 Diabetes	77
	2.5.14 Elderly	78
	2.5.15 Environmental pollution	79
	2.5.16 Epilepsy	79
	2.5.17 Eye diseases	79
	2.5.18 Family planning	80
	2.5.19 Feet	81
	2.5.20 Genito-urinary disease	81
	2.5.21 Handicapped	81
	2.5.21.1 Young chronic sick	82
	2.5.22 Maternity	83
	2.5.23 Mental illness	84
	2.5.24 Mental subnormality	88
	2.5.25 Nutrition	89
	2.5.26 Physique	92
	2.5.27 Rehabilitation	92
	2.5.28 Respiratory diseases	93
	2.5.29 Self-medication	93
	2.5.30 Sexually transmitted diseases	94

	2.5.31 *Smoking*	94
	2.5.32 *Terminal care*	96
	2.5.33 *Tuberculosis*	97

3	**Unmet Demand**	99
3.1	*Primary medical care*	100
3.2	*Accident and emergency departments*	101
3.3	*Referral to out-patients*	102
3.4	*In-patient care*	102
3.5	*Inappropriate care*	102
3.6	*Private care*	103

4	**Resources**	104
4.1	*Facilities*	106
	4.1.1 *Ambulances*	106
	4.1.2 *Acute bed provisions*	106
	4.1.3 *Day hospitals*	111
	4.1.4 *General practitioner hospitals*	112
	4.1.5 *Health centres*	112
4.2	*Medical and dental manpower*	113
	4.2.1 *Community physicians and community health doctors*	114
	4.2.2 *Consultants*	115
	4.2.3 *Dental practitioners*	115
	4.2.4 *General practitioners*	116
	4.2.5 *Junior hospital doctors and dentists*	117
	4.2.6 *Medical migration*	120
	4.2.7 *Student doctors*	120
	4.2.8 *Women doctors*	121
4.3	*Nursing and midwifery manpower*	121
	4.3.1 *All nurses and midwives*	121
	4.3.2 *Community nurses of all types in attachment schemes*	123
	4.3.3 *Health visitors*	126
	4.3.4 *Home nurses*	127
	4.3.5 *Hospital nurses*	129
	4.3.6 *Midwives*	130
	4.3.7 *Nurses in general practice*	130
	4.3.8 *Student nurses*	131
4.4	*Professional and technical manpower*	131
4.5	*Other resources*	132
	4.5.1 *Prescribing costs*	132

5	**Use of Services**	135
5.1	*General practitioner services*	137
	5.1.1 *Assessments by individuals of their contacts with general practitioner services*	137

5.1.2   *General practitioner workload and attitudinal studies*   138
     5.1.2.1   *All-inclusive studies*   140
     5.1.2.2   *Allocation of working time*   143
     5.1.2.3   *Appointment systems*   144
     5.1.2.4   *Deputizing services*   145
     5.1.2.5   *Family planning and abortion*   145
     5.1.2.6   *Home visiting and patient transportation systems*   147
     5.1.2.7   *Investigations*   148
     5.1.2.8   *Prescribing*   149
     5.1.2.9   *Referrals*   152
     5.1.2.10   *Sickness certification*   154
5.2   *Dental practitioner services*   154
5.2.1   *Assessments by individuals of their contacts with dental services*   154
5.2.2   *Dental practitioner surveys and workload statistics*   155
5.3   *Community health services*   157
5.3.1   *Assessments by individuals of their use of community health services*   158
5.3.2   *Referrals by doctors*   159
5.3.3   *School children*   160
5.4   *Hospital accident and emergency and out-patient departments*   161
5.4.1   *Assessments by individuals of their attendances at accident and emergency and out-patient departments*   161
5.4.2   *Accident and emergency services*   162
5.4.3   *Out-patient services*   164
     5.4.3.1   *Ad hoc studies of the purpose and function of out-patient departments*   164
     5.4.3.2   *Organization of out-patient departments*   168
     5.4.3.3   *Peripheral consultant out-patient services*   169
5.5   *Hospital diagnostic and pharmaceutical departments*   170
5.5.1   *Pathology and radiology services*   171
5.5.2   *Pharmaceutical services*   172
5.6   *Hospital in-patient services*   172
5.6.1   *Assessments by individuals of their contacts with hospital in-patient services*   172
5.6.2   *Ad hoc studies of the use made of non-psychiatric in-patient services*   173
5.6.3   *Emergency bed services*   175
5.6.4   *General practitioner hospital services*   175
5.6.5   *Mental handicap and mental illness services*   176
     5.6.5.1   *Censuses of mentally handicapped patients*   177
     5.6.5.2   *Census of mental illness patients*   178
     5.6.5.3   *Long-stay patients and case registers*   179
5.6.6   *Non-central government routine in-patient statistics*   179
5.7   *Day hospitals*   181
5.7.1   *Geriatric day hospitals*   181
5.7.2   *Psychiatric day hospitals*   182
5.8   *Other hospital services*   183

6	**Evaluation of Medical Care**	184
6.1	*Scope of the chapter*	184
6.2	*Techniques used in evaluating medical care*	185
	6.2.1 *Accessibility*	185
	6.2.2 *Facilities available for care*	186
	6.2.3 *Acceptability*	186
	6.2.4 *Process studies*	187
	6.2.4.1 *Diagnostic procedures*	188
	6.2.4.2 *Treatment*	188
	6.2.4.3 *Appropriate use of treatment facilities*	189
	6.2.5 *Outcome studies*	190
	6.2.5.1 *Mortality*	190
	6.2.5.2 *Morbidity*	191
	6.2.5.3 *Satisfaction of patient/family/staff*	193
	6.2.5.4 *Economics*	194
	6.2.6 *Complex studies*	195
	6.2.7 *Caveat*	197
7	**Information Systems—the Future**	198
7.1	*Four steps in establishing a H Inf S*	199
7.2	*Management requirements from information systems*	199
	7.2.1 *Classes of data required for management*	200
	7.2.1.1 *Trends in demand for services*	200
	7.2.1.2 *Trends in bottlenecks*	200
	7.2.1.3 *Use of resources*	200
	7.2.1.4 *Outcome of care*	201
	7.2.1.5 *Monitoring of innovations in health care*	201
	7.2.2 *Information requirements for planning*	201
7.3	*Towards a health information system*	202
	7.3.1 *Evolution of present activities*	202
	7.3.1.1 *Precise specification of aims*	202
	7.3.1.2 *Relationship of aim of study to possible course of action*	203
	7.3.1.3 *Improved relationships between the research staff, NHS staff, and management*	203
	7.3.1.4 *Enhanced quality of definitions*	203
	7.3.1.5 *Dual record systems*	204
	7.3.1.6 *Collection of data as a by-product of operational systems*	204
	7.3.2 *Gaps in presently available data*	204
	7.3.2.1 *Need*	204
	7.3.2.2 *Unmet demand*	205
	7.3.2.3 *Use*	205
	7.3.2.4 *Outcome measures*	206
	7.3.3 *The development of new methods*	206
7.4	*Some practical considerations*	208

Quick Reference List: 210
  Description 210
  Contents 212
  Abbreviation List 217
  Quick Reference List 220
  Quick Reference List Key 309

Bibliography 333

Subject Index 349

CHAPTER 1

INTRODUCTION

This chapter spells out the aim of this review and the potential readership. Consideration of these two issues leads on to discussion of the statistics that are relevant to this aim and readership and the boundaries that have been selected for the inclusion of material in the review. A section is provided on the organization of the National Health Service (NHS), with particular reference to the collection and presentation of statistics at local level. The main purpose of the review is met by the Quick Reference List (QRL); a section discusses the layout of the text and Quick Reference List. This is followed by further rules that have been used in deciding what statistics are eligible for treatment in the QRL and text within the specified boundaries that the review aims to cover. Though the text in each of the chapters gives some guidance as to the interpretation of statistics stemming from major studies, a general section on this issue is included in this chapter. This in no way attempts to replace the extensive treatment that has been published in other standard texts, but should serve as a guide to the major pitfalls in using 'shelf' material collected and presented by a range of workers. The final section in this chapter discusses the other published guides to available statistics and bibliographies of sources of statistics; these signposts to available material have proved invaluable in the preparation of this review and should be consulted by users wishing to satisfy themselves about the availability of other data.

1.1 Aim

The aim of this review is to provide an index to sources of statistics which quantify the health problems of the population in the United Kingdom (UK) and the use made of the health service. An earlier review has covered *Central Government Routine Health Statistics* [B 14]; this dealt with mortality and morbidity data, and statistics on cost, facilities, staff, workload in the health service—providing the statistics were published by central government in a regular series of reports. The fairly rigid criteria for entry into the previous review is contrasted with the much more difficult attempt in the present contribution to cover the remainder of published statistics relevant to the health and health services of the population. This is an open-ended commitment to consider all published statistics, however limited, providing they make a contribution to the general picture.

1.2 Potential readership

One important issue that influences the scope of the coverage and the treatment that the material is given is a consideration of the potential readership (of course the time available for the review and the length considered suitable for the text are equally important considerations). It is suggested that a reference work such as this should be aimed predominantly at the casual or non-specialist user of the statistics; it is important therefore that the layout attempts to guide the user towards relevant material, whatever the particular issue is that he wishes to study. It is anticipated that the review will be of interest to those concerned with population's health and the health-care system in this country. Such individuals may be personally involved in studying the organization and delivery of health care, by virtue of being employed in health-service management and planning. The review should also be of interest to those who are learning about the delivery of medical care, whatever their ultimate field of work. Because of the attempt to provide coverage over such a broad span of literature the detail on any particular issue may limit its value to experienced staff working on health services research—though even for such individuals the QRL may be of use when they are looking at problems outside their specific field of interest. At the same time the text should provide in a fairly concise form a description of the method used to collect the data, particularly in order to warn any potential user of the statistics about problems in their interpretation. Section 1.6 explains that not all studies indexed in the QRL are covered in the text.

1.3 Boundaries to coverage

The review does not attempt to cover clinical studies *per se*—even though it is recognized that innovations in techniques for diagnosis and treatment can have major implications for delivery of health care. The review also does not deal with the steadily growing literature on tactical OM/Work Study projects that reflect on desirable changes in the organization of care. There is an important difference between the previous text which reviewed regularly published tables of statistics and the major extension that is involved in the present work; this is to a great extent referring to books, reports and articles scattered through the scientific literature. Apart from the difficulty created by lack of a clear-cut boundary of work relevant to this review, there is considerable variation in the text accompanying some of the published statistics. Some reports contain both tables of statistics and a detailed description including interpretation, usually written by the research worker. Others only provide a cursory indication of the aim, method, sample selection, data collection, analysis or pitfalls in interpretation.

1.4 Organization of the National Health Service

1.4.1. The organization of the National Health Service (NHS) is related to the development of different systems for the collection, transmission or presentation of various sets of statistics. This section examines this issue briefly and draws attention to the influence of NHS reorganization in 1974.

1.4.2. The source of statistics that have been screened for potential relevance for this review falls into a number of different categories. The main set of health statistics that were excluded was statistics published as a routine by central government in the UK (this was the source material dealt with in the previous review—[B 14]); however, there was a range of other central government publications that are relevant, i.e. all those published as a result of surveys and other special enquiries. The principal sources in this category are indicated in the following section.

1.4.3. The next category to be considered was the regular publications from non-central government health agencies. The main time span covered by the present review is 1948–76 inclusive; this overlaps with major administrative reorganization that occurred on 1 April 1974 for both local authorities and the NHS. In the period 1948–74 there was a tripartite health service consisting of the Hospital Service, the Local Health Authority (LHA) and the Executive Council (EC). In general, hospitals were administered in groups at local level under a Hospital Management Committee (HMC). The HMC was responsible for the functioning of its constituent hospitals and a number of HMCs were collectively administered by their Regional Hospital Board (RHB); fourteen RHBs in England and one in Wales reported direct to the Ministry of Health (MoH—later Department of Health and Social Security—DHSS). The main exception to this structure was for teaching hospitals, which were grouped under Boards of Governors (BG) in England and Wales, which reported direct to the DHSS. This latter arrangement did not apply to Scotland or Northern Ireland, where teaching and non-teaching hospitals were under RHBs.

The LHAs were organized in a single-tier system, these authorities being responsible for providing community services for a county or a county borough, apart from London with boroughs within the Greater London Council (GLC). Some of the larger counties operated a divisional system with a varying degree of delegation to the divisional authority. The LHA was responsible for the provision of district nurses, district midwives and health visitors; the staff operated from health clinics though in some authorities the staff have been attached to general practitioners. The local Health Departments also provided the school health service either directly or in association with the Local Education Authority (LEA).

The ECs formed a single-tier system, with each council being located at LHA level. The ECs were responsible for the general administration of the general practitioners, dentists, pharmacists and the supplementary ophthalmic services in their own area.

This structure is described because it is linked to the collection and presentation of statistical material on the functioning of the health service. In general HMCs, RHBs and ECs acted as agents for central government collecting statistics for standard returns and submitting these at appropriate intervals for central processing. Some RHBs and individual hospitals (particularly teaching hospitals) produced a statistical report, though the detail included was not only restricted to the patients treated at that hospital but usually did not incorporate the range of variates handled by the Hospital In-patient Enquiry (HIPE—see [B 14]). Quite different was the arrangement for producing an annual report by the LHA. The tradition had commenced with the work of Simon in the middle of the nineteenth century; the Medical Officer of Health (MOH) had a statutory duty to prepare and present an annual report to his authority and submit a copy to the appropriate central government department. Copies of the last reports produced for each LHA in the UK have been examined; though these provide an illuminating description of the health problems of individual localities and the arrangements made to tackle these, they have been excluded from coverage in the review by the restricted geographical nature of the material. The consolidated data are available via central government reports and were covered in the previous review [B 14]. Chapter 5 discusses the content of MOsH reports (5.3).

1.4.4. Reorganization has resulted in a 'unified' management structure; each country is divided into regions, with a Regional Health Authority (RHA) within which there are a variable number of Area Health Authorities (AHA). Within areas there are a variable number of districts, with a District Management Team of full-time officers plus representatives of the hospital consultants and family practitioners. The main exception to this structure is the absence of a regional tier in Wales, whilst the areas are responsible in Northern Ireland for welfare services as well as health services. The post of MOH has been replaced by that of Specialist in Community Medicine (SCM), with posts of Area Medical Officer (AMO) and District Community Physician (DCP); for the matching local authority there is an appointed officer responsible for advice on environmental health. The policy for preparation of reports at district, area and regional level is presently under review; the new legislation [B 347] has not transferred the statutory responsibility of the former MOH to produce a report, to the Area or Regional Medical Officer (RMO) in the new structure. In due course, a series of statistical publications may emerge at local level, though the emphasis is likely to concentrate on the collation of statistics for 'internal' examination as part of the annual planning cycle whilst central government continues to collate, process and publish routine national statistics. Some areas have produced annual reports for 1974 and 1975 with a combination of statistics and narrative, but covering the complete range of services for which an area is responsible (i.e. hospital, family practitioner and community health services).

1.4.5. Another (potential) source of routine health statistics is the occupational health services—either those of major employers within large industries or locally organized 'group occupational health services'. The material that is collated and published is relatively sparse; again the bulk of statistics of occupational health (accidents, prescribed disease and sickness absence) is handled by the appropriate central government departments.

1.4.6. The final source of statistics is publications stemming from special studies and research projects. These complement the other sources—and have usually been carried out for the very reason that the other sources of statistics are inadequate to resolve a particular problem. The method of publication is unrelated to the structure of the health service and any 'available' statistics should have been considered for inclusion in the review, whether appearing in books, regularly published journals, *ad hoc* supplements to journals, or independently produced reports that are available from the sponsoring authority either at cost or free of charge (these latter have only been included as available if copies have been circulated to the principal libraries throughout the UK). Special studies may be carried out by health authorities (whether by staff at district, area or regional level), university departments of community medicine or designated medical-care research units, other university departments or research units, voluntary and other agents and organizations. The location of the team doing the work may alter the arrangement for presentation and publication of results. Alderson [B 17] has drawn attention to the tendency for academics to publish, whilst health-service staff may carry out essential studies whose results are acted upon without any attempt at formal publication.

1.5 Layout of the review

Both the text and the QRL have been ordered, wherever possible, in the same way; they cover statistics on:

Chapter 2   Population Needs for Health Care
Chapter 3   Unmet Demand for Health Care
Chapter 4   Resources
Chapter 5   Use of Services
Chapter 6   Evaluation of Medical Care

The table of contents (p. 9) shows in considerable detail the ordering of the text for the complete review; there is also a table of contents preceding the QRL.

If a user of the review cannot immediately locate an entry on the QRL relating to the statistics in which they are interested (using the contents list as a guide, or directly scanning the QRL) it must be remembered that some published statistics cover several topics. It has not always been possible or feasible to include multiple entries to one piece of work in several localities of the QRL. For example, an issue discussed in the text is that data on 'workload', when classified by diagnosis, may have to be used as an indication of prevalence of disease in the absence of appropriate population surveys. However, not every study included in Chapter 5, 'Use', has been also indexed in the Chapter 'Need', even though it can be argued that they give some indication of the distribution of health problems of the population that requires care. As indicated in Sections 1.6 and 1.8, rather different considerations determined coverage of a particular piece of work in the text and QRL; some studies included in the text are not indexed in the QRL and vice versa. As a general rule, within any particular field of activity in the Chapter 'Need' general studies are treated first and then specific studies ordered alphabetically by topic. Chapter 3, 'Unmet Demand for Health Care', and the accompanying QRL section are ordered in the way a patient may pass through a sequence of contacts with the health service from initial contact with the family doctor, referral to out-patients, wait at out-patients, waiting list for hospital admission, and then wait for discharge back to the community. Conceptually there is overlap between some measures of unmet demand (such as did the patient wishing to have an abortion obtain one?) and many of the aspects of evaluation (e.g. patients' opinion as to whether they have obtained the level of care they expected from the health service). This again is an example of where complete multiple entry has not occurred between Chapter 3 and Chapter 6 QRL entries.

Chapter 4, 'Resources', covers facilities, manpower and other resources; these topics form separate sections within which the material is arranged alphabetically. In Chapter 5, 'Use of Services', the sections are ordered in the approximate sequence of services a person would encounter upon entering the health-care system. Most sections commence with a subsection describing reported assessment by individuals of their use of that particular service, while the later subsections are organized alphabetically. Generally, studies covering the largest geographical area take precedence within each subsection. Where there are two or more with similar geographical coverage, the earlier study is inserted first.

The QRL entries relating to Chapters 4 and 5 follow the same ordering of sections and subsections as the text. Chapter 6 provides the main exception to the parallel ordering of text and QRL. This is because the text provides a general (and fairly brief) review of the method of evaluative studies. This uses an accepted classification of method that is not linked (or linkable) to a sensible order of studies by topic. It was decided after considerable deliberation to organize that text according to a method axis (for one of the main aims of the text is to indicate the present state of development of studies on evaluation)—whilst the QRL has been ordered by topic (for the potential user of the QRL will approach this with a subject in mind, rather than wanting references to a technique which may be applied to a wide range of health service activities).

Whilst reviewing all available statistics the authors were led to a consideration of the present gaps and deficiencies in: national studies, statistics provided by regional and local authorities, and the contribution of research studies. This issue was mentioned in the previous review [B 14]; it is more relevant to the present work, where the balance between routine collection of statistics and presentation of *ad hoc* studies has been assessed and a judgement made about the present deficiencies in the overall picture that is available. These issues are explored in Chapter 7, 'Information Systems—the Future'.

1.6. Material covered in the text

In general, the principal surveys and studies included in the QRL will have some coverage in the text, the length of treatment depending partly on the size and scope of the study and a judgement of its contribution to the general picture. Each major study that is discussed will normally have the aim of the study, the method, the potential uses and the problems of interpretation of the data described. There are some examples where the discussion of the study design or problems of interpretation have not had a specific mention in the text—either because of the very parochial nature of the work or the fact that studies of similar design have already been described. However, it is not practical to repeat, for each study discussed in the text, the same issues related to the validity, interpretation and use of published statistics. A number of general points are therefore dealt with in the following section.

1.7. The application of published statistics

The successful use of someone else's results is fraught with danger. However, it is not appropriate to deal at length in this review with this important topic, which has been tackled in a variety of ways in standard texts in the fields of applied statistics [Armitage, B 24; Stuart, B 428], epidemiology [Abrahamson, B 2; Alderson, B 18], and the social sciences [Belson and Thompson, B 43; Moser and Kalton, B 342; Oppenheim, B 362]. The following text draws attention to some of the difficulties in: study design and sampling; accuracy of data; clarity of the report; interpretation of the material.

1.7.1. *Study design*

This must incorporate a clear-cut aim, which is feasible and appropriately linked to the design used in the study. A vital aspect of this is the identification of the target population and a suitable approach to sampling that will enable extrapolation from the specific results to a wider sphere. Relatively few studies will have involved a carefully selected national probability sample; this therefore indicates the importance of all reports to clearly indicate the sampling frame, the method of selection from this and the intended and attained sample—with consideration of any hidden non-response. The method of data collection is also of crucial importance and is dealt with in the following subsection. However clearly thought out is the study design, it is always advisable that 'piloting' has occurred before definitive data collection.

1.7.2. *Accuracy of data—general considerations*

It is important that the user of any set of published statistics has a clear idea of the accuracy of the data prior to attempting to use the material. This section discusses the common sources of error and bias and the various ways in which they may be identified; consideration of these issues should facilitate correct interpretation of data. When commenting upon the accuracy of any particular 'instrument', it is usual to distinguish the reliability of the data collected from the validity. The reliability is the extent of the agreement between repeated measurements; this is a compound of variation in the item being assessed plus the error introduced by the observer collecting and processing this information. The validity of the technique is the extent to which a method provides a true assessment of that which it purports to measure.

Wherever possible a research worker will use an 'instrument' that has already been standardized and validated; even so, in any major study it is important to check on the accuracy of the data collected by such means. However, in many projects, particularly those tackling new problems, specific methods for collecting relevant and accurate data will have to be developed. This may necessitate lengthy method studies, as a preliminary in order to develop suitable ways of collecting data—this is especially so when the field survey involves large numbers of subjects and requires a simple technique for collecting data on attitudes, habits, symptoms, signs or results from investigations. The following indicates the range of 'instruments' that have been developed: Cochrane and his colleagues [B 109], when studying the prevalence of respiratory disease, refined a standard questionnaire to elicit symptoms of respiratory disease, whilst Rose [B 392] was responsible for developing and validating a questionnaire to detect the presence of cardiovascular symptoms; Marr [B 304] described a tested method of obtaining data on dietary intake; Yasin *et al.* [B 490] devised and validated a questionnaire to assess habitual leisure activity. Many epidemiological surveys involve recording of physical signs and a lot of work has been done on the method of eliciting valid material from clinical examinations: Rose and Blackburn [B 393] describe the steps to be taken to reduce the errors in the collection of data from cardiovascular surveys; as a specific example of work in this field Rose *et al.* [B 394] describe the work that led to the production and testing of a new machine for recording blood pressure. As an example of the improvement of the reliability and validity of data from investigation, Blackburn and his colleagues [B 54] standardized the technique for recording and interpreting electrocardiogram (ECG) tracings obtained in surveys; Warren [B 455] has validated interview surveys of handicapped persons against their general practitioner's notes and recollections.

Some of the error introduced in data collection will be random; this may result in mis-classification of individuals, or the recording of high or low values for continuous variates. It is important to have some guide as to the degree of this random variation; having quantified this variation, there are statistical techniques for overcoming the influence of random variation in the interpretation of collected data. A rather separate issue that has to be considered is the introduction of bias into the data collection; particular ways of phrasing questions, consistent faults in the technique of examination of patients, or errors in the method of analysing investigations may introduce a bias into the results so obtained. The use of more than one observer often introduces differences in the bias of the results whilst the degree of bias may vary between subgroups of the subjects in the study; this complicates the interpretation of the material more than the presence of random error. In assessing the reliability, validity and bias in the data collection system it is usual to consider (1) the innate variability in the subjects being observed, (2) the error or biases introduced into the subjects' responses by the experimental situation and (3) the contribution of observer error or bias. Where a particular investigation is used to categorize individuals into 'healthy' and 'diseased' subgroups, it is usual to consider the sensitivity and specificity of the test that is used. The sensitivity is a measure of the extent to which the method gives results free from false negatives (i.e. fails to pick up as diseased those individuals who suffer from the conditions). The specificity is a measure of the extent to which a method gives results free from false positives (i.e. the degree to which the technique falsely classifies as diseased subjects that are in fact healthy).

It is essential that the error rate of various 'instruments' used in epidemiology are known before data collected by them can be interpreted. This is a similar approach to any other scientific work—it is essential to calibrate a new instrument before it is put into action and subsequently necessary to recalibrate the instrument at appropriate intervals. The word instrument may be used in the epidemiological field in a rather broader sense than in the general scientific world. It can refer to the techniques for collecting (1) written or verbal information from people, (2) observations as a result of examination of subjects or (3) data from the investigation of patients. Only when one has a precise indication of the accuracy rate of the measures used in a study is it possible to interpret results with certainty.

1.7.3. *Accuracy of subjects' responses*

When questioning subjects in any survey, information may be obtained about (1) current symptoms, (2) habits, characteristics, knowledge and attitudes, or (3) previous history and practice. It is important to consider these three facets in a rather different light. Some of the early work carried out on the recording of symptoms in population surveys was in the respiratory field; Cochrane and his colleagues [B 109] reported significant variation in the proportion of miners reporting various symptoms (cough, sputum, pain in the chest, dyspepsia) when interviewed by different observers. A planned study clearly showed the influence of a standardized respiratory questionnaire in improving the consistency in the answers. Fairbairn *et al*. [B 183] have shown that health visitors obtain as reliable results as doctors using the questionnaire. Further use of the questionnaire shows a relationship between positive responses and measured evidence of impaired respiratory function [Sharpe *et al*., B 412; Fletcher and Tinker, B 194; College of General Practitioners—CGP—B 112].

Histories may be obtained by interview with or without a standard questionnaire, or the questionnaire may be completed by the respondent either under supervision or only guided by written instructions. Each of these approaches has been carefully studied and the validity of the data collected assessed and related to the costs. There is documented evidence that the attitude and manner of the interviewer, and even the sex of the interviewer, can affect the respondents' responses [Kannel *et al*., B 271; Colombotis *et al*., B 115]. Milne and Williamson [B 323] warn that automatic administration of a questionnaire may generate a 'response set' where a positive answer to a series of questions is the first alternative. (Having answered yes correctly to the first question or two, this response may then be given incorrectly to succeeding questions.) Use of self-completion questionnaires has the disadvantage that it is difficult to be sure that the appropriate individual has completed the form (and not some anonymous alternate).

Considerable work has been done on the collection of information from patients about their current habits and characteristics; for example, a lot of effort has been invested in the collection of data on smoking habits. No direct validation study of such questionnaires has been carried out, though Doll and Hill [B 162] and Todd [B 436] have reported on the reliability of statements about smoking habits. Indirect validation of the questionnaires has been demonstrated by the relationship between reported smoking and assessment of respiratory functions [e.g. Bewley *et al*., B 51; Holland and Elliott, QRL 329]. Even for relatively simple matters such as age, there is a tendency to report this inaccurately; first is the tendency to round age to certain terminal digits, with preference for recording ages with a terminal digit 0, 5 and 8. This was observed by Farr [B 189] when examining the tabulations by single year of age of the national mortality data, and has again been noted in the 1961 census [B 213]. A rather different aspect is the tendency for certain subsections of the population to introduce bias; some women approaching middle age consistently understate their age, whilst there is also a tendency in the elderly and very elderly to exaggerate their age.

There is evidence that it is considerably more difficult to obtain information from certain subgroups of the population such as the psychiatrically disturbed. For example, Murray [B 345] suggested that those persons habitually consuming large quantities of analgesics are emotionally disturbed and very likely to fail to report their over-consumption of analgesics in a survey. When asking patients about their previous history (either their exposure to aetiological factors, or their health in the past), due consideration has to be given to the influence of the current situation and recent past; this may stimulate or depress recall of past events. When questioning patients about their previous health, it has been shown that the validity of responses deteriorates with the increase of the period over which attempts are made to collect information. In the Survey of Sickness carried out in this country some 30 years ago [Stocks, B 426, 427], subjects consistently reported a higher prevalence of illness in the 4 weeks preceding interview than in the period 4 to 8 weeks before; this finding was observed whatever the months of interview (it was not therefore a genuine effect of secular variation in prevalence of disease, but an effect of loss of data due to memory bias). The General Household Survey (GHS) [QRL 510] has some evidence that there is a drop in recall even when using a short reference period of 2 weeks. The relationship between use of hospital services reported on interview and actual evidence from an examination of hospital records has shown discrepancies in the recall of such events by the patients. Some studies have shown a modest tendency to under-report such events (National Centre for Health Statistics [B 346]; Vessey *et al*. [B 445]), whilst Palmer *et al*. [QRL 521] showed that a sample in North Lambeth tended in general to over-report. In the GHS [QRL 512] an attempt was made to identify the prevalence of long-standing disability; the question used in 1971 was split into two linked questions in 1972, and an appreciable drop in the positive responses occurred.

Detailed studies have been carried out in the psychiatric field, examining the large and persistent differences in the admission statistics by diagnosis between American and British hospitals. Cooper *et al*. [B 117] suggest that most of this difference is spurious and generated by variation in interpretation of symptoms and use of diagnostic labels. Further work in an international pilot study of schizophrenia, sponsored by the World Health Organization (WHO), has led to the development of standardized instruments and procedures for valid assessment of patients with mental disorder in different countries [B 487].

1.7.4. *Accuracy of examination findings*

When studying the influence of raised blood pressure upon health, a number of research workers became concerned about the accuracy with which blood pressure could be measured. Rose *et al*. [B 394] and Armitage *et al*. [B 25] showed, as well as the innate variation in blood pressure, there was error that occurred due to the instrument, and the observer. Gardner and Heady [B 207] have indicated variation in response of the blood pressure of subjects in the same situation, but in the presence of different observers. Other studies of the relationship between body build and cardiovascular disease required the measurement of skinfold thickness, which may be used as an estimate of obesity. An instrument was devised by Edwards *et al*. [B 178] which was suitable for survey work and provided consistent and valid measures of skinfold thickness. Ruiz *et al*. [B 399] have shown how the selection of the specific site for measurement affects the reading, even with shift of only a few centimetres.

Other facets of clinical examination to be studied in this way have been: examination of the heart [B 374]; physical signs in airways obstruction [B 217]; physical signs in ulcerative colitis [B 219]; the detection of absent pulses in the peripheral limbs [B 314].

1.7.5. *Accuracy of investigation results*

With the increase in the investigation of patients for diagnostic purposes and in order to control therapy, a considerable amount of work has been carried out on the accuracy of such measures. A number of studies have been mounted where different techniques for recording ECG tracings were used, and comparisons made of the interpretation of individual records by a number of observers [QRL 308]. Rose and Blackburn [B 393] have described a technique for reducing the inter- and intra-observer variation in interpreting ECGs. Work has been done on the accuracy of certain biochemical measures such as serum cholesterol (and its relationship to the prevalence or subsequent development of cardiovascular disease); there have also been a number of studies on the accuracy of haematological measures, such as the haemoglobin, the packed cell volume, serum iron, etc. Whitehead [B 461] has reviewed the development of quality-control techniques in laboratory services; by the adoption of standard methods and the monitoring of variation, the precision of the results may be improved. An earlier study by Whitehead [B 460] showed how different technicians could influence results, independently of technique and subject variation. Of particular interest to epidemiologists has been the observer variation in interpretation of X-rays [B 492] and the assessment of respiratory function [B 489]. With growing interest in the screening of 'well-women' for *in situ* carcinoma of the cervix, studies have been carried out on the reliability and validity of cervical cytology [B 493].

1.7.6. *Bias introduced by non-response*

In any survey it is important to obtain an adequate response rate, as the non-respondents are likely to be a biased segment of the study population. Poor response is often associated with advancing age, restricted educational level, semi- or unskilled manual occupations and residence in rural areas. The important issue to consider is whether these effects can introduce bias into survey results. For example, because of the close relationship between age and advent of disease, it will often be the fact that the non-respondents by virtue of their age distribution are likely to be less healthy than the respondents.

The bias introduced into surveys by non-respondents was clearly reviewed by Cochrane [B 107]. In presenting results from surveys carried out in South Wales, he showed a rather complex bias; the prevalence of pneumoconiosis was highest in those who came most readily for examination, whilst the prevalence of tuberculosis was higher in those reluctant to respond. Cochrane commented on the general phenomena, which holds for many diseases, that those most likely to be affected come forward less willingly for investigation; this phenomenon has been reported in relation to a number of other population studies and screening investigations, such as for malignant disease, chronic respiratory disease, coronary artery disease, developmental abnormality of children and hearing defects in children, etc. A specific example is the examination of 'well-women' for early carcinoma of the cervix; a number of authors (MacGregor *et al.* [QRL 426]; Osborne and Leyshon [QRL 518]; Sansom *et al.* [B 403]) have reported that the response rate is lowest in social classes IV and V, and this is the very group in whom there is a higher prevalence of positive cervical smears.

In order to assess the bias introduced into any study by non-response, it is essential to try and obtain some information about the individuals who initially fail to participate. Lambert [B 279] arranged for a sample of non-respondents in a large-scale postal enquiry on cardio-respiratory disease to be approached and interviewed; an attempt was made to find out about their characteristics, smoking habits and symptomatology. There was the expected variation in demographic characteristics, with over-representation of rural residents and those in social classes IV and V. The smoking habits and symptom prevalence in the non-respondents did not differ to an appreciable extent from the original respondents.

In the absence of definitive data on the characteristics of the non-respondents it is useful to analyse the data on those who do respond in relation to delay until reply and also the data for partial responders and reasons for non-response. In a number of her reports Cartwright [QRL 126, 127, 128] has used this approach to support the weight that can be placed upon the survey results.

In certain prospective studies, it has been possible to examine the mortality of the respondents in relation to the mortality of the non-respondents. Doll and Hill [B 163] and Horowitz and Wilbeck [B 252] found that the mortality rate amongst non-respondents was higher shortly after the initial survey (as one would expect if non-participation was due to being severely ill). However, the excess mortality did not disappear after a number of years of follow-up in any of the three studies. Doll and Hill suggested that this is an indication that there is general association between mortality and the tendency not to reply to an enquiry, whether the tendency is due to a deliberate refusal (which is rare), or a mere neglect of these things (which is frequent).

In three recent surveys on the elderly, determined efforts have been made to find out about the mental, physical and social well-being of non-respondents. Pike [B 371] surveyed the elderly in his own practice. Amongst a small representative sample of these non-participants (twenty-one men and twenty-two women) there was evidence of clinical or social need in only a few cases. Milne and his colleagues [B 322] approached a sample of nearly 1000 men and were able to examine 65 per cent. They used routine general practitioner records to compare the general health of respondents and non-respondents. There was significantly less documentary evidence of hospital care, vascular disease and peptic ulcer in the male non-respondents; significantly less hospital care, hiatus hernia and urinary tract infections amongst the female non-respondents. Akhtar [B 9] studied fifty-two non-respondents amongst 286 subjects invited to participate in a detailed investigation of the health of the elderly; he visited them in their own homes and was able to contact all but two. After a brief interview he concluded that mental abnormality was rare and physical disability conspicuously absent amongst those who initially did not participate.

The general weight of evidence suggests that extreme care is required in interpreting studies where the response rate is low. Many studies have found that the non-respondents represent a biased segment of the total study group—biased not only in respect of demographic characteristics but also in the prevalence of disease and subsequent mortality.

1.7.7. *Items required in a report*

Any usable report must cover some details of the general method of the study (target population, sampling, data collection, validity of material); response (including information about the non-responders); definitions of all the items included in the study, with details of the coding system used (where this is not a standard national or international system some guide must be given to the structure of the coding system and the possible error rate of coding); presentation of the results (this will usually be of greatest use if the raw material has been included, rather than tabulations presented of grouped data or analyses by derived variates); an indication of the degree of manipulation that has occurred is helpful, plus a specification of availability of the raw data for transfer to enquirers wishing to carry out further analyses themselves. The provision of a copy of the questionnaire used in the study is an advantage as the opportunity to examine such forms provides the user with a further guide on some aspects of data capture and permits cor.sideration of the cross-tabulations that are feasible within the complete data sets.

1.7.8. *The problems of routine data*

The preceding section indicates in a fairly general way the items that should be covered in a statistical report in order for it to be read and the results applied by the reader to his own problem. There is a great difference in the stringency with which standard survey methodology is applied in different studies. This varies from one piece of research to another, but also there is a considerable difference between a piece of research carried out with adequate funding and a reasonable time scale, to the quick scavenging for some statistics in the health field by someone neither trained in scientific discipline, nor provided with appropriate facilities to carry out the work, nor given the time in which to plan the study, pilot the system for data collection, or write up the results with care. Alderson [B 13, 16] has discussed some of the problems of routine data-collection systems (in brief the difficulties with completeness of coverage, delay, accuracy, retrieval, applicability, flexibility, acceptability and confidentiality). This string of issues is not intended to suggest that all routine statistics are poor and all research surveys are good; this point is taken further in Chapter 7, where the appropriate balance between routine and *ad hoc* sources of data are discussed (see Subsection 7.3.3). There is an important contrast between routine statistics and those derived from a specific survey; the former often has to collect fairly simple items over a wide range of interests, whilst the research study may amass a large volume of detail—but directed at so specific a point that the material is inadequate for application to a slightly different issue in a different part of the country.

1.7.9. *Interpretation and application of published statistics*

This is of course the key question, and the hardest to deal with in a short (or long) space. However, the following brief note indicates the main points that need to be considered in this activity.

The first issue that must be considered is the validity of the basic data; a guide to this aspect has already been covered in the subsections above that deal with study design and accuracy of data. Often, in the absence of clear information about some of the relevant issues in the published report, the user will have to make some judgement about the weight that he can put upon the material. A particular aspect of this will occur when there are two or more sets of published data that conflict. This may be because there are fundamental errors in some of the work, or that the method and samples were not comparable, there were hidden differences in the definitions or classifications used, or the sample sizes are small and associated with wide confidence limits in the results. Often consideration of these points will require some conclusion whether the data, imperfect as it is, can be used with caution as giving a better indication of the real state of affairs than guesswork. (This will be the issue when time/money/facilities are not available to carry out a further tailor-made survey.)

1.8. Contents of QRL

In order to be considered for entry into the reference section of this work—the QRL—the statistics have to contribute to the national picture. Because the surveys that have been considered range from multi-national on-going surveys to limited local studies, there are rather different reasons for accepting some published statistics as eligible. There is obviously no doubt about a survey involving England, Northern Ireland, Scotland and Wales, where the sample has been selected to provide representative statistics across these four countries. There is an intermediate category of study that may cover more than one region in the country, where the data collection has not been organized on an appropriate sampling basis and the statistics cannot be readily extrapolated to national levels; however, it may still be felt that in the absence of other data the material contributes to the national picture. The other extreme is where a small local study has tackled an issue for which no other statistics of a more general nature are available. The QRL distinguishes the extent of the survey by indicating the geographical cover and sample size (the latter grouped into five categories); this immediately provides a warning of the faith that can be placed upon the material by the potential user. Another important issue is the time span over which the statistics are thought to be still of relevance. In general, the studies have only been included in the QRL if they relate to material collected since the initiation of the health service (i.e. 1948 onwards). It must be remembered that: (1) the steady change in the patterns of disease affecting the community, (2) alteration in the availability of the health and welfare services (including their organization) and (3) trends in use of these services will have resulted in material that may have been collected 5 years ago being unrepresentative of the present picture.

The previous review [B 14] attempted to index in the QRL individual tables from reports; because of the scope of coverage of the present work this approach was not feasible. For some of the major works that have been included this level of detail has been covered. However, because of the vast number of tables of statistics that can be published in a single survey report it has been found essential to group up the coverage of tables and indicate the range of variates that have been tabulated but not the specific items nor the specific cross-tabulations.

1.9. Data-collection forms

The previous work [B 14] was also able to provide samples of the data-collection forms for the national mortality and morbidity systems. Again, because of the much larger number of questionnaires used it has been found impossible to present copies of data collection forms. The QRL indicates which publications include copies of the survey forms in the report, as it was thought important at least to identify those studies where there appears to be no data-collection form presented in the original publication.

1.10. Guides to available statistics

In an investigation on the way in which research papers in certain subjects were distributed throughout the journal literature, Bradford [B 57] found that the journals in each subject area could be manipulated to form three groups, so that each group contained about one-third of the total number of research papers in the subject. The first group consisted of a small number of journals containing a large number of relevant papers—core papers—the second group contained an intermediate number of moderately productive journals, whilst the third group contained very many journals that contributed a few relevant papers. This is now known as Bradford's Law and seems to be of general application to information retrieval in many fields. The present review has attempted to be as comprehensive as possible. However, as already indicated, difficulty has been created by (1) the absence of clear-cut boundaries to references that are potentially eligible within the coverage of the review and (2) problems in deciding for these references within the coverage whether they are of sufficient merit to index. Another important consideration is the difficulty in maintaining a review such as this in an up-to-date fashion; because of these considerations the following section has been inserted as an indication of other guides to available statistics. It is assumed that a full-time research worker will usually be familiar with the material directly relevant to his own on-going research; even such a worker is likely to have a boundary to his present awareness, and this review attempts to provide one source of further guidance. There are, of course, many other very different ways of accessing retrievable literature. The present section has categorized available guides under the headings of abstracts, bibliographies, indexes, lists of on-going research work, and statistical archives.

1.10.1. *Abstracts*

(1) DHSS—Abstracts of Efficiency Studies in the Hospital Service.
(2) DHSS—Hospital Abstracts.
(3) *Excerpta Medica*—this consists of forty separate monthly abstract journals covering the international literature in most areas of medicine and health; particularly relevant are likely to be Section 17: Public Health, Social Medicine, and Hygiene; Section 35: Occupational Health and Industrial Medicine; Section 46: Environmental Health and Pollution Control.
(4) The Royal College of General Practitioners (RCGP) Library Services provides periodic lists of abstracts within specific topics.

1.10.2. *Bibliographies*

(1) Central Statistical Office (CSO) *Guide to Official Statistics* [B 95]. This compilation provides a detailed guide to statistics that are available from all official and

important non-official publications and an attempt has been made to make it as comprehensive as possible. It covers nearly 800 topics in some 300 pages; around 2500 sources are identified. The guide deals with regular publications but also special reports and articles with significant statistical content that have been published over the last 10 years.

(2) Edwards, B., *Sources of Social Statistics* [B 177]. The aim of this book is to provide an effective yet critical guide to official sources of statistical material of social concern. It is restricted to standard regular publications and does not cover reports of specific research projects.

(3) Gauvain, S., *Occupational Health—A Guide to Sources of Information* [B 210]. Twenty leading experts in the field have contributed to twenty-two chapters which provide discussion of textbooks, journals, other publications, articles and other sources of information relevant to occupational health. Each chapter is not given standard treatment and there is some overlap between contributions. Also the index is not fully comprehensive and therefore the volume is not the easiest text into which to dip to find an appropriate reference. However, it provides a most useful guide providing it is read with care.

(4) Pickett, K. G., *Sources of Official Data* [B 369]. The aim of this book is to provide a guide to some principal sources of statistical data which are published on a regular basis; it provides considerable discussion on population and census material and also data on the labour force and education. Some information is given about secondary sources of such material but its overlap with the field of interest of the present review is negligible.

1.10.3. *Indexes to publications*

Government

(1) *Government Publications*, HMSO, London. This appears as a monthly catalogue with an annual consolidated volume which contains details of all items published by HMSO during the year (except for statutory instruments) and covers publications for England and Wales, Scotland, Northern Ireland and the appropriate government departments within these countries.

(2) *List of Principal Statistical Series Available*, HMSO, 1972. This was published in two parts, the first of which provided details of the scope, frequency and primary source of government statistics and the second a listing of 275 sources of official statistics. Though this list is now out of date it is supplemented by a regular amendment list in the quarterly *Statistical News* prepared by the CSO and published by HMSO.

(3) *Statistics*—a new subject catalogue first published in October 1975 which will be produced as a regular series. It provides details of all statistical reports that are in print and wholly or mainly statistical in content. It covers publications from January 1970 and will include reports provided by international agencies and other organizations for which HMSO acts as an agent.

DHSS

A series of monthly listings of current literature on various topics are produced and circulated to libraries and other users throughout the country. These include Current Literature on Cancer, Communicable Disease, Community Health, General Health Topics and General Medical Practice.

Index Medicus

This is published monthly with annual accumulations—*The Accumulated Index Medicus*, by the National Library of Medicine, United States of America (USA). It serves as one of the most comprehensive and up-to-date listings of articles appearing in approximately 2250 of the world's biomedical journals. It provides indexes by both subject and author, together with a useful 'bibliography of medical reviews'. MEDLARS is a tape service corresponding to *Index Medicus* and available for off-line computer enquiry; a retrospective search on this tape service would normally cost £50 to £100, though this cost may be met by the library providing the service. An on-line information retrievable service accessing a comparable data base is MEDLINE; this is for both retrospective and current awareness literature searches in the general field of medical science. Use of the service is free, but users are expected to complete an evaluation form. The service has been made available to a number of users as part of a national experiment sponsored by the British Library to investigate the future potential of on-line searching. A sub-set of this specialized data base is CANCERLINE which again is made available from the USA National Library of Medicine together with the USA National Cancer Institute.

Science Citation Index

This is an indexing service selectively covering the complete range of the world's significant scientific and technical journal literature (including technical reports) which uses the method of literature searching by tracing a subject back through citations. Access may be via (1) known key papers (books or other publications are of course suitable), (2) an appropriate subject or (3) searching for an author or organization known to be working in the field of interest. These different ways of accessing the data provide a powerful retrieval service. There are quarterly issues with an annual accumulation; the publications date from 1961 onwards.

1.10.4. *Indexes to research in progress*

There have been an increasing number of indexes of research in progress produced over the past few years; a recent count indicated that there are already at least forty-five research registers in the government sector alone [B 373]. The following indicates some of the indexes of research that are likely to be relevant to the area covered by the present review:

(1) Research in British Universities, Polytechnics and Colleges (formerly Scientific Research in British Universities and Colleges). This is now to be published in four volumes, the third of which covers medical sciences and the fourth social sciences. This, of course, has a restricted source of research locations, and depends on the enthusiasm with which the returns from the constituent research units have been completed. The problem in the past has been that many of the entries failed to precisely identify active research.

(2) Department of Environment's Research Register—this covers a rather restricted field of limited interest to the present review, though some studies on the interplay of environment and health are included.

(3) DHSS 'Annual Report of Departmental Research and Development'. This includes an indication of research carried out by the funded full-time research units and again depends on the way the material has been obtained and indexed.

(4) *Portfolio for Health, 2*, published by the Nuffield Provincial Hospitals Trust (NPHT—[B 358]), contains a detailed review of DHSS funded research.

(5) A survey control unit has recently been set up within the CSO, which has now established a computerized record system; no definitive plans for publication of details of individual surveys on specified subjects have yet been released. The notification of surveys conducted by health service authorities is currently under discussion, and at present very few surveys are notified by health service authorities to the Survey Control Unit.

(6) The annual or periodic reports of other funding authorities indicate the work carried out under their auspices, i.e. reports from the NPHT, the Medical Research Council (MRC), the Social Science Research Council (SSRC), etc.

(7) Details of medical-care research carried out in England and Wales appear as news items in *Health Trends*, and for Scotland in the equivalent *Health Bulletin*.

(8) At an international level a number of indexes are coming into being, for example, 'Directory of On-going Research in Cancer Epidemiology', International Agency for Research on Cancer, 1976. A European Economic Community 'Group on Biomedicine' within the Committee for Information and Documentation on Science and Technology is exploring the possibility of preparing a permanent index of research projects in biomedicine—but this is not near the publication stage at present.

1.10.5. *Archived statistics*

This entry is included for completeness' sake, though at the moment relatively limited material relevant to the present review has been archived in accessible national systems. The SSRC Survey Archive (which is held at the University of Essex, Colchester) aims to collect, preserve and make available for secondary analysis any machine-readable data collected or compiled by British academics, or any machine-readable data which would be of interest to British academics for secondary analysis. The archive will provide any British academic with a copy of magnetic tape of any requested data free of charge, subject to certain restrictions on obtaining the depositor's approval or undertaking to provide reports of analyses made. A main index of statistics held in the archive up till 1975 has been published together with supplementary sheets showing subsequent additions. There are eleven main classes of survey indexed, of which 'Social Surveys' is likely to be of the greatest interest to readers of this review. Information about the archive is held in every University and Polytechnic Library in Great Britain.

Even though a survey has not been lodged with the SSRC archive, it is always worth considering whether (1) unpublished tabulations are available or (2) special tabulations can be produced from data stored by the research workers. This will particularly be worth considering for major government surveys. The published reports will often indicate whether further data may be obtained and, if so, whether a charge is levied for this.

CHAPTER 2

NEED

2.1. Introduction

'Need' is a term that is bandied about a lot; for example, many of the documents on reorganization of the health service have stressed the importance of identifying the health-care needs of the population and redeploying resources in order to more appropriately meet these needs. Before discussing studies that have been used to assess need it is appropriate to spell out what is meant by this concept. Acheson and Hall [B 6] in their contribution 'Epilogue' have suggested that the concept of 'need' has some of the qualities Macbeth ascribed to the dagger—the false creation that proceeded from his oppressed brain. They feel that it exists yet it eludes the clutches of those who attempt to define it.

Bradshaw [B 59] has identified four types of need: normative—which the expert or professional defines as need; felt need or want; expressed need—felt need turned into action; and comparative need—obtained by studying the characteristics of people in receipt of a service and defining those with similar characteristics as in need. Cartwright [B 89] pointed out that this taxonomy provides a helpful framework but that the problem remains of establishing criteria within the different categories. She indicated that this could be studied by looking at 'measurements' of need (both 'hard' and soft measurements such as feelings of isolation—both may be normative ones), identification of whether services reach those in need, and whether services are distributed in ways that relate to people's needs. Twaddle [B 442] states that the process of health status designation can be seen as consisting of an interaction between an individual and his status definer, in which normative standards of adequacy are applied to the individual in the context of a specific situation, to assess his capacities for role and task performance. Other sociological opinions on this topic have been expressed by Parsons [B 366] and Mechanic [B 315, 316, 317, 318].

In a pragmatic contribution Fry [B 203], who used a different definition of 'wants'/'needs'/'resources', distinguished six levels of health and disease: health; pre-symptomatic phase; phase of symptoms; general practitioner care; specialist care; ultra-specialist care. He emphasized that actions and decisions have to be taken at each threshold and that these depend on the individual's attitudes and family background, local cultural habits, the organization of medical care, and social and administrative issues. In a similar vein, Garfield [B 208] emphasized that health and sickness are not clear-cut divisions, but a spectrum from well, worried-well, early sick, to sick; people are uncertain of their exact location on the spectrum and constantly change from one state to another. Two specific examples of differing opinions between 'people' and the 'professionals' are (1) Morris [QRL 490] who observed that many subjects in his study thought that decayed teeth were normal (see Subsection 2.2.2.1), and (2) Holland and

34

Waller [B 248] who report that 'smokers' cough' was thought to be normal (see Subsection 2.2.2.4). Phrased slightly differently Clarke [QRL 146] commented that chiropodists' estimates of unmet need (a normative measure) exceeded not only people's demand for attention but also their perceived need (want); some people did not identify a requirement for treatment where this was thought to be indicated by the chiropodists. Culyer, Lavers and Williams [B 130] discuss health indicators and distinguish Measures of State-of-Health, Measures of Needs-for-Health, and Measures of the Effectiveness of Health-affecting Activities. They are using 'Need-for-Health' as target levels set by the 'Minister', who has assessed what society needs for each of a variety of States-of-Health.

For the purposes of this review the categorization of need described by Alderson [B 18] is used. In this need is divided into a health need that is unperceived by the individual, and a health need that is perceived. The former is a condition that is unrecognized by an individual or his family, but is potentially discoverable by a practitioner on careful investigation of the total physical, mental and emotional well-being of the individual, using standard techniques and accepted criteria for investigation. Such a condition may warrant intervention (when it is thought that prevention, management or specific therapy would be of benefit), but will also include those diseases for which currently available forms of intervention are of little benefit. A health-care need is perceived when the individual or his family identify an 'abnormality', which they acknowledge is usually brought to the attention of the medical profession. Subsequently they may (1) take no action whatsoever to seek medical care, (2) make use of one of the informal agencies including self-medication or (3) contact one of the conventional branches of the health service. Not all perceived need will be accepted by the medical profession as being correctly identified—and in certain circumstances this may be labelled as over-demand or neurosis. Matthew [B 311] used a very similar approach; however, Williams [B 469] commented that 'need' is, in this context, a supply concept and that some people may be sick, but since there is nothing we can do for them, the implication is that they are not in need. This *reductio ad absurdum* incorporates a very peculiar view of the total activities of the health services when caring for an irreversible fatal condition; it serves more to indicate the pitfalls and blind alleys that can be approached when attempting to define need.

Another important aspect is consideration of the application of research or statistics on need. Edmonds [B 176] criticizes much research on need, suggesting that as demand will always outstrip supply (which means that many measures of need are merely a reflection of supply) it is more appropriate to assess the benefits from increments of the various resources in relation to the present mix of resources. This will guide the decision maker where to spend (or save) £10,000 next year.

Even though there will obviously be argument about the appropriateness of the above classification, there is even greater difficulty in identifying published material which contains statistics that are directly relevant to this issue. This is predominantly due to the lack of definitive studies and the tendency to use other data as 'indicators' of need. It will be obvious that a lot of the assessments of need are subjective—determined by the views of the patients or professionals. A number of authors have discussed the use of indicators of need, which are often derived from routine data, *faut de mieux*. Rosser and Watts [B 396] tested a method for assessing the health status of patients on admission to and discharge from hospital. They make no strong distinction between a health-status index and a measure of health outcome, since the conceptual and practical problems of devising either type of measure are similar. Chapman and Coulson [B 97] have indicated the improvements in the ability to identify the health of a community by examining data for small localities and combining examination of mortality for specific causes, infant mortality, hospitalization data, illness in and absence from school, response to immunization programmes, use of other state health services and census data. Chen and Bryant [B 100] advocate a classification model for sorting various health status indices into homogenous groups; this takes into account the source of data whether these apply to individuals or population, and their orientation (function, symptoms, general view of health, or combinations of these). They stress the difficulty of devising an index that is reliable, valid and feasible, and provide a critical review of a number of indices.

Dunlop [B 169] has reviewed the ways of assessing need for care amongst the elderly in the USA; apart from direct estimates from surveys, pointers come from data on utilization of services, queues for care, and informal care by friends and relatives. He stresses that a major determinant of use of institutional facilities is the availability or lack of family and financial resources. In a WHO International Collaborative Study of Medical Care Utilization it was necessary to select indicators of morbidity for defining levels of health; Kalimo and Rubin [B 270] present some analyses from this study showing the interrelationship between the indicators and specific symptom states. The interest in the topic of indicators is demonstrated by the establishment of a Clearing House on Health Indexes by the USA National Center for Health Statistics; this had identified over 1000 relevant publications by 1975.

It has been suggested in a series of papers published on the reorganization of the health service [B 143, 144 and 145, 153, 407] that any redistribution of health service facilities should be associated with a careful review of the health-care needs of the population; it is not immediately clear how this could be done. As an over-simplification, if the main determinants of health need in a population were the proportion of very young and elderly it would be a relatively simple matter from a decennial (or preferably 5-yearly) census to estimate the total facilities required; it would also be possible to check whether the present use of the services was greater, equal, or less than the expected in any particular locality. The dream of the medical administrator is that a relatively simple index of health need could be derived from assessment of a restricted range of parameters. However, the preceding paragraphs have indicated the complexity of the problem; the 'norms' for provision of care have often been based on incomplete studies and require careful interpretation in their application to any particular locality (see Subsection 2.3.3).

This chapter covers the literature on need in three main sections: population studies; morbidity statistics from the NHS; problem specific studies. There are two main classes of population study; national studies are dealt with first and local ones second. For inclusion, local population studies must have involved a sample of the total population or a very broad age group and have tackled a wide range of medical problems. Various methods of identifying an appropriate sample may have been used, including access to lists of individuals in particular occupations.

Statistics from the NHS include (1) data from health screening, (2) morbidity statistics from general practice, and (3) morbidity statistics from hospital care.

The remaining material in the chapter relates to studies that have explored specific issues. Some of these studies have been based upon nationally drawn samples but are included in this problem-orientated section of the chapter because they have focused upon a specific health problem (in contrast to the entries under population studies, which involve surveys each covering a wide range of problems). An exception to this general rule is the inclusion of studies that deal with particular client groups, such as children or the elderly; the relevant studies have often dealt with a range of medical problems, including physical, emotional, mental and social. It has been found easier to locate these studies primarily under the designation of the person being studied rather than have multiple entries under all diseases involved.

In order to simplify the presentation of the text and the QRL, an arbitrary decision has been made about the relevance of certain categories of data. This was referred to in the previous chapter (Sections 1.6 and 1.8). The following two subsections amplify these earlier comments and indicate the considerations that have taken place in order to decide which sets of published statistics are relevant. In particular, this requires consideration of the rather different ways in which measures of need may be obtained. Though these ground-rules were developed, consideration of space conflict with the wide range of studies had to be considered; the coverage has, of necessity, remained somewhat eclectic.

2.1.1. *The value of data from population studies*

One approach to identifying health-care needs is to interview a sample of individuals and ask them questions about their social setting, their recognition of signs and symptoms of disease, their attitudes to sickness and health care, and perhaps their contact with health services in the recent past. This approach, usually designated as a Health Interview Survey (HIS), may be applied to a representative sample of the total population, a sample drawn from carefully selected locations throughout the country, or subsets of the population chosen by locality, age, occupation or other characteristics. The virtue of an HIS is that data from a fairly large sample of respondents may be obtained with limited expenditure of resources (compared with the use of medical and other staff to investigate the subjects). In certain circumstances by obtaining an indication of the knowledge, attitudes and practice of members of the population a more appropriate picture of their health care needs may be obtained, compared with information derived from other approaches. In particular, the respondents' answers indicate how much ill-health they perceive, their reactions to this, and the reported incapacity from the ailment. Though there are important variations in the method, by which such information may be obtained, this is a subsidiary issue compared with consideration of the major options in place of an 'interview' survey.

Data may be obtained from subjects by a variety of methods, such as the use of self-completion questionnaires, direct interview, group interviews or diary records; it is important to consider the validity of data obtained from such approaches. Obviously, because a question has been asked and an answer given, the resulting information cannot be immediately accepted without question. Many of the studies that are covered in this review have been carefully carried out, with great care taken to check on the quality of the data. Even when independent checks have been carried out and estimates of error rates produced, caution must be taken in handling the published results. There are likely to be errors from: random sampling errors; bias from failure to respond or incomplete response; misunderstanding; memory errors; inappropriate attempts to quantify vague or imprecise notions; deliberate distortion; processing errors in recording, coding, analysis and retrieval. The sources of error in surveys have been reviewed by Abrahamson [B 2], Alderson [B 18], Bennett and Ritchie [B 47] and Moser and Kalton [B 342]. It must be emphasized that this text cannot identify all the problems of interpretation and application of the statistics covered in the QRL; the text tries to indicate some of the general principles involved and the extent to which certain classes of material are appropriate for particular uses. The reader should bear the above general warning in mind and must examine the details of the method given in the original publication before using a particular set of data.

An alternative strategy to an HIS is the collection of data from examination and investigation of the respondents or a sample of these. Some data will have to be collected by questioning the subject, but the aim is to cover quite different issues by direct examination or complement any responses with observations (for example, measuring the blood pressure explores issues rather different to simply recording whether the subject is under treatment for raised blood pressure). The introduction of this examination, usually referred to as a Health Examination Survey (HES), raises considerable problems in the design of the study. Apart from the obvious effect on the resources required to carry out the examination and investigation, the knowledge that this is to be done may have a marked effect upon the response rate. In addition, though indirect validation of the results may be obtained by use of standard procedures and duplicate examination, it is equally necessary to consider the accuracy of examination and investigation results as responses from subjects. Error may be due to the subject's variation in response to the situation, the instrument being used, the observer, or interaction between these different aspects of the measurement. There is an extensive literature on measurement error, which has been reviewed by Alderson [B 18]. It is important to remember that the material contributes a rather different view of the health needs of the population from an HIS. For example, by identifying variation from physiological and psychological normality the investigator can quantify the 'morbidity' in the population which is not recognized by the subjects themselves or their families. This general remark is not meant to suggest that assessment of abnormality is straightforward; even with the measurement of blood pressure, there is a considerable 'grey area' between normal levels and levels at which treatment is definitely justified. The delineation of abnormality in the psychiatric field is even more open to differences of opinion. It must also be borne in mind that no general treatment of such unperceived morbidity will be initiated without either alteration (1) in the knowledge, attitude or practice of the population, or (2) the development of screening programmes to detect and treat such conditions.

An HIS or HES, as indicated above, may be directed at a representative sample of a total population or aimed at a highly specific subgroup of the population. In the text and QRL, reference is made to the few classic complete population studies that have been carried out in this country; the majority of the studies have been aimed at subgroups of the population. The next category of study considered in the text is those that have used geographically defined populations. The remaining categories have involved either age-specific subgroups of the population or have used a variety of subsamples of the population in order to tackle specific medical problems; no attempt has been made to classify these studies, but they have been dealt with alphabetically by category of medical problem involved.

2.1.2. *The value of mortality and morbidity data*

The published material derived from interviews or examination of samples of the population only covers a fairly restricted range of health problems. In the absence of appropriately collected and published data there has been a tendency to use mortality and morbidity data as a substitute. This can be defended where there is a clear suggestion that the data being used are related in a known way to the incidence and prevalence of the disease in the population. For example, with a disease that is rapidly fatal for all patients affected (and assuming accurate certification and analysis of mortality data) a valid picture of the distribution of the disease in the population will be obtained from mortality data; in contrast, such material is of little value in assessing the burden placed upon the patient and his family by a chronic disabling disease with low fatality. A rather different aspect is that in the past there has been a tendency to use material on the overall mortality of the population to provide some guidance as to their general health; another approach has been to use infant mortality, expectation of life or some other product of mortality data as an indication of the healthiness of a locality. When examining the health of specific occupational categories, the Registrar General's decennial supplement on occupational mortality has been invaluable. These data were discussed in detail in the previous review [B 14].

In the recent past there has been a major extension of the collection of morbidity data in the United Kingdom. Historically, notification of infectious disease was the first system to be established, but this has now been followed by a systematic collation and publication of data on: abortion; cancer registration; congenital abnormalities; handicapped persons; hospital in-patient data for admission to acute and chronic hospitals, and those for the mentally ill; infectious disease; morbidity in school children; sickness absence from work. Other sets of statistics relate to specific problems such as Industrial or Road Traffic Accidents. The bulk of this material is published as routine reports from the DHSS and Office of Population Censuses and Surveys (OPCS); as with the mortality data, these have been covered in the previous review [B 14]. The main source of data recently added in this field has been the second National Morbidity Study (NMS); this has collected data on the reported ailments for a sample of about 300,000 people contacting their family doctor over a period of a year. There is no suggestion at the present time that this collection of morbidity data from general practice will become an established routine system funded and supported by central government; it therefore comes within the general scope of this review. It is also complemented by a wide range of separate publications produced by those enthusiasts in general practice who have invested their own time and effort into examining and publishing data for patients under their own care. A report from a single-handed general practitioner on the disease for which patients consult him may provide a very biased estimate of morbidity in the community; this issue is dealt with in Subsection 2.3.2.3. One major advantage of studies in a stable practice is the opportunity to observe the 'natural history' of disease and the influence of treatment.

Rather different is a consideration of the value of hospital morbidity data for those conditions where it is thought that any patient with the disease in question is referred to hospital. This particularly applies to malignant disease; only a very small proportion of patients thought by the family doctor to have this disease are not referred on medical grounds, or because of refusal of the patient to attend hospital. Alderson [B 10] found only 1·1 per cent of 540 patients dying from malignant disease had not been referred to hospital. There is still the problem of identification of the presence of the disease, but the progress of malignant disease is such that deterioration in a patient will usually lead to hospital referral; however, Heasman and Lipworth [B 243] have demonstrated appreciable discrepancies between clinical and post-mortem diagnoses for patients dying in hospital. On these grounds it is argued that relevant hospital morbidity data may provide a good indication of the distribution of the cancer in the population; many years ago it was concluded that population surveys were a less efficient method of collecting data on cancer patients [Dollinger, B 165]. For many other chronic diseases this is not so; even for patients suffering from acute stroke, there may be strong pressure from the patient or the family to nurse the patient at home. It is therefore difficult to tell whether hospital morbidity data provide a meaningful indication of the load of the disease carried by the community; obviously, if appreciable proportions of patients are cared for outside hospital, the statistics will become increasingly unreliable.

An important bias in the morbidity statistics from hospital and general practice is that they reflect the use made rather than the objective 'need'. Titmus [B 435] commented that the higher income groups know how to make better use of the service; they tend to receive more specialist attention; occupy more of the beds in better equipped and staffed hospitals; receive more effective surgery; have better maternal care; and are more likely to get psychiatric help and psychotherapy than low-income groups. Though this view has been disputed by Rein [B 381], strong support has come from Alderson [B 12], Hart [B 234], Marsh and McNay [B 306] and Cartwright and O'Brien [B 91]. A rather separate source of error exists when studying conditions in which there is an appreciable proportion of sudden unexpected deaths. Hospital morbidity data are inadequate to reflect the true statistics for coronary heart disease; the value of (and necessity for) using data from coroners' autopsies (Crawford and Morris [B 120]) and records from insurance companies (Morris, Heady and Barley [QRL 492]) has been clearly demonstrated.

Hospital morbidity statistics as generally published refer to 'events' occurring to patients. For example, analyses may show the number of spells of in-patient care there have been for conditions such as coronary heart disease; it is not possible to convert the data to estimates of prevalence of a condition in the population, because the number of readmissions of individual patients is not known. Acheson [B 4] has discussed this issue at length and shown how the organization of a system for record linkage can lead to cumulative records of events occurring to individuals in a defined population and thus generate statistics of much greater value.

Rather separate to the contribution of routine statistics on hospital treatment morbidity to the understanding of the 'health' of a community is consideration of studies on the need for hospital care (by direct access investigation, out-patient attention, day care or in-patient treatment). Up until now the statistics have been considered from the point of view 'What do they convey about the distribution of disease in the population?'; the converse of this is a search for statistics that tell us about the appropriate level of care required by individuals suffering from particular diseases (taking into account the patients' circumstances). The development of a method for assessing the requirement for hospital care is described in Section 2.3.3; as with population studies in general there is a lack of definitive studies and method problems in the handling of available data. Forsyth and Logan [QRL 243] and Airth and Newell [QRL 11] have indicated that there is a close relationship between use of hospitals and availability of hospital facilities—the more acute beds in a district the higher the admission rate and longer the length of stay. Vanaanen [B 443] has suggested that emergency admissions are a reflection of population structure whilst planned hospital admissions vary in relation to the facilities available. Change in hospital morbidity data may therefore indicate change in facilities rather than any underlying alteration in the distribution of the disease in the population, or change in the social factors influencing requirement for institutional support.

As an alternative to a population survey (HIS or HES) the extent of a health-care problem can be assessed by the collection of available data from different facets of the health-care system. Gillum and his colleagues [B 214] have reported a study of cardiovascular disease, indicating the value of data on 'hard' end points such as fatalities or hospitalization.

2.2. Population studies

This section first discusses national surveys that have been mounted to assess the health of the population and then deals with a few local population surveys. The main characteristic that distinguishes some of the latter work from studies discussed in Section 2.5, Problem Specific Studies, is the use of a population sample and the study of a range of health problems. Those surveys that have used national probability samples, but only tackled one specific medical problem, have been inserted into Section 2.5.

2.2.1. *National population studies*

2.2.1.1. *The survey of sickness.* Before the outbreak of war in 1939 there was no single source in England and Wales from which a complete picture of the nation's sickness experience could be gained. During the early part of the Second World War there were indications from various sources that the health of the civilian population was not as good as it had been pre-war. The GRO suggested that about 2500 people aged 16–64 could be questioned each month, and limited data obtained from them in order to derive an index of morbidity. The first interviews began in January 1944. The method of sampling was adjusted by leaving out Scotland, limiting the number of districts used in each region and taking clusters of addresses within selected rural districts. A multi-stage stratified sampling system was used with the national register (the population index set up at the beginning of the war) as the final sampling frame. From February 1945 an interview survey was carried out each month until March 1952; from December 1944 persons aged 65 and over were included and the sample size increased to 3000 a month and later 4000 a month. From July 1949 the questions were restricted to health in the 2 months preceding interview instead of 3. A standard schedule was used, though this was modified slightly with supplementary questions being added; a copy of this is provided in the report. The coded material was punched on to cards and handled mechanically.

The final report of the survey [QRL 407] had a considerable section devoted to some of the problems of the survey, with a detailed examination of the bias introduced by the memory factor. This is followed by a general critical appraisal which considered the validity and general usefulness of the data that were obtained. One interesting issue is the comment that the tables that were provided became heavily weighted with data on minor and trivial illness, and in particular it was unrewarding to examine for time trends. For example, during the severe influenza epidemic in the first quarter of 1951 the level of reported sickness attained 75 per cent, compared with 71 per cent during the epidemic-free corresponding quarter of the previous year, the increase in morbidity being swamped by the high level of background minor illness. Apart from a number of comments about interpretation of the data it is emphasized that the surveys' positive contribution was to identify the large amount of ill health which people suffer, that does not lead them to seek medical advice. It was suggested as a final conclusion that the main contribution of such a survey is not to provide a permanent operation identifying the total load of ill health, but to contribute as the need arises particular items of information on illness and its effects that cannot be readily obtained in a routine way. Due to the development of other routine systems for obtaining morbidity data (see [B 14]) and shortage of funds the survey ceased in 1952.

2.2.1.2. *The General Household Survey.* A major alteration occurred in the collection of data in Great Britain, with the initiation of a GHS in 1971. The aim of this survey was to provide a substantially improved flow of social statistics to complement the wide range of routine material currently processed by central government, and to develop an instrument to examine the interaction between different policy areas. The intention was to create a survey that was developed in close collaboration with a number of government departments, such that the material collected was closely linked to their needs for information on housing, employment, education, health and social services, transport, population and social security. Consideration of the predominant objective of the survey indicated that a very long interview would be required with all respondents; at the same time there were constraints on resources available. These two factors markedly influenced the study design. It was essential that respondents cooperated willingly in order to obtain the detailed answers called for in the interview.

A nationally representative sample was required and it was decided to use a three-stage sampling technique. The sample is obtained from a frame of local authorities stratified into standard region, and within region by type of area and rateable value. Each stratum includes about 300,000 people, and one primary sampling unit is selected from each of the 168 strata every 3 months. Each selected unit is used four times at 3-monthly intervals and in any 1 month 56 units are being used; 14 for the first time, 14 for the second, third and fourth times. The samples have been designed to be representative of the adult population living in private households (i.e. persons over 15 in 1971, 16 in subsequent years). The sampling is similar for the whole of Great Britain, but the number of households contacted is doubled for Scotland in order to provide the minimum of precision thought necessary for separate analysis. There is a close parallel between the sample design for the GHS and that used for the Family Expenditure Survey (FES); these two surveys now continue throughout the year, using the same primary units. This will enable information from the two surveys to be related. The sampling procedure identifies addresses from the electoral register; the interviewer converts the list of addresses to the identification of households. For multi-household addresses a maximum of three households at any given address are interviewed; with more than three households present a sample is taken. Following interview at a multi-household address, an appropriate number of further addresses are deleted to prevent over-representation in the sample. The initial report provides considerable detail on the sampling error of the survey.

This Social Survey uses a detailed structured interview for the study, which was tested in pilot trials during the development phase; the interviewers have been carefully trained and supervised. The intention is always to change the items included in the study in response to users' requirements; at the same time there will be an effort to reshape the interview so that it becomes easier and so that questions of dubious validity are deleted.

The minimum response rate (i.e. completely co-operating households) in 1971 was 71 per cent; including all partial response a maximum rate of 85 per cent was achieved. There appears to be marked stability in the response rate from month to month, but modest variation across the country. (There was a consistently lower rate in the conurbations and higher rate in the rural areas.) Throughout the report there is referral to the quality of the information provided. The simplest checks that can be carried out on the data are by comparison with other material or by examination of internal consistency of response. Comparison of the survey with 1971 Census data suggests that the GHS provides good representation of the population in private households. However, an appreciable proportion of the morbidity in the total population is amongst residents in institutions.

The health section collects data on activity limitations caused by sickness, consultations with doctors, use of health and personal social services, and visits to hospitals. The questions on activity limitation endeavour to identify those with chronic handicap: these depend upon the respondents' subjective impressions of 'typical' activity levels. All this material is collected by direct questioning and at the present moment no independent verification of the data takes place. This might be possible by detailed investigation of a subsample, including examination of health service records from community and hospital care. Comparative analyses with the second NMS are also desirable (see Subsection 2.3.2.2). Work with the earlier Survey of Sickness (see Section 2.2.1.1) showed that there was considerable variation in reported sickness where a 2-month recall period was used, between the first and second month. It was decided to restrict questioning on acute illness to a 2-week reference period; preliminary analysis suggests that there may even be a consistent variation in sickness and use of facilities between the first and the second week. This is due to a tendency to enhanced recall of recent events. There are doubts over the interpretation of data on use of community services; it is felt that respondents do not clearly distinguish the agencies involved. The material for 1 year also produced relatively small numbers of events for certain activities of health care.

The first year's study carried out in 1971 collected data from nearly 12,000 households and nearly 35,000 individuals. There is obviously a tremendous amount of material that is potentially derivable from the completed questionnaires; apparently over 1000 tables were produced and only a restricted set of these appear in the published report. Much more information was released and discussed with individual central government departments; attention is also drawn to the fact that the OPCS welcome requests for access to the data from research workers, providing confidentiality is not broken. It is also suggested that 'special populations of interest' may be identified and followed up.

A second report of the GHS has been published [QRL 512]. The sample design was precisely the same in 1972 as that used in 1971. There has been some change in the method with the introduction of new topics into the questionnaire that is used; additional data were collected on housing costs, medicine taking and smoking. In order to provide independent verification of the results, data collected for the GHS in one quarter were compared with the 1971 Census returns for the same households. In general, there was good agreement between the findings of the two surveys (where they were comparable). It is suggested that GHS under-represents individuals of late middle age and the elderly (particularly males) with over-representation of the very young and young adults. Small households are under-represented and large households over-represented with the self-employed heads of households being prominent among the non-responders.

One of the important issues is the identification of the presence of chronic sickness; the wording used to establish this was altered for 1972, by splitting the question into two subsidiary questions. The second of these stated explicitly 'Does (it) limit your activities compared with most people of your own age?' There was a considerable drop in people answering this in a positive way, particularly amongst the elderly. It is not clear quite how the phrasing of this question has been interpreted by these responders, but it is likely that many of the elderly felt that the limitation was of the order to be expected at their age. It is a moot point whether it is more important to identify long-standing illness or disability that limits activities or only if it is considered to limit the activities to a greater extent than would be expected for persons of that age. The wording for this question was again altered for the 1973 survey; there was little difference in the distribution of responses and analyses were produced for pooled data for $2\frac{1}{2}$ years. There appears to be no change as far as the questioning on acute sickness is concerned. The data on consultation with general practitioners could, however, be compared with the material available from the NMS (see Subsection 2.3.2.2); this provides a useful check on the distribution of answers by the respondents and to a certain extent gives an indirect estimate of the validity of the material.

Data were collected as usual on use of 'services' from local authorities and other agencies. There appears to be no tabulation of this material in the report and no explanation of the missing analyses in the text.

In the fourth quarter of 1972 additional questions on medicine taking were inserted, chiefly designed to measure the basic patterns of consumption amongst people taking analgesic medicines including the extent to which these were self-prescribed. The questions were asked on supplementary schedules on behalf of the DHSS in an attempt to identify the use of medicines known to produce adverse side effects when taken over prolonged periods or in heavy doses. Comparison of this material is made with the survey by Dunnell and Cartwright [QRL 220]; there were some differences in the way the questions were phrased, the reference period, and the length of the prompt lists used (the GHS asked about analgesics, whilst the other study covered all medicines). This probably accounts for the main differences observed between the two sources of data.

The DHSS and the SHHD asked for questions to be inserted in the GHS so that any changes in the smoking habits of the population could be monitored, and questions were included in the survey. Inclusion of the smoking section in the survey provides at one and the same time an example of the advantages and flexibility of the survey and an illustration of the limitations the nature of the survey imposes. The advantages are, of course, that the responses on smoking can be related to other important socio-economic variables; however, the GHS framework means that the data have to be interpreted with caution. The data only relate to private householders and exclude those in institutions; particularly important may be the exclusion of (1) those in the armed forces, other than living in married quarters, and (2) students; this is likely to bias the data for the young, by exclusion of these groups. Interviewing at the family fireside is also likely to affect the validity of data for young people, if they are interviewed in the presence of their parents. The questions on smoking follow a lengthy section on chronic and acute sickness and this is likely to influence the extent of smoking reported. Comparisons were made with GHS and Tobacco Research Council reports on smoking in the population. It is suggested that the GHS understates the tobacco consumption, particularly amongst the young.

The only additional issue covered in the health section in 1973 was the introduction of questions about health-centre usage. Additional tables were provided on consumption of medicines and smoking habits.

2.2.2. *Local population studies*

Relatively few population studies have been carried out in this country. The first one to be included is inserted because it was carried out in 1939 and thus warrants consideration from the point of view of development of method. A wide-ranging series of studies have been carried out in South Wales (with some collaborative work elsewhere) and a section reviewing the series of these studies is included. This is followed by two contributions on residents in the immediate catchment area of London teaching hospitals.

2.2.2.1. *An early study.* In 1939 the employees in a Midland corporation were examined [QRL 490]; the author drew attention to the deficiency of morbidity statistics in the country: 1592 workers were examined, 1352 men and 240 women; due to the small number involved, women were excluded from the published results. The subjects filled in a questionnaire, which covered their own and their family history. A full medical examination was then carried out; many of the men were seen twice and a few three times, to complete the investigation. About sixty were sent for a second opinion to consulting staff of the local municipal hospital; the pathological and X-ray facilities were freely used, though it was not possible to do routine radiography of the chest.

In discussing his findings Morris pointed out that about 7 per cent had major disorders, whilst minor disorders were legion. Most of the major disorders were symptomless or did not interfere with the daily work. The minor disorders usually were quite obvious—they were seen, but not perceived. Although 50 per cent of the men had seen their doctor within the past 2 years, most of the major disorders would have benefited from medical care, whilst the minor ones were largely avoidable and unnecessary. The author suggested that the findings demonstrate the value of routine medical inspection of adults, such as is taken for granted in school children. This study is described as it illustrates an early contribution to method, and indicates the degree of unmet demand that was identifiable.

2.2.2.2. *South Wales studies.* A major contribution to the method of such studies and the examination of a wide range of medical problems has been the work of Cochrane and his colleagues. The following note describes the development of the work of this MRC Unit, to indicate the way in which the method evolved over a 20-year period in response to changing problems; increasing attempts were made to standardize techniques and reduce observer error, though not all the studies relied on data-collection techniques which had been validated. A general review of the work in South Wales has been provided by Cochrane [QRL 149]; a large-scale epidemiological survey was mounted in the Rhondda Fach, to measure the factors influencing the natural history of coalworkers' pneumoconiosis [QRL 151]. The population was identified by the electoral roll and lists of school leavers; it was checked by home visiting during and after the survey; 91·7 per cent of the male population and 86 per cent of the female population were X-rayed. This excellent response rate was the result of extremely careful preparation prior to the survey and enthusiastic visiting of those who initially did not participate. Extreme care was taken in reading the X-rays; the definitions of abnormality were standardized and two observers read the X-rays independently.

In 1953 a private census was carried out at which identification particulars were recorded for everyone 5 years and over living in the valley; an occupational history was recorded, when appropriate. The community was again X-rayed [QRL 152]. This demonstrated that it was possible to follow-up a population of about 25,000 people; 95 per cent of those included in the 1951 survey were X-rayed again.

A random sample drawn from the 1953 Rhondda Fach census were visited in their own homes for measurement of systolic blood pressure. This was carried out by one observer using a standard technique; the arm circumference was measured for correction of the recorded pressure. Ninety-eight per cent of first-degree relatives living within 25 miles had their blood pressure recorded. This material has provided a very useful analysis of the inheritance of arterial blood pressure [QRL 464]. Another random sample of fifty-five were selected for investigation of the prevalence of coronary heart disease, using clinical history, examination and ECG [QRL 642]. The next survey was carried out in the Vale of Glamorgan, to provide comparison of an agricultural area [QRL 153], the population again being defined by a private census. Ninety-five per cent of those aged 5 and over were persuaded to participate—the best ever recorded for a voluntary chest X-ray survey. All persons attending this chest survey of the Vale were asked 'Have you ever suffered from goitre?' Those answering yes were seen by two observers and examined clinically, whilst one observer visited an equal number of controls matched for age and sex. A lay assistant subsequently visited the subjects and collected a detailed history; samples of past and present water supply were obtained for women with non-toxic goitres. Presence of goitres in parents and sibs was ascertained by history, but the relatives were not examined [QRL 660].

As each subject attended in the 1953 and 1955 surveys, he or she was questioned about painful swelling of the small joints of the hands and feet [QRL 462]. From this source, general practitioners and rheumatism clinics, lists were compiled and all those people with suggestions of disease interviewed in their own home. Suspect patients were then X-rayed and serological data examined; the diagnostic criteria were standardized.

An attempt was made to ascertain the numbers of patients with mental disorder in the Rhondda Fach and Vale of Glamorgan, from 1 January 1951 to 30 June 1956 [QRL 121]. The study was based almost entirely on documentary evidence, search being made of records in all mental and general hospitals serving the area. Evidence was also sought from general practitioners about cases of suicide and attempted suicide, but no attempt was made to interview patients in order to ascertain 'a true count' of psychiatric cases in the population.

A survey was then carried out on the 55–64-year-old population of Leigh, Lancashire [QRL 311], to compare the prevalence of respiratory symptoms and disability in miners with that found in men who had worked in other occupations. The electoral roll was used as a basis for a random sample of housing; samples of 100 houses from the whole of Leigh were chosen in succession and each sample was visited before the next was begun. After fifteen such samples had been visited, 245 men between 55 and 64 had been found and the sampling was stopped; just over 90 per cent of the men selected in the sample agreed to attend at a central hall for various investigations. Those failing to keep an appointment were revisited and either persuaded to accompany the visitor immediately or given a further appointment. Associated with the development of the survey technique a standardized respiratory questionnaire had been introduced and techniques for measuring respiratory function in a standard way; again, duplicate X-ray reading was carried out. This work in South Wales and England stimulated a comparable study in Scotland; a community X-ray survey was carried out in Annandale [QRL 148].

In order to extend the search for aetiological factors in chronic respiratory disease, a further population survey was carried out in Staveley, Derbyshire [QRL 307]. This town was selected as a considerable proportion of the population were foundry workers and it was then possible to examine the relationship between occupation and prevalence of disease. A private census was carried out. The electoral roll was used to check that all houses had been visited. In the age groups 25–34 and 55–64 four main occupational groups were identified: foundry and ex-foundry workers; miners and ex-miners; men who had worked in either or both of these occupations and some other dusty job; men who had never worked in dusty occupations. From four random samples respiratory symptoms were recorded on a standardized questionnaire, standardized techniques were used to assess ventilatory capacity, and a chest X-ray was taken. Whilst the survey of the men was in progress, one of the workers visited the wives of the older men in their homes, to complete a respiratory questionnaire and obtain measures of ventilatory capacity.

In the late 1950s a major extension of the study programme began. Further studies were carried out in the Rhondda Fach, with a detailed investigation of various sub-samples of the population who had been contacted in the 1951 survey. In these subsequent detailed investigations, the prevalence of ischaemic heart disease, rheumatoid arthritis and anaemia was measured. The next report published of this work dealt with the prevalence of anaemia in a sample of subjects investigated in the Rhondda Fach in 1958 [QRL 375]. As before, subjects were visited and invited to come to a centre for investigation; each person was directly questioned about injections in an attempt to identify those with Addisonian anaemia. A range of investigations were carried out on samples of blood (haemoglobin, packed cell volume, blood films, serum iron and serum vitamin B_{12} levels were estimated). Data on heights and weights were collected from a sample of subjects in the 1956 Vale Survey, and survivors of the 1954 Rhondda Fach Survey who were measured in 1958 using a standardized technique [QRL 33]; the first-degree relatives over 5 living within 25 miles were also visited. It should be noted that the subjects measured were not completely representative of the actual communities, because respondents from the Rhondda were the 'survivors' from the first survey, and their relatives living in the vicinity were included.

Higgins and his colleagues [QRL 308] published a report on the epidemiology of coronary disease. In this they describe the detailed reinvestigation of the Rhondda Fach sample of subjects and relate this to the findings from three earlier published surveys (one of the rural community of the Vale of Glamorgan, one of the rural community in Dumfriesshire, and a third survey of miners and ex-miners in the Rhondda Fach).

In 1963 the adjoining townships in the Rhondda Fach were involved in a survey of intra-ocular pressure. Residents aged 40–74 were included and 91·9 per cent participated; after a home visit a clinic appointment was made. After a history had been taken the anterior segment of the eye was examined by a slit-lamp, the pressure was read using two calibrated techniques, the optic discs were examined, and a third of the subjects had their fields of vision tested. Where necessary arrangements for treatment or further supervision were made [QRL 332].

In 1966 a return visit was paid to Staveley in Derbyshire and a 9-year follow-up examination was carried out [QRL 309]; at the same time, a co-operative study was carried out with a team who had surveyed a sample of subjects in mining communities in Marion County, West Virginia (Higgins *et al.* [QRL 310]). During the 1960s further diseases were studied in South Wales. In 1961 a survey was carried out in the Rhondda Fawr [QRL 723] in which a sample of women were invited to attend a clinic for a dental and medical examination which included venepuncture. The response rate (70 per cent) was lower than in other of the 'Cochrane' surveys. Each subject was given a self-administered questionnaire which covered the symptoms commonly attributed to iron-deficiency anaemia; samples of the women were then asked to participate in trials of oral iron therapy [QRL 231]. This study on anaemia was extended by three further trials carried out on two samples from the Rhondda and a sample of 14-year-old schoolgirls [QRL 229].

A hundred subjects were drawn at random from the Cardiff electoral roll and their first-degree relatives aged over 15 who were also resident in the city were contacted in a survey of varicose veins [QRL 704]. The majority of subjects were seen at a central clinic but seventy-two were visited in their own homes. A detailed standard questionnaire was used; one observer examined the patients standing up. It is pointed out that such an investigation needs standardization of room temperature and of physical exercise immediately prior to examination. Eighty-eight of the initial 100 sampled were examined and a further 201 (90 per cent) of first-degree relatives.

A sample of men and women aged 55–64 examined in the Vale of Glamorgan for arthritis in 1956 were followed up in 1967 [QRL 8]. A standard questionnaire was used to collect data on previous and current medical history, particularly on fractures sustained and the presence or absence of back pains; at the initial examination X-rays of the hands of men and women and the vertebral column of women were taken. These measurements were repeated under standard conditions in 1967 and a venous blood sample was taken; the X-rays were assessed under standard conditions using three observers for the hands and the same observer for the spine. Of the eligible sample remaining alive, 98 per cent of men and 92 per cent of women participated in the repeat investigation.

In 1968 a follow-up study was done on the subjects who had been initially examined in the community survey of the Rhondda Fach of 1958; 91 per cent of the survivors were re-examined [QRL 697]. Subjects were seen either at a central clinic or in their homes in the Rhondda; an attempt was also made to see those survivors living elsewhere. All subjects were examined for cardio-respiratory disease and arthritis; a sample of venous blood was taken, for haemoglobin and PCV estimation. This issue has been further examined by analysis of 3-year mortality of over 18,000 women initially examined in seven population surveys carried out from 1964 to 1969 in South Wales [QRL 228].

In 1967 all women in a defined area in the Rhondda Fach between 20 and 64 were asked to co-operate in a survey which included standard questions about urinary tract symptoms and consumption of analgesic tablets [QRL 696]. The 'analgesic group' were compared with controls for urinary tract symptoms and various indices of kidney function. The women in the analgesic group were visited a year later; a detailed questionnaire was completed on the consumption of tablets and items adapted from the Cornell Medical Index [QRL 695]. Murray [QRL 497] suggested that the habitual consumer of analgesics often had a psychological illness and failed to acknowledge their habitual consumption of analgesics.

In the late 1960s a random sample of voters in the Pontypridd area of Glamorgan were invited to complete a questionnaire asking about symptoms of headaches; over 94 per cent approached responded. A high proportion of those identified by the questionnaire as suffering from 'migraine' were diagnosed as having migraine in a clinical validation study. Waters [QRL 693] reported on an ophthalmological examination in relation to the headache data. Other data from the 1968 survey [QRL 694] included questions on current smoking habits and nine questions from the Cornell Medical Index (CMI) health questionnaire.

A survey was carried out in the Rhondda Fach in 1968–9 and a small coastal town in 1969, when subjects 65 and over were approached [QRL 227]. They were invited to attend a clinic (and a home visit was arranged where this was not possible); several simple tests of learning and recall were performed and a history taken of general health with specific questions about medicine consumption. Haematological investigations were carried out under standard conditions. As an extension to this study, general practitioners in Coventry identified a sample of Asian patients and a random sample of 'English' patients [QRL 226]. Only subjects 65 and over were contacted and invited to go to a clinic (again a home visit was paid where appropriate). Height, weight and skinfold thickness were measured and a brief dental examination carried out. A sample of blood was taken to assess red blood cell values, B_{12}, folate levels, ascorbic acid, protein, calcium and cholesterol. There was some difficulty in getting an adequate response from the Asian subjects due to their mobility; only one Asian refused to participate, whilst 30 per cent of the English subjects declined.

The first study reviewed in this section was the 1950–1 radiographic survey of the Rhondda Fach [QRL 151]; this population has been followed up and studied on many occasions. Cochrane [QRL 150] reported a 20-year follow-up of the initial survey group; the location was unknown for only ten of the 7713 included in the initial population study. The death certificate was obtained for all those subjects that had died.

2.2.2.3. *Bermondsey and Southwark*. A rather different issue was studied by a research team based at a London teaching hospital, who looked at the health problems of the population in the immediate catchment area; the aim of this survey was to obtain a detailed and accurate picture of the health of the population around Guy's Hospital (Wadsworth, Butterfield and Blaney [QRL 669]). An attempt was made to identify the subjects' perception of illness and their use of services in the urban community. This was as background to understanding demand for care; two earlier studies had focused upon the functioning of out-patient services [QRL 669].

The survey was carried out in the two London boroughs of Bermondsey and South-wark in 1962 and 1963. Five samples of 500 names each were drawn randomly from the electoral registers in order to spread the sample over the whole area and over a complete calendar year. A standard questionnaire was devised, to collect data on symptoms or complaints, diagnoses or causes of illness, medicines and measures taken and other background data. Care was taken to identify the issues which could be accurately reported by respondents; discussion of 'socially unacceptable' conditions was excluded. In addition to minimizing memory error by a 2-week recall period, an appropriate frame of reference was provided in order to stimulate memory.

Two or three days before interview a letter of introduction was sent to each subject. The overall response was 87 per cent, with 2163 completed interviews. Information was incomplete for 335 subjects in the sample; the major reason for non-response was movement out of the area or absence for other reasons. Only forty-five subjects refused to co-operate. The sample was representative of the two boroughs, though there was slight overrepresentation of the elderly and a deficiency of those 20–30, with slight excess of divorced females and small households. Some of the items on the questionnaire were pre-coded whilst others were coded shortly after completion; the data were punched on to tape for computer analysis.

2.2.2.4. *Lambeth*. In the absence of adequate information from official statistics to serve as guidance for planning purposes, it was decided to carry out a survey in the locality of St. Thomas' Hospital to study the prevalence of certain clearly specified diseases in the defined population [B 248]. The intention was to measure the prevalence of four common conditions (cardio-respiratory disease, functional disability, skin disease and duodenal ulceration). At the same time, the amount of medical need being met by the medical services in the area was assessed. Some of the published work stemming from the series of studies required for this exercise are particularly relevant to this review from the contribution that they make to the development of method.

An important feature was the use of a preliminary survey to identify the population served by the hospital. The addresses of a 10 per cent sample of in-patients and 5 per cent of out-patients were examined; this showed that a third of these patients lived in Lambeth [B 248]. The subsequent surveys concentrated solely upon this borough. A 20 per cent sample of households was drawn, in order to provide a reference population, for the subsequent calculation of rates; the adults in these households were used in the next phase of the study. Part of the research involved the use of different methods to identify the base population; comparisons were made between the private census, the EC lists, the Electoral Roll and the GRO 1966 sample census.

Cardio-respiratory disease was initially identified by sending a questionnaire to a sample in the borough; a further sample was then drawn of those with positive and negative responses to this questionnaire, in order to check whether the initial data were valid. The selected subjects were asked to complete the full MRC respiratory questionnaire [B 319] and the WHO angina questionnaire [B 392]; other social, occupational, educational and housing data were also collected. The subjects were then examined and data recorded upon medical care in the 6 months preceding the survey [QRL 10]. The second condition studied was chronic functional disability; a validated interview schedule was used to identify the subjects with chronic disease and disability [QRL 62, 258]. The third condition studied was skin disease, which was identified by medical or nursing interviewers who recorded the patients' symptoms and carried out a limited physical examination [QRL 556]. Finally data were sought about the prevalence of duodenal ulceration using tested questions; a sample of subjects positive to the questions were called for radiological investigation if the diagnosis of duodenal ulceration had not previously been made. An essential part of the study design was the identification of those with recent hospital contact; samples of those reporting and not reporting such contact with the hospitals were checked against the hospital records; Palmer *et al.* [QRL 521] showed a tendency to over-report in-patient experience; there was more accurate reporting by the young women in the sample and those in higher classes.

Full information was obtained from 5499 (99·2 per cent) of the dwellings eligible for enumeration; this yielded a population of 18,347 individuals. The next phases of the study were restricted to those aged 15½ and over; 13,903 of these subjects responded to the self-completion questionnaire (over 99 per cent).

2.2.2.5. *Miscellaneous epidemiological surveys.* It is difficult to know where to draw the line in the location of a large number of epidemiological studies. However, apart from the separate description of the above population studies the remainder have been included in the section of this chapter dealing with specific medical problems. This has been a relatively arbitrary decision, but has been taken in an attempt to distinguish the few major studies that have attempted to identify the general health needs of a population from other studies aimed at specific aspects of health care or disease. The studies that have provided relevant statistics are indexed in the QRL, but the majority of them are not discussed in the text; where relatively standard methods of cross-sectional, retrospective or prospective studies have been implemented space has necessitated omission of the description of many valuable studies.

2.3. Morbidity statistics from the NHS

The general issues of the value and appropriateness of routine or survey data of morbidity treatment in primary medical care or hospital as a measure of need have been commented upon in Subsection 2.1.2. This section provides some details of the specific sources of data (both from general practice and hospital) that are covered in the QRL. It begins with a short subsection on the data that are available from screening programmes.

2.3.1. *Screening*

Since the beginning of this century there have been certain subgroups of the population who have received regular health checks in order to detect disease before it is noticed or brought to the doctor. This particularly applied to children under 5 attending an Infant Welfare Clinic, and school children. Data from these schemes (which have been carefully reconsidered recently by the Court committee—[B 119]) are published in the appropriate central government statistical volumes and have been covered in the previous review [B 14]. Over the past few years there has been increasing interest in detecting chronic disease in adults by mass screening campaigns; an early example was the search for tuberculosis (see Subsection 2.5.33 which discusses mass X-ray campaigns). More recently there have been enthusiasm and controversy [B 298] over screening for various cancers, heart disease and other chronic diseases.

The method of a screening campaign is comparable to an HES, though the target population and the aims are rather different. A screening programme will often be aimed at a high risk subgroup of the population, who will be encouraged to come with the 'hope' that any detected disease will be identified early and appropriate curative treatment instituted. Two rather different approaches have been used; the first concentrates upon one specific condition (such as carcinoma of the cervix) and tests for the prevalence of early disease in the general population or the incidence in women who are rescreened. The second (multi-phasic screening) searches for the presence of early signs of a range of diseases, usually using history, examination and investigations to detect borderline or overt abnormality.

The prevalence and incidence of the various diseases, their speed of progression, their response to early and late treatment, the validity of the screening tests, the harm done by missing actual disease or falsely labelling someone as 'positive' all require to be considered before deciding whether screening is justified on financial and other grounds. This is a complex subject, but it comes into the terms of reference of the review as any screening study may generate data about the distribution of untreated disease in the population. The value of the data will depend on the representativeness of the respondents, the validity of the screening techniques and the range of conditions included in the campaign.

The controversy surrounding screening has been indicated in this subsection; this suggests that the prime activity in this field should be carefully planned projects, so designed that evaluation will be feasible. This suggests that the major activity in this field is likely to be research projects, rather than routine work carried out by the NHS. However, because of the major activity in this field of many LHAs prior to reorganization, it was decided to locate this entry within Section 2.3, Morbidity Statistics from the NHS, rather than under either population or problem specific studies.

2.3.2. *Morbidity statistics from general practice*

Reference has already been made to the value of morbidity statistics as an indicator of population health needs (see 2.1). It was there argued, in the absence of a continuous national HIS/HES, that it was appropriate to use morbidity data from general practice as one source of relevant material. In setting up schemes for the collection and presentation of such material a lot of thought has been given to the mechanics of the system; this has perhaps diverted attention away from the important issues of the validity of the recorded data and the actual relationship between diagnosed ailments of patients contacting their general practitioner and the total illness of the population served by the practice.

The inception of the College of General Practitioners (later Royal College—RCGP) provided a boost to research in general practice. A series of papers have been published on the organization of medical records for research purposes [B 204, 179, 77, 278, 378, 423, 5, 125, 218, 382, 186]. A considerable body of advice was provided in the book, produced for the college, on research [B 180].

The College of General Practitioners [B 111] developed a coding system to be used in recording morbidity in general practice, which has been further refined [B 113]. Morrell [B 335] has discussed the serious limitations that are imposed on research workers in general practice when they are restricted to conventional diagnostic codes in labelling the problems that are presented. Hull [B 257] advocated a rather different approach to disease coding, which identified the system involved, the disease process and the organ involved. Morrell [B 335] noted a rather unexpected relationship between the symptoms presented to the general practitioner and the diagnoses subsequently recorded; this was further discussed by Clark [B 105], in relation to problem-orientated medical records.

On a wider issue the College Research Unit has issued a glossary covering recommended definitions for the whole range of primary medical care. The following two examples indicate confounding factors that can distort comparisons in the absence of precise definitions. Marsh and McMay [B 305] have demonstrated the appreciable contribution to primary medical care that can be made by nurse and health visitor. Variation in availability and use of such staff, together with different reporting systems, could bias the morbidity data generated. A number of authors [e.g. B 465, 306] have noted that newly registered patients generate more contacts than established patients; this again could cause bias in morbidity statistics, unless appropriate allowance is made.

A vital element is the calculation of the list size of the practice(s) over the period of the study. Lees and Cooper [B 287] identify problems of definition, inflation and net change in practice list. Various authors have used: those staying on the list throughout the study period, those ever on the list during the study, those on the list at one point in time, or the mean of estimates from several totals such as quarterly counts. The first NMS had an inflation of 1·1 per cent, which was reduced to 0·7 per cent after investigation; seven of the 106 practices had an excess of over 4 per cent. Discrepancy between the EC lists and counts of patients for whom the practitioner is actually responsible have been estimated at 20 per cent by Backett *et al.* [B 31] and 18 per cent by Morrell *et al.* [B 336]; Farmer *et al.* [B 187] discuss the reasons for these discrepancies. One approach to circumventing this issue has been suggested by Marshall *et al.* [B 307] for use when comparing consulting patterns. There may also be a steady alteration in list size; for example, McGregor [B 297] documented a net increase of 5 per cent over 2 years in a relatively stable population.

Last [B 281] used data from national statistics, general practice studies and a range of epidemiological surveys to quantify the disease present in an average-sized general practice in a year. He drew attention to the likelihood that there was a considerable amount of undetected disease, which might be found without adding greatly to the burden of the day's work. This undetected disease will result in a gap between recorded morbidity and true prevalence of disease in the community. The prevalence of self-care has been indicated by Horder and Horder [QRL 333]; Cartwright [QRL 127]; Wadsworth, Butterfield, and Blaney [QRL 669]; and the GHS [QRL 510, 512, 513]. Further light is thrown on this issue by Kessel and Shepperd [QRL 370]; they showed that about 15 per cent of patients on a doctor's list were non-attenders over a 2-year period with only 3 per cent not attending over a 10-year period. The non-attenders appeared to have the same amount of trivial illness as other patients, they worried less about their health, had a lower score for emotional disturbances, considered themselves healthy, did not use other medical care or self-prescribing to replace contact with their general practitioners, were not neglectful of their health, but tended to be more critical of the services of their doctor. Hannay and Maddox [B 231] provided an important contribution on method; they examined the symptoms for which patients (1) sought advice from pharmacist, relative, friend or acquaintance, or (2) consulted their general practitioner. They separated the types of problem into 'medical' and 'social' and scored each event on the degree to which the action was incongruous. This approach identified those problems of a serious nature that were not being brought to the family doctor and those trivial issues that were.

A series of papers have been published on the validity of data recorded by general practitioners. In considering the accuracy of the analyses one must bear in mind the possible errors in capture, coding and processing of the material. The general accuracy of records in primary medical care has been discussed by Morrell and his colleagues in a series of papers [B 335, 336, 337, 338, 339], Clarke and Bennett [B 106], Dawes [B 135], Munro and Ratoff [B 344] and Farmer *et al.* [B 187]. Hannay [B 230] commented upon the inaccuracy of addresses held by health centres, whilst Kay [B 272] showed that a trained clerk had a considerably lower error rate in coding social class than practitioners. The second NMS preliminary report [QRL 509] indicates that processing may have introduced some errors into the computer file.

Sidel *et al.* [QRL 611] have drawn attention to a constellation of ageing, single-handed doctors in an inner London borough working in isolation from inadequate premises and by-passed by many of the innovations in the delivery of medical care. It seems likely that such major variation in attitudes, background and practice organization could distort both the pattern of treated morbidity and reporting habits. What is not known is how 'typical' are the volunteers who participate in morbidity surveys. Crombie [B 124] has suggested that the diagnostic fashions and differences in the case mix that a family doctor draws towards him can have some influence; providing the number of doctors is sufficiently large, the overall population that is served approximates closely to the general population. It is thus possible to obtain fairly accurate statistics on morbidity within the population. In the absence of data from population surveys, morbidity data from primary medical care have two main advantages: first, they relate to conditions that may not warrant hospital care nor cause fatality (i.e. will not be represented in the main national statistical systems); secondly, the patient will often be followed up over many years, thus enabling the doctor to record progress, response to the treatment and interaction of the patients and his condition with the environment. There remain a number of difficult issues of study design and interpretation of results. Morrell and Kasap [B 338] reported a study on the effect of an appointment system on demand for medical care. Data were collected for demand for (and provision of) medical care in a London general practice during two seasonally matched periods of 6 months in successive years. Though significant differences in the pattern of medical care were observed, it was not possible to establish to what extent these reflected a change in the prevalence of or severity of illness in the population (or stemmed from organizational changes in the practice).

Unfortunately the general approach used in many of the published studies varies, which means that many of the interesting publications cannot be readily compared. Details of the actual practice are often not given, whilst there are variations in the way the data are recorded. Some studies exclude different categories of patient contact and there is of course the major problem of deciding whether the prime cause for a contact in general practice should be recorded, or all morbidity about which the patient asks the doctor during a single consultation. There are also problems of definition of an episode, particularly with an intermittent chronic disease. Different ways of handling such material can provide quite different counts of 'events'; this creates difficulty in calculating a specific rate. A new approach to this issue has recently been suggested by Marshall *et al.* [B 307]. The user should bear these points in mind and as with any other set of statistics interpret the data with due caution. Hart [B 233] had indicated how the health of South Wales mining communities is very different from that of the country as a whole, and the way in which this is reflected in the statistics from general practice.

2.3.2.1. *The first National Morbidity Study.* A study was launched in 1951 to pilot a method for collecting and analysing medical records kept by a small number of general practitioners. There was increasing interest in the GRO and MoH to test to what extent general practitioners' clinical records could be used as a source of morbidity statistics. Ten practitioners were visited and the system for recording discussed with them; only one or two had previously made any attempt to record their consultations in a form suitable for statistical analysis. A small sum of money was made available to reimburse those doctors who found it necessary to provide extra payment for their secretaries for the additional work imposed.

The doctors counted the number of patients registered and compared this with the total list size provided by the EC and with one exception there was fairly close agreement. For each consultation the doctors were asked to record: date of consultation; place of consultation; certificate issued; type of referral if appropriate; diagnosis or other reason for consultation.

The interim conclusions from this work, *General Practitioners' Records: An analysis of the clinical records of eight practices during the period April 1951–March 1952* [QRL 404], was that a small group of practitioners had been able without exceptional difficulty to keep records over a 12-month period, suitable for statistical analysis. Various methods of recording were favoured by the different doctors, but the advantage seemed to lie with a specially modified NHS continuation card. The doctors were allowed complete freedom of terminology in recording diagnoses, which were then coded using the ICD. It was stressed that this was a new venture and the optimum method of classifying and tabulating morbidity statistics from general practice was only just being explored.

The pilot study was then extended for a further 2 years. The second report, *General Practitioners' Records: An analysis of the clinical records of some general practices during the period April 1952 to March 1954* [QRL 262], provided a very brief discussion of the relative value of the rates for consultations and patients consulting. Attention is drawn to the fact that some morbidity is not brought to the attention of the family doctor and other problems are referred to hospital. The other factors, such as idiosyncrasy in use of medical terminology, which cause variation within the practice are briefly discussed.

During the time of the pilot study discussed in the above paragraphs the College of General Practitioners was founded and their members quickly declared their interest in furthering research by general practitioners. Meetings took place between the CGP and the GRO and agreement was reached about launching a morbidity study. The object was to measure, in total and for each disease, the amount of sickness encountered in general practice. After considerable discussion 106 practices involving 171 doctors participated in the survey; two doctors withdrew during the year, though their partners continued. All practices used a standard method for recording limited particulars about each patient contact—this involved identifying the patient by name and address, recording sex, date of birth or age, the diagnosis, dates of consultation, and admission to hospital if this occurred. The recording began in May 1955 and lasted for 12 months. The report has been published in three volumes—*Morbidity Statistics from General Practice*: Volume I, *General*; Volume II, *Occupational*; Volume III, *Disease in General Practice* [QRL 408, 405, 564].

A special card was designed and used by all participating practices. Usually a duplicating system was used with patient records and survey cards, but a few doctors used only the survey card. This was submitted for processing and then returned to the doctor for use in patient care. Standard instructions and definitions were provided for recording each patient contact, and only at the end of the year was the material sent to the GRO for processing.

It was agreed desirable to include an occupational enquiry in the survey, with the aim of providing information on the relationship between morbidity and occupational factors—such information not being available from other sources. One hundred and twenty of the doctors agreed to record the additional information required; this involved completing record cards for all patients on the list, including those who did not consult during the study year. The occupation of patients was recorded on the survey record card for all men and women over 15 years of age; for children under 15 the occupation of the father or guardian was entered. A standard system was used to distinguish full-time and part-time workers, those not paid, and women who were engaged in home duties. Where the doctor was in any doubt the industry was recorded as well as the occupation.

At the end of the 12 months' survey the record cards of medical contact were coded as already described; in addition the occupations had to be classified—using the Registrar General's (RG) classification developed for the 1951 census. Where there was doubt during the coding, an enquiry was sent to the general practitioner for further information. Those practices with more than 12 per cent of the patients having no occupation stated were excluded (three practices).

2.3.2.2. *The second National Morbidity Study*. The aim of this study was to collect morbidity data from general practice in a form that was compatible with the 1955/6 survey. In addition to collecting morbidity information it was decided to collect data about use of facilities, both in the community and from hospital; the intention was also to identify patients' consulting patterns—see *Morbidity Statistics from General Practice, second national study, 1970–71* (OPCS [QRL 509]).

It was decided to use the diagnostic index E-book—see Eimerl and Laidlaw [B 180]; there were a number of practices in the country using this system, which was therefore already well tested. For each face-to-face contact the date of first consultation, the episode type, the name, and date of birth were recorded. For any episode up to six consultations could be coded with a facility for a continuation entry. A system for coding referrals to other agencies was also used. It was thought that about forty practices were regularly using diagnostic indexes and the intention was to accept into the study sufficient practices to include a quarter of a million people. In the main study fifty-four practices were initially involved, though one withdrew during the survey (this was fortunately from an over-represented area). A table indicates that the coverage across the country is very close to the OPCS estimate of population distribution. Of course, such a selection of volunteer practices does not guarantee their representativeness. In particular, the doctors were below average age for the country, more of them tended to work in health centres, and they had above average levels of support from nursing staff. It was essential that the practice register was up to date throughout the survey year; a considerable effort was invested in checking the practice-held registers.

Unlike the previous survey coding of diagnostic and other information took place at practice level, rather than centrally; this was a consequence of use of the 'E' book. The Royal College of General Practitioners' classification used was derived from the seventh revision of the ICD, though the eighth revision had come into general use; this created some problems with the use of the classification, which was modified in order to bring it up to date. The DHSS designation of the practices as being urban or rural was used; this is not a code consistent with other OPCS classifications of local authorities as urban/rural and makes comparison with other sources of statistics difficult.

There were two different aspects to processing the data: first was to accumulate a computer-based practice register; second was to input the morbidity data. The confidential morbidity data did not leave the practice in a form that it could be directly identified by patient name, whilst the output from the system was reduced to statistical tables. (At one stage there was fierce criticism of the study in the press and Parliament, particularly voiced by Enoch Powell; however, he was reassured and his attempt to close the study was averted.)

The success of a study such as this depends in part on careful preparation, and close liaison between the central processing and co-ordinating services and the individual practices. Considerable effort was invested in piloting the study, and amending the guidance and instructions given to each practice. However, it was also essential that a considerable investment of effort goes into checking the validity of the data. The checks that were carried out were upon the accuracy both of the practice register, and of the morbidity data. A detailed check of a sample of the registers was carried out, for persons with no recorded morbidity in the study; this indicated an error rate of about 3·4 per cent. However, two-thirds of the study population proved its presence by consulting and therefore it is estimated that the true inflation was nearer 1·1 per cent of the total population. An attempt was made to check the completeness, accuracy and standardization of the morbidity data. A check of the coding was carried out which indicated some particular diagnostic problems and also variation between practices; it was suggested that coding errors resulted only in marginal errors in assessing morbid processes. A print-out of a sample of morbidity data was also checked against the actual practice records. It appeared that about 3·5 per cent of consultations and 2·4 per cent of episodes recorded on practice records were not identified in the computer records, whilst 0·35 per cent of events on the computer files were not recorded in the practice notes. There was no independent check of the actual diagnostic labels used for specific contacts in any of the practices. There is no evidence from the study that recording errors could account for the appreciable variation in consultation rates by sex, age, urban, rural or regional location.

Comparison of the national studies of morbidity statistics from general practice is bedevilled by differences in recording practice, definitions, disease classification and use of ancillary staff. Taking these factors into account, Crombie *et al.* [B 126] have examined the variation in morbidity by cause between the two studies. They suggest that increases are mainly due to a reduced threshold of awareness and consultation for perceived illness; in addition, there appeared to be real reductions and marked increases for some conditions (and these are in line with other indicators of the secular trend of disease prevalence).

2.3.2.3. *Other studies from general practice.* In addition to the national systems for collecting data from family practice there have been a number of pioneer efforts where individual doctors or groups of doctors have invested effort in order to provide material on the patients that they see. Many of these studies, particularly when published by a single doctor and relating to patients under his own care, will not be relevant to the general review—because of the restricted nature of the population covered. Other studies have concentrated more on the organization of the general practice rather than on the morbidity of the patients; these studies appear therefore in the section on workload in Chapter 5 (see Section 5.1). There remain a number of studies which require mention, either because of their pioneering nature, or because they have involved the collection of data from a larger number of doctors, and thus present material of greater substance.

Pemberton [B 367] recognized the contribution that data from general practice could make to study of general morbidity, whilst Pickles [B 370] had clearly demonstrated that advances in knowledge could be made on specific diseases. A major study as far as method is concerned was published by Horder and Horder [QRL 333]; they provided data on the patterns of illness presented to an individual general practitioner for a thousand patients seen in the winter and a thousand patients seen in the summer. In addition an attempt was made to determine the nature and extent of illness which (a) by-passed the family doctor and reached some other medical agency without his knowledge and (b) never reached any medical agency at all. Ninety-eight families were visited and 300 persons questioned about illness in the 3-month period prior to the visit. For those patients reporting illness details were obtained about the type of problem and the action taken.

John Fry has been responsible for an extensive series of papers about the patients in his Beckenham practice; these warrant mention because of the time-period over which the data have been collected and the detail with which they have been presented [QRL 250, 251, 253]. More extensive data have been published in *Profiles of Disease* [B 201] and *Common Diseases* [QRL 254]. Comparable data have been published in *Towards Earlier Diagnosis—a guide to general practice* [B 246]. This book was based on the clinical material from his own practice; the distribution of type of disease was related to Dr Hodgkin's earlier experience in hospital.

In 1964 seventy-seven general practitioners, out of 280 volunteers in the south-west England regional faculty of the RCGP, were selected on grounds of age, location and type of practice [QRL 726]. Out of the seventy-seven, sixty-eight participated through-out the year of the study. Data on each practice were collected by questionnaire and for 1 week each quarter from September 1964 to July 1965 details on all consultations (a total of 51,140).

In 1965–6, sixty-eight doctors in South Wales collaborated in a study of general practitioners' workload [QRL 713]. Again the emphasis was on workload rather than morbidity treated, though analyses are given by type of problem and thus some material is available on morbidity treated by the family doctor. A comparable study endeavoured to collect complete data on use of the health services in Exeter during the period November 1966 to October 1967. Ashford and Pearson [QRL 37] collected detailed data on the patients cared for by sixteen practices including forty-nine doctors. The material related to just over 50,000 patients; details were collected of these patients' contacts in general practice, out-patients consultations, and spells in hospital during the year. Some of this material is more relevant to a consideration of use of the health services, in particular the sophisticated mathematical manipulations that have been carried out on these data. Since 1968, 1400 general practitioners and some 46,000 'married' women aged 15–44 have been involved in a long-term study of the effects of oral contraceptives upon the health of those taking them. The preliminary report provides a wealth of detail about the morbidity occurring in these women [QRL 365]; though collected for a very specific purpose, the report can be used as an indicator of illness in this section of the community and by virtue of the sample size and geographical coverage provides data of value.

2.3.3. *Morbidity statistics from hospitals*

In planning a health service it is essential that information is available on the need for various forms of specialist care [B 16]. This may be need for investigation and diagnosis (direct access, at out-patients, or as an in-patient) or for treatment (as an out-patient, day case or in-patient). Assessment of the incidence and prevalence of morbidity in the general population is one approach to the estimation of need; the examination of statistics on the use of hospital facilities may provide some indication, but as with morbidity statistics from general practice there are a number of problems with this approach. The general issues have already been discussed (see Subsection 2.1.2).

Airth and Newell [QRL 11] showed a close relationship between provision and use of beds in the ten non-metropolitan regions in the country. Other authors have com-mented on the relationship between provision and use, suggesting that these are more closely related one to the other than to any objective measure of need [B 191, 53, 244]. As indicated earlier (Subsection 2.1.2) the use of norms for provision of hospital facilities is likely to reflect historical development of the service, rather than objective assessment of need.

In 1941 the Minister of Health launched a survey to assess the availability and adequacy of hospital facilities. With the help of the Nuffield Provincial Hospital Trust teams were appointed to visit the ten areas of England and Wales; background statistics were collected and, with support from a number of official bodies, information was gathered from health staff in the areas. In addition, numerous hospitals were visited to gain local views. A series of reports were published [QRL 469]. Though the statistics are now of limited interest, the general approach is worth noting; it was recognized by the authors of one report [QRL 284] that 'any exact measure of the adequacy of hospital services is almost impossible'.

Since this time the Nuffield Trust has funded a series of further studies exploring this issue. Two in Scotland looked at statistics of available facilities and their use, and the variation in use in relation to overcrowding and occupation [QRL 504, 505]. This was followed by comparable studies in Northampton and Norwich [QRL 506], Tees-side [QRL 11] and Barrow [QRL 243]. The latter study endeavoured to cross-check on the relationship between need and met demand by collecting statistics on mortality in the community, prescribing and use of direct-access investigations, delay for out-patient appointments, fluctuation of waiting lists, opinions of the effect of waiting lists upon referral patterns and assessment of the requirement for hospital care for a sample of in-patients.

Bearing in mind the above points, the QRL for this chapter contains reference to a number of major studies on hospital activity, where it is felt that these contribute some indication of requirements for specialist care stemming from a defined population. These studies are discussed in greater detail in Chapter 4, 'Resources' (see Subsection 4.1.2). This material is complemented by the detailed analysis published from the HIPE; this was included in the previous review [B 14].

2.4. Morbidity statistics from industry

A further source of data about the distribution of illness in the community is statistics of recorded absence from work. Though this only relates to a segment of the general population (that is the working population), the material can be used as a useful pointer to the incidence and prevalence of acute and chronic disease. At the same time some statistics relate to identifiable morbidity from industrial injuries or a defined list of industrial diseases. The statistics of certified incapacity have to be interpreted with caution; Alderson [B 11] suggested that apart from any direct effect of occupation on health, incapacity rates in the current situation may be influenced by several over-lapping factors: the place of residence of the worker, including the influence of environment and availability of medical care; the multiple processes of selection of an individual 'into' or 'out' of a particular occupation, which are in part related to the physical or psychological demands of a job; the financial and social consequences of declared illness, including membership of a sick-pay scheme; the completeness of notification of incapacity (for example, certain professional workers may not be required to produce certificates unless incapacity is prolonged); the general and particular unemployment situation; the morale within an industry and other little under-stood subcultural factors also surely play a part.

Sickness absence statistics for the country as a whole are handled by the Social

Security branch of the DHSS who publish a regular series of reports. These were reviewed by Whitehead [B 459] in the earlier volume of this series. These data are complemented by statistics produced by a number of other central government departments for particular groups of workers (see bibliography prepared by Gauvain [B 210]). These publications are beyond the terms of reference of the present contribution, but relevant to this text are the equivalent statistics published by major employers as a routine, or as a result of some special exercise. Though the requisite data are recorded at source (i.e. documentation of characteristics of each individual and details of the 'problem' for which he consults) for many industries the collation of such data for the organization as a whole is rare, let alone tabulation and publication. The material that has been published in the past is indexed in the QRL.

2.5. Problem specific studies

This section deals with a very wide range of studies, with the common characteristic that each has examined a specific medical issue and provided statistics that contribute to our knowledge of the population's health needs. The classification used in the QRL and the order of the text is alphabetical by 'problem'; within this the individual studies are ordered from major to minor by geographical cover, and then from earlier to recent work.

Two rather separate categories of problem have been interleaved in the one alphabetical order; these relate to specific medical issues, such as 'blindness', and definable categories of patients, such as 'children'. This approach was selected as it aligned with the study designs that have been used; surveys usually either concentrated upon a specific medical problem or dealt with a range of issues in a defined group of patients. It is obvious that some studies on population subgroups may deal with several different diseases. Where the emphasis has been, for example, on the study of the health of children this is felt to be the correct location of the reference; if the study has concentrated upon the nutrition of children, it has been included with other nutritional studies. In case of difficulty in locating an entry into the QRL, users should consider the different approaches that might have been used in placing the entry within the framework identified in the QRL contents list.

In order to establish some limit to the text, entries either involve a major national study, or provide an example of a new approach to collecting relevant data even when this has been applied to a restricted sample. It has not been the intention to describe every epidemiological and sociological study whose findings are indexed in the QRL; this means that specific warnings about the interpretation of statistics reported in any particular study cannot be given. Some of the general points raised in the previous chapter (Section 1.7) about interpretation of routine statistics and information collected in surveys must be borne in mind when using published data; a number of these points are reinforced in this section, in discussion of particular studies. In general, attention must be paid to the representativeness of the particular study population, the bias arising from methods of sample selection and non-response, the validity of the data (depending on respondent, observer and instrument error or bias), the errors or limitations imposed by the data processing and presentation, the confidence limits due to sample size and random errors.

2.5.1. *Abortion*

Routine statistics were covered in the previous review [B 14]. A major study was carried out by Cartwright and Lucas [QRL 131] of a sample of women having an abortion in 1971; the respondents were contacted in institutions licensed for abortions. There were problems with sampling, as only two-thirds of the institutions approached agreed to the study; 272 (89 per cent) of the eligible women having abortions in the participating institutions provided interviews. The enquiry documented the characteristics of women seeking and obtaining an abortion. Not all women requesting an abortion have their pregnancies terminated. This is discussed in the following chapter (Section 3.1).

2.5.2. *Accidents*

In 1960 a British Medical Association (BMA) working party [QRL 92] co-ordinated a study of non-fatal domestic accidents. For a year hospitals and general practitioners in seven areas of Great Britain (with a total population of over half a million) were asked to notify such accidents; the MoH then arranged for a health visitor to complete a standard questionnaire at a home visit. Only half the doctors in the areas participated, though all the hospitals agreed; it was thought that data were obtained for less than half the home accidents. A comprehensive study of home accidents occurring in Aberdeen has been published [QRL 442]; a number of other studies have dealt with other subgroups involved in accidents such as the report by Murdoch and Eva [QRL 496] which was restricted to injuries to children.

The Government Social Survey carried out an investigation on motor-cycle accidents in 1958, *Accidents to Young Motor-cyclists—statistical investigation* [QRL 595]. The aim of this study was to attempt to classify accident rates occurring to motor-cycle riders by age and riding experience, using data directly available through the police information which was transferred to the Ministry of Transport. The initial data available from the accident statistics were deficient in a third of the records and a laborious process of following up the gaps was undertaken and ultimately 94 per cent of the records were adequate. The analysis was based upon 4790 accidents. The Social Survey attempted to obtain a denominator for the accidents by drawing a sample of motor-cycle owners from the licensing authorities in a two-stage probability process. A very simple questionnaire was sent to each of 10,221 owners; 95 per cent responded.

A contributory factor to morbidity from motor-cycle accidents is the absence of a crash helmet. The issue has been examined by Scott [QRL 594]. This study was carried out for the Road Research Laboratory (now Traffic and RRL) in order to investigate the factors affecting the wearing of crash helmets. After a pilot survey the main survey was carried out in five towns in England. A police constable stopped individual motor-cyclists and directed them to the interviewer at the roadside; the interview, which was confidential, did not take place within the hearing of the policemen. A standard interview schedule was used.

One thousand one hundred and fifty-four were interviewed; about 15 per cent refused. It must be emphasized that this study did not attempt to obtain a representative sample; the sample was weighted by the number of miles driven (which increases the likelihood of being stopped) and the sampling only took place on a few restricted hours and days in five chosen towns.

2.5.3. *Addiction*

Reference was made in the earlier review [B 14] to the statistics of known or registered addicts; the value of these statistics has been discussed by Bewley *et al.* [B 52; QRL 65]. These national figures have been supplemented by a number of publications on the prevalence of drug-taking; because of the present legal position the collection of valid data on this issue is extremely difficult and the favoured approach has been to establish an informal network of sources of information in order to obtain the best estimate of community prevalence [QRL 15, 380]. Some data have been obtained of the prevalence of drug-taking amongst students, using anonymous questionnaires; despite the high response, the validity of such data is unknown [QRL 67, 429]. Harder data have been obtained for patients attending the Edinburgh Regional Poisoning Treatment Centre [QRL 242].

Other forms of 'addiction' warrant consideration, because of their impact upon health—alcohol consumption and smoking. The latter has a special subsection devoted to it (2.5.31). The prevalence of alcoholism is difficult to identify; some indication is given from mortality data or as a diagnosis responsible for admission to (mental) hospitals [B 14]. Kessel and Walton [B 274] have discussed various sources of morbidity statistics; data may be derived from available information on: psychiatric patients, attempted and successful suicides, attendance at family doctors, involvement in accidents, or from surveys of prisoners. Some fairly hard data are available on road accidents, including raised blood alcohol in fatalities and positive breath tests [QRL 185]. The statistics from hospital and primary medical care are suspect, as it is likely that a considerable proportion of alcoholics are not recognized or recorded.

2.5.4. *Adverse drug reactions*

It is well recognized that a proportion of patients who are treated by conventional therapy will develop an adverse reaction [B 260]. This issue is discussed in Chapter 6 (Subsection 6.2.5.2), as this is predominantly an issue of evaluation of medical care. However, an understanding of the problem is a small but essential component of the assessment of total medical needs (as advancing age is a determinant of health-care requirements, so is the fact of conventional medical treatment by generating a sequence of untoward effects which require further care and rehabilitation). The major source of data appears in the 'Need' chapter of the QRL, but a number of other studies are indexed in the 'Evaluation' chapter.

2.5.5. *Alimentary disease*

A number of epidemiological studies of various specific problems have been indexed in the QRL. These studies do not include any particularly novel features in study design or method.

2.5.6. *Arthritis*

One epidemiological study has already been described (Subsection 2.2.2.2), whilst other less precise indications of the prevalence of this condition can be obtained from interview surveys such as the GHS. Wood [B 479] has discussed some of the method problems of epidemiological studies of rheumatic disorders, whilst he and his colleagues have reviewed the contribution of various routine statistics to this topic [B 480, 481, 482, 483, 484]. Data from other surveys are included in the QRL.

2.5.7. *Blood diseases*

The prevalence and aetiology of anaemia have been discussed in the subsection (2.2.2.2) on South Wales population studies. Another source of data on the distribution of anaemia in the population is multiphasic screening (Subsection 2.3.1). An early study instituted by the CGP involved informal notification of patients with pernicious anaemia in a number of practices; allowing for diagnostic and reporting errors this study quantified the magnitude of the prevalence [QRL 596].

2.5.8. *Cancer*

Relevant data to an assessment of need have already been covered in the previous review [B 14]; some additional material has been produced in occasional publications. McKenzie [QRL 433] produced a report with six detailed tables, the first five of which presented serial mortality data for malignant disease. This is, of course, a secondary publication of data that have already appeared in the RG's statistical review; the material has, however, been laid out in a new way, presenting trends over 50 years supported by a relatively brief commentary.

The appendix to this report contains additional material by Case and Pearson [B 93]; they prepared mortality tables from 1911 to 1955 showing the age and sex specific mortality for 5-year age groups, by 5-year calendar period for specific sites. Further publications in this series have been produced [QRL 136].

Hill *et al.* [QRL 312] published a special report *Cancer Incidence in Great Britain, 1963–66*; this is a collation of routine data, brought together in a form that is not otherwise available. The bulk of the material consists of diagrams supported by a number of tables showing the average registration rates for different malignancies for different parts of Great Britain.

Rather different to the above two reports is *Oral Cancer in England and Wales—A national study of morbidity, mortality, curability and related factors* [QRL 68]. This report contains information on neoplasms of the lip, tongue, rest of the mouth and salivary glands; there are some data on the smoking and drinking habits of the population. Though this is a collation of secondary material available from other sources, the method of presentation and the critical commentary make it a very useful publication on this specified topic.

A number of regional registries have published analyses of their local data, but this has now been superseded by the national publications. The national registration scheme has covered the whole of England and Wales since 1962. These sources were covered in the previous review [B 14].

The recent spread of schemes for screening the population (see Subsection 2.3.1) has resulted in some data on the incidence of various cancers, particularly breast and cervix, with improved delineation of the high risk groups.

2.5.9. *Cardiovascular disease*

The contribution on population studies in South Wales includes some surveys on coronary heart disease and hypertension (see Subsection 2.2.2.2). This is one of the topics for which a large number of epidemiological studies have been mounted; these are indexed in the QRL, but not discussed here individually, as the methods used have already been indicated in this earlier section. The principal variation in the different studies is the choice of population; some are geographically based, with or without an age/sex restriction. Others have used occupational groups, because of the advantages of a readily available sampling frame.

One particular form of cardio-vascular disease is that affecting the cerebral vessels. Bronte, Stewart and Pickering, writing in 1959 [B 68], suggest that methods of diagnosis are not sufficiently reliable or practicable for large-scale application to have enabled field work to be done. Since this time a number of prospective studies have identified the incidence or fatality from this disease, using varying techniques for identifying the diagnosis; these have included routine general practice records (see Subsection 2.3.2.3, study of the contraceptive pill [QRL 365]), clinical examination (studies in QRL section of cardio-vascular disease) or routine death certificates obtained in a prospective study [QRL 170].

2.5.10. *Children*

Over the past 30 years there have been a number of major studies of samples of children, with the common principle that they have identified a cohort at birth and followed them up over many years. This technique of cohort study has been implemented for a number of large national samples and for several smaller local samples (the latter usually collect a wider range of items under 'research' conditions). By virtue of the complex nature of a cohort study, data on incidence and natural history of disease is obtained and 'aetiological' factors may be studied; these studies will therefore make a major contribution to study of the determinants of need. This section deals first with these cohort studies and then turns to a range of cross-sectional studies on infants, children and school children.

2.5.10.1. *Cohort studies of children.* A survey was carried out in 1946 [QRL 210], *Maternity in Great Britain*, on economic aspects of child bearing partly as background to the remodelling of the health services, and also to examine whether the fall in fertility was in any way related to the financial costs of the birth of a baby. The main material stems from a survey carried out by health visitors throughout England, Wales and

Scotland, for those mothers delivered during the week 3–9 March 1946, the interviews being carried out about 8 weeks after birth. Of 458 local authorities 424 (92 per cent) agreed to participate. Two overlapping questionnaires were used; the first dealt mainly with use of the maternity services and the second with the cost of pregnancy and confinement. The local authorities in the study (and thus respondents resident in them) were allocated at random to receive either one or other questionnaire. Where possible attempts were made to trace mothers who had moved to a new address whether in the same or a different authority. The data were coded and then prepared for mechanical tabulation. Additional data were obtained on visits by Douglas and Rowntree in the summer of 1947 to five local authorities.

An estimate was available of the loss to the sample from non-co-operation of thirty-four welfare authorities and late notification of births. This was done by comparing estimates of actual registrations during the study week with the MOsH notification lists. It was then possible to look at the interviews which were missed. Successful interviews were carried out with 90·5 per cent of mothers on the lists. The main reason for loss was mothers being untraced (this was shortly after the war and there was considerable migration of mothers); there was difficulty in tracing unmarried mothers and the failure to interview was considerably higher in this group. Apart from this specific bias, it was suggested that underenumeration did not affect comparisons between social classes.

After the study of children born in 1 week in March 1946 had been carried out it was realized that follow-up of this national sample would provide a unique opportunity to describe the home environments in which young children are brought up and to throw light on a number of problems concerning their health and growth during the pre-school period. Though a number of local surveys on such issues had been carried out, the report Douglas and Bloomfield [QRL 212], *Children under Five*, deals with the national scale, and gets over the problem of the distorted picture that local surveys can present.

Thirteen thousand, six hundred and eighty-seven children were involved in the 1946 survey, but due to lack of resources it was decided to reduce the sample on follow-up by approximately half. Illegitimate children and twins were excluded, and a random sample was then made of one in four children from manual workers and self-employed (who had together comprised 72 per cent of the original maternity survey sample). The full numbers of children in the other social groups were retained, and in this way the number in the follow-up survey was reduced to 5386. The method of sampling gave approximately equal numbers in each of the social groups, but the original sample structure could be obtained by suitable weighting. The children were contacted by health visitors when 2 (in 1948) and $4\frac{1}{2}$ (in 1950). Using a tested standard questionnaire the health visitor called at the home to find out about illness and home conditions. In five local authorities a special check on the reliability of the data was carried out [QRL 212]. In the 1950 survey 90 per cent of the records were returned within 2 months, but after 7 months 2 per cent were still outstanding (the main difficulty was to trace families who had moved). The general standard of form completion was very satisfactory, but occasional questions were not answered and in others internal discrepancies were revealed. All such queries were referred back to the health visitors and most were answered.

On each occasion when the survey was carried out some losses occurred; these were unavoidable (death and emigration) and avoidable (untraced, refusal to co-operate, and other miscellaneous reasons). In 1948, 4742 mothers completed interviews (88 per cent of the initial sample) and in 1950, 4668 (87 per cent of the sample). The greatest number of losses was due to deaths and emigration (9·0 per cent); point-blank refusal was uncommon (1·1 per cent in the first survey, and an additional 1 per cent in the second survey). There was no clear evidence that the overall losses (which were greatest in the professional and non-manual subgroups) distorted the representativeness of the sample, but some mothers might have withdrawn their children to avoid revealing some particularly unusual family circumstance or abnormality of the child. Local authorities were asked to identify from their records, physical or mental defects of these children and whether or not the parents were living together. Again there was no evidence that there was a particular distorting effect from the loss of this material in the main survey.

The children in England and Wales were then followed through primary school education, to relate the influence of home and school upon educational opportunities of children—*The Home and the School* [QRL 211] and subsequently from entry to secondary school until they were 16½—*All Our Future* [QRL 213]. Teachers recorded school absences, behaviour and attitudes to work; tests of intelligence and attainment were given under supervision at 8, 11 and 15. Data on the children's health were obtained by the health visitors and school nurses; the children were examined at 5, 8, 11 and 15. Losses amongst the cohort have been small because the whole country was involved and children were only really lost if they died, went abroad, were untraced or their parents refused to provide information. By March 1957, by which time the children were 11, 4·9 per cent had died and 6·7 had emigrated with their families. This is not thought to be a biased loss, because they represent a 'natural' decrease in the survey population which could hardly be regarded as distorting the survey—even though the children who died tended to come from the manual working classes and those who emigrated from the middle classes. No arrangements were made to enrol children who migrated into this country from abroad—such as the West Indians. The sample therefore becomes progressively less representative of the national population of school children because of this factor. Only 81·5 per cent of the survey children who were at school in England and Wales in 1957 had taken tests at both 8 and 11 years—some of the children could not be traced, some were absent from school at the correct time, a few were too backward to be tested, a few had parents who refused to allow them to sit the test, and a few were at schools which could not set aside time for testing and supervision. A rather high proportion of the children not tested were at private schools, particularly small ones; this distortion was relatively small. There were also fewer boys largely from manual working-class families than would have been expected if the losses had been random. The social class bias is the only considerable distortion found. Another potential source of bias is keeping the children under observation; this may in fact have stimulated their attitude to work and affected their parents' interest in their school careers. There was no evidence that this was so when a comparison with data from control children aged 11 plus was made.

Out of the original sample of 5362, 4720 were in England, Wales and Scotland in 1962 (88 per cent). Out of this available sample complete information was collected for 76·8 per cent, test information on some of the years for a further 16 per cent, and no test information on 7·1 per cent. The children for whom full information was available did not differ significantly from the total sample, but those with no information included children who were in Educationally Sub-normal (ESN) classes.

Use of the statistics generated by such a major study must be tempered by consideration of the quality of the basic data. With a small core research team data have been gathered in from a wide variety of sources, usually depending on individuals completing the questionnaires on top of their usual daily activities.

Shortly after the national study had been launched by Douglas, a comparable local study was mounted in Newcastle. A group of babies born in 1947 have been followed to school-leaving age and three reports published [QRL 623, 468, 467]. The primary purpose of this investigation was to measure the frequency and extent of disease and disablement in a representative sample of Newcastle's children—with a view to a better understanding of the types and incidence of illness from infective causes and the conditions under which they occur. The scope of the study extended during its progress to the examination of the health service in relation to assessments of the needs of the children and their families.

The study population consisted of all children born to Newcastle residents in May and June 1947. In all 1142 infants were enrolled, of whom 44 died in the first year, 127 removed and 4 left the survey, leaving 967 resident in Newcastle (and members of the group) in June 1948. Data were collected by the midwives, health visitors who carried out a regular programme of visiting, and research doctors who examined the children when 1, 3 and 5. Hospital records were made available and family doctors provided information.

Contact with the schools grew slowly and it was not until the children were in the last year of primary school that systematic observations were made. Detailed information was made available about educational progress, behaviour, the development of character traits, leisure activities, and plans for further education and employment. The school health service provided all relevant records including height and weight for the children when 5, 9, 13, 14 and 15 years old. Mechanical sorting and analysis of the data were carried out.

Twelve years after the national study by Douglas, a further study of a sample of births throughout Great Britain was mounted. The aim was to study the factors associated with perinatal mortality; the main publications on this aspect of the cohort have been Butler and Bonham, *Perinatal Mortality: first report of the British Perinatal Mortality Survey* [QRL 111] and Butler and Alberman second report [QRL 110]. Records were completed for 98 per cent of 17,204 notified births in England and Wales and registered births in Scotland during the week 3–9 March 1958. Material was made available by midwives and doctors completing standard questionnaires. The intention was that this should be completed by the midwife in attendance at delivery, but should include documentation of all contact with medical personnel from the first antenatal visit onwards. Socio-biological factors were recorded such as age, occupation, social and family background, antenatal attendance and smoking habits. This material came from the mother on questioning. Data on past obstetric history and the duration and course of pregnancy were abstracted from the antenatal records together with information on the length and course of labour, the newborn baby's sex, birth weight and progress in the neonatal period.

The data on live births were complemented by collection of material on 7561 still-births and neonatal deaths throughout the 3 months March, April and May 1958. Again comparable information was obtained about the mother, the pregnancy, the labour and, where appropriate, the progress of the infant in the first few days of life. A detailed enquiry into post-mortem findings was carried out; pathologists working in a number of regional pathology centres examined all babies dying in March, using a standard necropsy technique and recording the results on prepared questionnaires. These included a full macroscopic examination and wherever possible histological examination of most of the organs. Deaths in April and May were examined at a number of co-operating centres using the survey pathology questionnaire; in addition the routine autopsy report was obtained for many deaths. There were 17,204 mothers delivered in the first week of March including 668 (4 per cent) perinatal deaths; 7561 mothers had one or more perinatal deaths in the 3-month period (there were the usual proportion of twins, triplets and quads). The results from this comprehensive survey have been published in two reports [QRL 110, 111]. The first report is restricted to an examination of data relating to singleton births. The second report provides further detailed examination of 'high-risk' maternities; the report consists of contributions from a number of different authors, presenting more complex data than in the first report and occasionally using different classifications and approaches to examination of the material.

In 1964 the opportunity arose to trace and study the 1958 cohort of 17,000 births; the National Child Development Study was set up for this purpose. The aim was to establish a longitudinal study of the cohort of children born in March 1958 in order to examine their health, physical development, behaviour, educational attainment and home environment. The information was gathered from three main sources: (1) from schools by means of a schedule completed by the head and class teacher (the educational assessment) together with a few specific tests and other assessments; (2) from mothers and sometimes fathers, who were interviewed, usually by a health visitor, using a structured interview schedule; (3) from the school health service, who undertook medical examinations and carried out some specific tests. The tests and schedules for gathering information were so devised that the questions were as objective and unambiguous as possible, relying as they did upon many different observers and reporters. The system for collecting the data was tried out in a number of local authorities before it was finalized; the documents were forwarded to the local authority and returned from them when data-collection arrangements had been finalized.

It was felt important that the material from the interviews should have as first priority collection of data on a child's development and environment. Some items of interest, such as reaching specific milestones, were curtailed in view of the possible errors in recall. Factual information was sought about the social background of family and the home. Other issues were the child's separation from his mother, pre-school experience in nurseries and play groups, periods in care, attendance at clinics, hospital admissions or specialist care and other medical history. Current information was sought about the child's behaviour, physical co-ordination and adjustment at school.

A comprehensive medical examination of each child was carried out not only to identify handicapping conditions but also to spot minor defects. Standard tests of function and examination of the special senses were carried out (vision, speech, hearing, motor co-ordination), and measurements of height, weight and head circumference. The results of the first follow-up, when the children were 7 years old, were presented in the report by Davie and his colleagues [QRL 179]; the main report was published as a paperback with only limited factual data presented and in hard copy with an appendix of statistical tables. A special study of a representative sample of 200 children in the original cohort who were adopted involved comparison of the development of these children at 7, compared with controls including illegitimate children remaining with their natural mothers [B 410]. A preliminary paper on the children aged 11 has also been published [QRL 532]; this is based on data from questionnaires completed by the child's teacher, health visitor and school medical officer. A major report on the children when aged 16 has been published, but the material on health is of limited interest compared with the sociological issues including educational progress [QRL 241].

The National Birthday Trust has sponsored a further study of all babies born in the week beginning 5 April 1970. As before, data were collected on standard questionnaires, completed by the responsible midwife. In addition to details of the mother, her pregnancy, and the delivery, particulars were recorded about the first week of life for live-born children. Babies born dead after the twenty-fourth week of pregnancy were also included. The first report [QRL 141] deals with the first week of life of the sample; a second report on the obstetric care of the mothers is in preparation. Again the intention is to follow this cohort through school life, but no results have yet been published.

Obstetricians and paediatricians are becoming increasingly concerned about the quality rather than the mere quantity of the survivors of the perinatal period. The concept of a continuum of reproductive casualty has been proposed by Lilienfeld and Pasamanick [B 289], though Barker and Edwards [QRL 50] found no marked impairment of performance at age 11, in relation to obstetric complications recorded in birth records. Neligan and his colleagues [QRL 500] describe two interrelated studies. The first was a community survey of a geographically defined population—the Newcastle Survey of Child Development. This was a longitudinal prospective study of a 3-year birth cohort, whose obstetric and perinatal information had been published by Russell [QRL 585]; over 13,000 survivors of the first month of life were enrolled and followed through to school age. Quite distinct was the hospital study of all the survivors of a range of relatively rare adverse factors present in children born in hospital from January 1961 to May 1970. The intention was to assess their neurological and intellectual development, up to the age of 8.

The present data on the community study relate to 13,203 singleton legitimate births in the 3-year birth cohort. Basic information on mothers' social background, past obstetric history and pregnancy, and each child's birth and condition in the first month of life was available from the Newcastle maternity survey. The original and following observations were made by medical, nursing and teaching staff responsible for the children, but the recording was standardized to some extent. Due to the prospective nature of the study the number of children for whom material is collected has varied, one factor being whether or not the specific item or set of data was collected; this varies from episode to episode throughout the follow-up period. In addition there is loss of children due to mobility. Where possible limited material has been obtained by postal follow-up. By the age of 5 information was only available for 9626 children (73 per cent) and by 10 for 9000 (69 per cent).

The infants included in the hospital study were 218 survivors of one or more of six very severe adverse factors (cardiac arrest; delay of more than 20 minutes in establishing regular respiration; birth weight of 1360 g or less; apnoeic/cyanotic attacks; convulsions; cerebral irritations requiring sedation for more than 7 days). These index cases and 200 controls were identified from the routine neonatal records of the maternity hospital. The index cases were examined at ages determined by clinical indications and practicability, and the following recorded: (a) standard clinical/neurological examination; (b) assessment of gross motor system development; (c) STYCAR hearing test; (d) STYCAR vision test; (e) Denver development screening test. The report does not describe how the controls were selected.

2.5.10.2. *Congenital abnormality*. The national system for notification of congenital abnormalities produces valuable statistics [B 14]. More detailed data are available from local/regional studies; the method of establishing a congenital abnormalities registry has been described by Smithells [B 417]. A survey of congenital malformation was conducted in South Wales in 1964–6 [QRL 567] and statistics from this are included in the QRL. Elwood and Nevin [B 181] have described how much improved material can be obtained by combination of data on: births in the population from the Northern Ireland Record Linkage Project [B 99]; stillbirth and infant deaths recorded by the health department; deaths from the RG; voluntary notification of congenital abnormalities; hospital records of genetic counselling; autopsies. The Oxford Record Linkage Study [QRL 236] has also provided data, whilst the cohort studies described in the preceding section include data on this topic.

2.5.10.3. *Infancy*. The four studies discussed in this subsection all examine various aspects of mortality in infancy—a relatively rare outcome of care of children under 1 year of age. The justification for including them in this chapter is that they have explored the factors associated with high risk of death—and thus contribute to understanding of 'need'. The studies already discussed in the preceding section have contributed a lot of information on the health problems of infants; they are located elsewhere because of differences in method. Heady and Heasman [QRL 304] used routine mortality data to examine the social and biological factors affecting infant mortality and stillbirth rates. The study was feasible because the Population (Statistics) Act, 1938 had provided for the recording for confidential statistical purposes only of the mother's age, number of previous children and date of marriage. It was possible to relate these biological factors (and others which had been recorded for many years) to social data derived from information given at birth registration.

The basic data were obtained and linked from the draft entry completed by the Registrar at registration of birth, and the information recorded by the Registrar at registration of death. All children born in 1949 and 1950, who had died under the age of 1, were included (the study was subsequently extended to those dying under the age of 2). The combined data from these two sources of information were used to compare the characteristics of the mother at the time of the baby's birth with data on the age, place and cause of death of the infant. The main advantage of this study is that it was prospective in nature and calculated rates based upon events occurring to a defined population. A number of papers were published from this mammoth study, which analysed data on some $1\frac{1}{4}$ million births and the related stillbirths and deaths in the first year [QRL 304]. Including the second-year deaths amongst children born in 1949 there was a total of some 80,000 deaths and stillbirths for analysis. The GRO report did not contain a commentary, but published as much of the original material as practicable; even so, selection of the tabulated data had to be made. For some aspects of the analysis a technique for standardizing the multi-variate data was used, which enabled examination of the influence of one factor upon outcome with the other factors held constant.

A subsequent analysis of national data was prepared by Spicer and Lipworth [QRL 624]. The aim of this study was comparable to the previous one and carried out in order to provide more up-to-date data on the trend in stillbirths and infant mortality, and on the influence of regional and social factors. Again the basic tables were published as quickly as possible with only a very brief commentary in order to release the data while the results were still topical.

The factors examined were social class of father, parity and age of mother and region of birth. Where appropriate certain groups of causes of death were examined, depending on the numbers available. The method adopted was similar to the previous report. The investigation covered the period 1 April 1964 to 31 March 1965. As before, the infant deaths were traced to the birth record and from these records the birth and death entries were linked. The population at risk required to provide a denominator for the analysis was a 10 per cent sample of the births registered in the period 1 July 1963 to 30 June 1964. The report does not explain why this was not for an exactly matching period of births; also it is not clear whether the period of investigation defined the period of birth or the period of death.

The crude rates in the analysis present a picture of the experience of a single recent year, but there is some difficulty in separating the effects of individual factors at work because all of them are intercorrelated. The influence of region and social class were examined by standardization; the statistical technique aimed to isolate the effects of the main variables on the assumption that there are no interactions. This assumption is an oversimplification, and though the statistical model gives a good description of the stillbirth mortality it is less satisfactory for the neonatal and post-neonatal deaths.

A rather different approach was a special enquiry carried out by the DHSS, *Confidential Enquiry into Post-Neonatal Deaths, 1964–1966* [QRL 187]. Study of mortality statistics in 1963 suggested that infant deaths in the post-neonatal period (i.e. deaths between 4 weeks and 1 year of age) were not continuing to fall, as were deaths in the first 4 weeks of life. A limited survey of post-neonatal deaths was conducted in order to see what factors were involved, whether lessons could be learned that would help in saving infant life, and to give some indication of the possibility of further enquiries.

Two country boroughs and one county in the same region were involved in the study; this involved 679 infant deaths between the ages of 4 weeks and 1 year in 1964–6 in the three authorities. Information was obtained from the parents, the general practitioner and the hospital doctors concerned. Two senior paediatricians each provided an opinion as to the cause of death and whether there was any avoidable factor in the clinical care, administrative management or social setting of the infant's life.

There is no comment in the text about the validity of the data apart from drawing attention to the fact that the designation 'avoidable factor' was a subjunctive judgement that there has been some departure from the accepted standards of care in its widest sense.

A much more specific issue was explored by the MoH, *Enquiry into Sudden Death in Infancy* [QRL 472]. Professors Bedson and Camps [B 42] drew attention to the problem and suggested a scheme for investigating it; examination of statistics suggested that there were about 1500 sudden deaths in young children every year, i.e. about 20 per cent of all deaths in this age group. Selected areas of the country were involved in the study (twelve London boroughs and the administrative county of Cambridge). The coroners agreed that post-mortem examination would be carried out in all such cases and histology and bacteriology obtained according to a set protocol; in addition, examination for viruses was to take place periodically on a sampling basis. Information was also obtained by the coroners' officers and the health visitor. The report covers the period 1954–63 and is based upon the analysis of data from 224 infant deaths and 400 control children, matched for age, sex and place of residence.

2.5.10.4. *Children: non-accidental injury.* Diggle and Jackson (1973) [B 158] suggested that the incidence of child abuse is unknown; they described a monitoring system for identifying child injury in a defined geographical area, but present no statistics derived from this. They emphasize that the technical problems are small compared with the 'political and organizational' issues linked to confidentiality, security and legal restrictions. Local systems for ascertainment have been described by Parry and Seymour [B 365], Diggle and Jackson [B 158], Hall [B 229], and Arthur *et al.* [B 26]. The advantages and disadvantages of mandatory reporting were raised by a study group [B 200].

2.5.10.5. *School children.* A number of the cohort studies (see Subsection 2.5.10.1) followed a defined group into and through their school life. In addition to these studies, a number of other major studies on the health and medical needs of school children have been reported. An overlapping series of epidemiological surveys were carried out on the Isle of Wight (Rutter *et al.* [QRL 588]). The aim was (1) to describe the extent and nature of the intellectual, psychiatric and physical disorders amongst the child population; and (2) to demonstrate some of the pointers to causes of conditions by identifying interrelationships and association with background factors. In 1964 a survey on intellectual and educational retardation was carried out on the children in the Island, and in 1965 surveys on psychiatric disorder and physical handicap. Children 9–11 were involved in the first survey and those aged 10–12 in the second two. The survey covered the total population of children in these age groups whose homes were on the Island. In general, mass screening methods were used to identify children with one or more conditions in which the survey was interested; screening was carried out by group tests and questionnaires completed by parents and teachers. The initial screening was to identify as many of the handicapped children as possible and the screening measures were so adjusted to include all the ultimate positives; this resulted in the designation of a fairly large number of false positives. All the children selected in this way, together with a randomly selected control group, were then individually examined and further information was obtained from teachers, parents and the children themselves. In the second stage of the enquiry information was obtained by interview with the mothers about the children, their health problems, their problems with other children and their material and social circumstances. The survey was only looking for chronic or recurrent conditions, which had been present for at least 1 year preceding the survey. The term handicap was used in the broad sense of any disability which impeded the child in some way in his daily life; precise operational criteria for each type of disorder were drawn up. A rating scale was drawn up to identify the degree of severity and a study was made of the various ways in which children may be handicapped by each condition. Examinations, tests and questionnaires were standardized; the reliability and validity of the data were checked and details of this are provided in the report.

After considerable discussion and planning in the first week of June 1964 group tests on intellectual and education retardation (devised by the National Foundation for Educational Research) were administered to all Island children born between 1 September 1953 and 31 August 1955. As a result of this the children were chosen for individual examination in the autumn; in addition, all children in ESN schools, those missing the tests, and 159 controls were studied further. Six hundred children were chosen for the general medical, psychological and neuropsychiatric examinations. The parents were asked to agree that their children should participate in psychological testing, complete the medical and social questionnaire and have a general medical examination. The psychological and neuropsychiatric examinations were performed by mainland specialists recruited and briefed for the purpose.

The 1965 surveys involved a preliminary screening following by individual examinations and interviews for those thought to have emotional and behavioural difficulties or physical handicaps. The whole school population born between 1 September 1953 and 31 August 1955 was again screened using questionnaires completed by teachers and parents. All the local authority schools participated willingly, and some of the independent schools on the Island. There was the problem that the LEA had no record of children resident on the Island who attended independent schools on the mainland.

The school health services register of handicapped children was checked and expanded and was the basis of selection of those with physical handicaps; records were reviewed from special schools and clinics and of all children seeing a paediatrician in the previous 3 years. A special request had to go to independent schools asking them to identify children with any form of physical handicap. Parents and teachers of these children completed a special health questionnaire. For each of the children so identified a schedule of interviews was organized involving social science graduates, psychologists and psychiatrists.

A detailed study of the rearing of children in Nottingham has been carried out by the Newsons [B 348, 349, 350]. Their initial study of infant care [B 348] involved lengthy interviewing of 709 mothers within a fortnight of their child's first birthday; their report provides a comprehensive sociological account of infant care, but no material on health or care of sickness (other than limited data on diet). The second phase of this longitudinal enquiry involved further interviewing of the mothers about the time of their child's fourth birthday [B 349]. In addition to children from the original cohort other mothers were recruited into the study. The third stage has involved contact with the mothers when their children were 7, in order to report on the process of child rearing through the eyes of the ordinary mother [B 350].

A range of routine statistics on the health of school children were covered in the previous review [B 14].

2.5.11. *Deafness*

Stevenson and Cheeseman [QRL 629] attempted complete ascertainment in Northern Ireland of all children born deaf or becoming deaf by their sixth birthday. After contacting all medical and welfare staff to obtain a list of potential subjects, a home visit was made by a doctor or health visitor to obtain a detailed history and access to medical notes. Selected subjects had a medical examination and audiometry. Fraser [QRL 247] studied a sample of profoundly deaf children in special schools in the British Isles, though it is not possible to relate the statistics provided to the population. An indication of the prevalence of deafness is a survey by Hinchcliffe [QRL 315] of random samples of the population of the Vale of Glamorgan and Annandale. Rawson [B 377] commented on the paucity of data on this topic.

2.5.12. *Dental health*

A national survey of adult dental health was carried out in England and Wales in 1968 [QRL 282]. The aim was to provide information about the dental health of the community generally and to establish whether there was regional variation in dental health.

The enquiry involved an interview, followed at a later stage by an examination in the subjects' homes. In order to identify regional variation, the sample was so selected that it was representative of four major divisions of England and Wales: (1) the North, (2) the Midlands and East Anglia, (3) London and the South-East and (4) Wales and the South-West. A two-stage sample was used; the first stage involved the selection of fifty constituencies out of 547; samples of about sixty-six people were then drawn from the electoral register in each chosen constituency. The initial list of subjects was also used to identify a sample of persons 16–20 and those aged 21. Where the named person was the head of the household, this household was entered into the subsidiary sample, and any person aged 16–20 was interviewed (this approach corrects the bias in the identification of large households, the likelihood of which will be proportional to the number of people on the electoral roll). The interview attempted to obtain information about dental attitudes and habits; the information was collected by trained interviewers using a standardized questionnaire set. This involved an introductory questionnaire to determine whether the people had entirely natural teeth, some natural teeth and partial dentures, or no natural teeth. Depending on the dental status an appropriate subsidiary questionnaire was then used; the questionnaire was planned to involve about a half-hour interview. At the end of the interview the respondent was invited to have a dental examination; if the respondent agreed the same interviewer returned at a convenient time with a dentist. The dentist carried out the examination and the interviewers then recorded the information called out by the dentist. It was felt essential that these examinations were carried out in the person's homes to maximize response; this automatically limited the extent of the inspection. The dental examiners were trained in a standard form of examination using minimal portable equipment and without X-rays. Forty-four dentists were involved in the survey; during their training comparisons were made of different examiners' findings on the same subjects. Some data are presented in the report on examiner variability.

About 3000 subjects were in the initial sample of adults living in private households, who were interviewed in May/June 1968; 85 per cent participated and 75 per cent had an examination. It appears that non-response was higher amongst the elderly, the 'less dentally aware', and those with a poor dental state. It was also felt that the sampling method used had not achieved adequate representation of those aged 16–21. The schedules were precoded where possible and used after definitive coding as data input documents for computer analysis.

In 1971 the Scottish Home and Health Department (SHHD) asked that a survey be carried out in Scotland to assess the dental health of adults that would be similar and comparable to the material collected for England and Wales in 1968. This has been reported by Todd and Whitworth [QRL 652]; the main design was similar to the England and Wales survey, but an improved technique was used for checking on gum condition and oral hygiene. The sample drawn was thought to be deficient in young persons (perhaps up to 21, and obviously for those who were not eligible for the electoral register). Because of the particular difficulties in delivering dental care to sparsely populated areas, the sampling fraction for the Highlands and Islands was inflated five-fold compared with the rest of Scotland. This specific technique gave more reliable data for this group of interest, but enables appropriate weighting to be applied to give results for the whole of Scotland. These data were supplemented by a search of the records in the Scottish Dental Estimates Board, to check on recent treatment; however, there was considerable difficulty in matching the records. Out of the eligible sample no interview was obtained in 10 per cent of the Highland and Island sample and in 12 per cent from the main sample; 81 per cent of the Highland and Island and 80 per cent of the main sample who were eligible had an interview and examination completed.

A complementary study was then carried out on children aged 5–15 in England and Wales by Todd [QRL 650]. The aim was to collect information about the dental health of groups of school children through a national survey, and to examine the factors which might influence the level of dental health. A large sample was required in order to be able to estimate the pattern of dental development at all ages. Originally it was proposed to include 11,000 children (1000 in each age group) but the Welsh Office request for information relating specifically to Wales led to the sample size for Wales being increased three-fold to give reliable information. Thus, the total sample size was increased to about 13,000.

It was decided to limit the study to local authority (LEA) maintained schools. As a first stage in sample selection, all secondary schools in England and Wales were grouped into 4500 'secondary units', each containing between 400 and 1000 pupils. The number of units in each LEA was counted and accumulated and the authorities ordered geographically: from this list, eighty-nine secondary units were selected for inclusion in the survey. The sixty-nine LEAs responsible for these units were then identified, and all primary schools in the selected areas were then allocated to secondary units. To avoid any bias due to prior knowledge of the actual units selected, all primary schools within the areas were allocated and only then were the selected units identified. (This procedure was followed in order to avoid the mammoth task of allocating all the vast number of primary schools in the country to secondary units.) Because of the large number of primary schools, half of the primary schools in each selected unit were excluded at random and the sampling fraction in the remaining schools doubled in order to reduce the dentists' travelling time. Thus, in the secondary schools one child in eighteen was interviewed and in the primary schools one in nine. The sample was based on all children aged 5–15 in the selected schools on 31 December 1972; individual children were identified from school registers. The dental examinations took place during January and February 1973 and as individual children were chosen in October

1972, early school-leavers in the 15-year age group were lost. As a result of this, the sample of 15-year-olds was biased—it was felt that the early leavers would present a different dental picture to those remaining at school.

The local authorities involved in the survey were asked to nominate one or two dentists to carry out the survey according to the workload in each area. Sixty-nine dentists participated in the survey; these nominated dentists attended a 1-week training course. The dental examination was standardized and lasted between 3 and 4 minutes. The examination collected information about the effects and consequences of decay, the evidence of trauma, the condition of the soft tissues and the orthodontic condition of the child. In general, the measurements of filled and missing teeth were very reliable; measurements of decayed and crowded teeth, and the need for orthodontic referral, showed some examiner variability. As in previous studies, the greatest variability occurred in the measurement of gum conditions.

Ninety-five per cent (12,250 children) of the original sample were examined.

In addition to the examination, the mothers of all the 5- and 14-year-olds and half of the 8- and 12-year-olds were invited to have an interview. Trained social survey interviewers collected information about the child's contact with dentists and previous dental treatment, including conservation and extraction. Information was also obtained on accidents and other dental problems and the child's reaction to contact with the dental services. In addition, background information was obtained about feeding, use of dummies and thumb-sucking in early childhood, opinions about dental hygiene and dental visits were recorded, and details about the kind of food usually eaten, including consumption of sweets and biscuits. The family background was also explored. As in the case of the examinations, the response rate of the interviews was high; altogether 3137 were interviewed, 91 per cent of the selected sample.

2.5.13. *Diabetes*

Wilkerson and Krall [B 467] described a population survey for diabetes in 1946/7; 3515 persons (718) in Oxford, Massachusetts, provided a history, urine and blood samples for screening purposes, with detailed investigation of those with abnormal values.

Tunbridge [QRL 661] discussed the national problem of undetected diabetes in this country and suggested how this could be tackled. An early attempt to screen a population sample for diabetes was carried out as part of a mass X-ray campaign in Salford [QRL 107]. This approach only taps the biased 'volunteers' in a population; Redhead [QRL 558] examined the urine of a one-fifth sample of his 10,000-patient practice. Since these pioneer ventures many studies have been carried out, using different samples of the population, different methods of contacting the population to obtain a urine specimen, and different criteria for identifying 'diabetes'. Careful examination of the method is required before comparing the statistics from the studies covered in the QRL.

The first major survey of a total population was organized by the Birmingham Diabetes Survey Working Party of the CGP [QRL 70]. Ten practitioners around Birmingham participated with an eligible list of 19,412 patients; 18,532 (95·5 per cent) tested their urine. A home screening test with glucose-oxidase paper strip was performed, with 95 per cent of the 493 positive patients having an interview, examination and Glucose Tolerance Test; a control sample of negative patients was also investigated in the same way. The patients were followed up and a subsequent report commented [QRL 71] upon the natural history of this condition, the influence of intervention and the value and limitations of diabetes surveys. The investigations were repeated on 382 of the patients after an interval of 10 years from initial screening; a further report [QRL 72] elaborates on the progress of the sample.

2.5.14. *Elderly*

Many studies have been carried out on the needs of the elderly, some of which are discussed in the sections on handicapped (2.5.21), nutrition (2.5.25) and terminal care (2.5.32). The health problems of the elderly merge into social and welfare issues; where studies have concentrated upon the latter aspects they have had to be excluded from the following discussion.

In 1945 a social survey was carried out on samples of the elderly in seven localities in England and Wales [B 397]; the survey in Wolverhampton was followed by a medical enquiry. Sheldon [QRL 608] visited the sample in their own homes and took a history. A more detailed survey was carried out in Sheffield [QRL 321]; following a social enquiry the respondents were examined in their own homes and dental, ophthalmic and X-ray examinations took place at hospital. An interview survey took place in Northern Ireland of a representative sample of those 60 and over, living at home and in acute or chronic hospitals. Many other local studies of the elderly have been carried out in the UK and some are indexed in the QRL; following an enquiry in East London [QRL 656], Townsend collected data for a large sample of residents in homes for the elderly throughout England and Wales [QRL 657]. Townsend and Wedderburn [QRL 658] interviewed a random sample of persons 65 and over in Great Britain to identify disability and self-evaluation of health. No validation was carried out of the survey data, though Pasker and Ashley [QRL 529] have suggested that there was an overestimate of the proportion bedfast, due to the wording of the question on this. A follow-up study (Tunstall [QRL 663]) collected, by interview, data from persons 65 and ones living alone in four areas of England. Similar studies have been carried out in Great Britain by Harris [QRL 296] and in the Scottish border country by Gruer [QRL 286].

As an example of more detailed investigation Isaacs [QRL 350] has looked at some of the problems of the elderly. This report presents the results from two studies; the first sought to identify the geriatric patients attending the hospitals in Glasgow, how they differ from other medical patients, and why they were not cared for in the community. The main study was a systematic medical and social analysis of 612 patients referred to one of the two consultants in the Department of Geriatric Medicine at the Glasgow Royal Infirmary from 1 October 1966 to 31 December 1967. A control group was selected from the general population by choosing from the referring general practitioner for each patient a person of the same age group and sex; these patients were interviewed by the social workers. Further control interviews involved 250 patients 65 and over admitted consecutively to the general medical ward at the Glasgow Royal Infirmary.

The second study involved collection of data about a sample of the general population of old people (over 65) usually resident in Glasgow who had died in Scotland; this was to identify how many had died in hospital, how long they spent in hospital before death, and to contrast their care at home prior to admission with that of patients who actually died at home. Basic data were collected on 7607 deaths; a subsample of 240 of these was studied in more detail, and an interview with the bereaved relatives was carried out (ten of the relatives refused to participate). This study, interesting as it is, does not discuss problems of validity of data, bias from the sample, or confidence limits of the material presented. Recently Isaacs and Neville [B 261] have described a method of assessing the needs of old people; this involved grading disability in relation to frequency of requiring help and frequency with which potential sources of help were spontaneously available.

2.5.15. *Environmental pollution*

Eleven government departments and research councils are presently involved in 100 projects monitoring the environment [B 139]. This involves collection of data on five separate topics: (1) air-pollutants are measured at source, along their pathway and when they cease to be airborne; (2) land-levels of pollutants are measured in soil and crops, and pesticides and metals are monitored in wild life, foodstuffs and man; (3) radioactive substances—fall-out in rain is monitored, and uptake in milk, drinking water and marine foodstuffs; (4) fresh water—emission of pollutants especially through sewers and discharge from industry are monitored; (5) marine pollution—this is checked additionally to the items already mentioned.

Though these systems for collecting data are rather beyond the scope of this review, they deserve brief mention as excess pollution is a risk to health. A comprehensive set of statistics are available on the above issues, predominantly collected by surveys sponsored by central government departments. The major sources of such material are briefly indicated in the QRL.

2.5.16. *Epilepsy*

Pond *et al.* [QRL 545] point out that nearly all the knowledge of the prevalence of epilepsy comes from hospital statistics, whilst a proportion of patients will never be referred to hospital. However, the majority of epileptics will be known to their GP, in order to obtain appropriate medication; a social worker visited all patients notified as suffering from epilepsy by practitioners in fourteen practices in South-East England.

2.5.17. *Eye diseases*

Sorsby [QRL 622] has provided detailed material on the blind in the country in the period 1955–62 and consolidated earlier material into the overall picture for 1948–62. This report is the last published by this author in a series of four (see also [QRL 619, 620, 621]). The classification used was based on data recorded on the old form of certification, being analysed by the clinical entities shown on the form. Since 1955 a double-entry has been recorded showing the site of the lesion and its aetiology. The data so derived in the 1948–54 period lent themselves to comparison with the more recent material, though there were difficulties with several entries—such as optic atrophy and congenital defects. Apart from a single page on the scope of the survey, there is no general review of the method or the problems with interpreting the data—though Brennan and Knox [B 60] have recently been very critical of the quality of the data available from the blind register.

A common cause of blindness is glaucoma; studies of this condition have been mentioned in Subsection 2.2.2.2. In addition to such population studies, Gray and Todd [QRL 281] have interviewed a random sample of those registered as blind, to determine the influence this has on (1) immobility and (2) the ability to read.

2.5.18. *Family planning*

Cartwright [QRL 128, 129] has described some of the obstacles to the use of effective contraception in England. She attempted to find out how people can be informed and helped to have the number of children they want at the time they want. The role of the family planning services was the main concern.

The study design involved selecting a sample of parents to whom a live-born child had recently been born. This, of course, does introduce a bias as such parents are likely to have a greater proportion of people who are failing to use effective contraception than in the population as a whole. The study involved twelve areas in England and Wales. The GRO selected 180 legitimate births in each area; an attempt was made to interview 150 of the mothers and a random sample of thirty of the fathers. Ultimately 83 per cent of mothers and 71 per cent of fathers so identified were successfully interviewed; basic information was recorded about the child and the previous pregnancies, the family intention and then details on contraception. In addition to interviewing parents the name of the family doctor was obtained and 76 per cent of those identified were interviewed or completed a postal questionnaire. Selection of doctors through the parents led to an excess of doctors in large population areas and a bias towards doctors with large practices or a low proportion of elderly in their practice. In nine of the twelve areas the MOH agreed that health visitors could be interviewed.

A further survey had been carried out by Bone [QRL 76]. This study, commissioned by the DHSS, assessed the adequacy of the existing family planning services in England and Wales as a guide to future development. A random sample of the population was interviewed. Two rather different samples were drawn: (1) married women (including separated, divorced, widowed and co-habiting) aged 16 to 40; (2) single women aged 16–35—the aim being to include 2500 of the former and 1000 of the latter subjects. A four-stage multi-stratified design was used resulting in the identification of 11,000 addresses. The specific categories of respondents were identified from these addresses by postal enquiry. Two thousand five hundred and twenty married women and 974 single women were eventually interviewed successfully; this was 86 per cent of married and 77 per cent of single women found to be eligible on age at the selected addresses.

It is possible that the inclusion of widowed and divorced affected the responses of the married women; it was not considered feasible in an official enquiry to ask single women whether or not they were sexually experienced, which automatically excluded some of the desirable analyses. In a further publication Bone [B 55] has elaborated upon methods of assessing the effectiveness and use of contraceptives.

2.5.19. *Feet*

Clarke [QRL 146] carried out a survey to find out the kinds of trouble people have with their feet and to estimate the unmet need and ummet demand for professional treatment.

Two complementary studies were carried out; the first was an interview of subjects by trained interviewers using a structured questionnaire; a subsample of these subjects was then examined by a professional chiropodist using a standardized record of the foot examination. Twelve study areas were selected at random (with probability proportional to population) and in each area 125 people were selected at random from the electoral register and visited; 1096 (73 per cent) were appropriately interviewed. Seventy adolescents were identified by asking if there was someone between the ages of 16 and 20 living in the dwelling; fifty-eight were successfully interviewed. The final sample was deficient of persons aged 21–24 and 65 and over, with an excess of skilled workers. A random half of the main sample were asked to have their feet examined by a chiropodist visiting them in their own homes; the reliability of the two state-registered chiropodists was tested in a separate study. Two hundred and eighty-five adults had their feet examined; a further seventy-six made appointments but failed to keep them, whilst the remainder (37 per cent) refused. Of those who were invited to have an examination those who did so reported more trouble (72 per cent of them) than those who did not have an examination (58 per cent).

2.5.20. *Genito-urinary disease*

Some of the surveys in the South Wales series of population studies have examined the prevalence of genito-urinary disease (see Subsection 2.2.2.2). These and other relevant data are included under the specific problem heading of genito-urinary disease in the QRL.

2.5.21. *Handicapped*

In 1953 Banks *et al.* [QRL 49] estimated the number of handicapped persons in one local authority in East Anglia by interviewing respondents in a 10 per cent sample of households. A major contribution to method was made by Jefferys and her colleagues [B 263], who described the development of a series of tests to be administered by an interviewer to quantify motor impairment. The reliability of these tests was assessed, but not the validity. In addition they used a simple postal questionnaire to identify motor difficulties and examined the validity of positive and negative responses against the interviewer-administered tests.

An extensive survey, *Handicapped and Impaired in Great Britain*, was reported by Harris *et al.* [QRL 297]. The aim was to identify the number of handicapped persons over 16 living in private households and relate this to local authority provision. The initial sample was a two-stage stratified random sample of households in England, Scotland and Wales. Approximately 250,000 addresses were selected from the electoral register: 100,000 of these were used to produce a sample of subjects with handicap

(Sample A) and 150,000 were approached to identify those so severely handicapped to need constant care (Sample B). Of the 249,259 households approached by post in June/August 1968, 85·6 per cent responded—the response rate was studied day by day to see if the proportion of impaired had progressively decreased over the response period (i.e. were the late and non-responders the healthy people?). There was no evidence of this and therefore it was assumed that the non-responders did not differ with regard to impairment.

Sample A identified 13,451 households with one or more persons claiming to be impaired—a total of 15,096 persons. Approximately half (58 per cent) of these were 65 and over; it was decided to interview all those under 65 and one in four of those over 65. The percentage interviewed out of the possible sample was 89 per cent (including abbreviated and proxy interviews). It was obvious from the response to the Sample B questionnaire that a certain amount of misunderstanding had occurred and some people had been falsely identified as requiring constant care. Despite scrutiny of the positive response it was found on interviewing that 1518 persons were not eligible. Out of the eligible sample of 1128, 85 per cent were interviewed. An appendix to the report gives information about the non-responders, but there is no clear indication of any gross bias from non-response.

The initial questionnaire that was distributed seems very simple; the respondent predominantly had to answer 'yes' and 'no' to the main questions. The interviews were a very different issue. The main schedule which was used for Sample A is a tremendous document, with 150 questions; in addition, tests of motor capacity of the upper and lower extremities were carried out. Those permanently bedfast/chairbound or needing a lot of help had to complete a 'wheelchair schedule', and an eight-page special-care schedule. An important issue, of course, is the validity of the data. This was discussed, if somewhat indirectly; particular attention was paid to the definition of impairment, and the limitations that are present in the sample. No attempt was made to check with doctors' records that the correct diagnosis was reported and it must be remembered that a few of the informants may have had the nature of their conditions withheld. Tests developed by Jefferys *et al.* [B 263] were modified to a certain extent, and then applied by the trained interviewers. The Social Survey drew up a classification of handicap for which definitions are available; they identified those who were very severely handicapped (needing special care) and then divided the degrees of care required into eight categories.

A separate volume from the study dealt with the impact of disability upon: difficulty in obtaining or keeping a job, temporary sickness absence, premature retirement and the need for sheltered employment [QRL 104].

Many local authorities have carried out local surveys to estimate the prevalence of handicap or actually identify each handicapped individual. However, due to the method used and the presentation of the data it is difficult to generalize from the findings [B 437], [QRL 614]. Gray [B 222] and Harris and Head [B 232] have produced guides to method for such surveys, which should improve the comparability of the data.

2.5.21.1. *Young chronic sick.* A report from the Scottish Home and Health Department [B 406] referred to the fundamental difficulty of forming an estimate of the total number of young chronic sick. Some information was obtained in England and Wales from a survey of all long-stay young persons in non-psychiatric hospitals. MacLennan [QRL 437] obtained names of young chronic sick from twenty-eight GPs near Glasgow; though detailed data are presented for the persons so identified, it is not clear how this approximates to the true prevalence.

In addition to the general studies on handicap in this section, other specific disabilities are dealt with in the subsections on Children (2.5.10), Deafness (2.5.11), Elderly (2.5.14), Eye Diseases (2.5.17) and Mental Subnormality (2.5.24).

2.5.22. *Maternity*

An important issue in examining the maternity services and need for care involves measurement of maternal mortality, i.e. outcome of care; this provides a vital element in the consideration of need/use/outcome. Some studies have already been introduced that come into this field—the cohort studies on defined groups of newborn children and perinatal deaths (see Subsection 2.5.10.1). This section deals with another aspect of outcome—detailed studies of maternal deaths.

There was concern in the late 1920s that maternal mortality had been approximately stable since 1911. A committee brought together by the MoH to look at this issue suggested the establishment of an investigation into maternal deaths; this was a confidential enquiry for public health and scientific purposes that was neither for specific criticism of individuals nor to initiate disciplinary action. An interim report on maternal mortality and morbidity was published in 1930, including the analysis of confidential reports on some 2000 maternal deaths; particular attention was drawn to avoidable primary causes of death which were felt to have occurred in 48 per cent of the events. The system of a confidential enquiry continued up until the advent of the National Health Service in 1948, with an analysis of material being presented in the annual reports of the Chief Medical Officer (CMO) of the MoH. In 1952 a slightly different system was introduced, with the same aim as the preceding enquiry; though this special exercise has continued over this period, it is quite different from the routine statistics published by DHSS and thus not covered in the previous review (CGRHS). Since 1952 an analysis of the material has been presented at 3-year intervals (see [QRL 676, 677, 678, 679, 29, 30, 31]).

The enquiry is initiated by the MOH (now Area Medical Officer, AMO) of the (local) health authority who usually learns of the death through local hospitals, local health authority staff or through certification (the latter being either from the local registrar of births and deaths or through the OPCS). In initiating the enquiry as much information as possible is obtained by discussion from those in the domiciliary service concerned with the care of the patient. The standard form is then forwarded to the consultant obstetrician at the hospital who provides full clinical details of any care which the patient received including if possible the post-mortem report. The form is then returned to the MOH (AMO) who transmits it to the regional assessor—a senior obstetrician in the region. The regional assessor records his views about the cause of death and whether there was any avoidable factor in the clinical care or administrative management. Since January 1973 deaths associated with anaesthesia have been made subject to special enquiry by newly appointed regional assessors in anaesthetics. The regional assessor then sends the report to the CMO at the DHSS and the final assessment and classification rests with the Department consultant advisers on obstetrics (and in appropriate cases the adviser on anaesthetics). The enquiries cover all deaths directly due to pregnancy and childbirth, and deaths due to other causes occurring in association with pregnancy and childbirth. (Now any patient can be included in the study if the pregnancy or childbirth is thought to materially influence the death and this has occurred within 1 year of childbirth.) During the period 1967–9 attempts were made to increase the coverage of the enquiry; the RG reported to a medical officer at the DHSS all deaths due to or associated with pregnancy, where this was mentioned on the death certificate. The regional assessors were informed of these maternal deaths to initiate enquiries if they were not already in progress. The CMO also receives a confidential report, through the Secretary of the Coroners Society for England and Wales, of deaths amongst women who were pregnant or who have been recently pregnant. From these three sources of material it is possible to estimate the minimum number of maternal deaths and it is suggested that the enquiry for 1970–2 covered 91 per cent of the known maternal deaths. This coverage has increased over the past 9 years from 79 per cent.

An important aspect of the enquiry is the assessment of avoidable factors. It is not suggested that where these are thought to be present death could have been prevented; the presence of an avoidable factor is regarded as an indication that the risk of death could have been at least materially lessened. With an improvement in education and health of the community and in maternity care the number of deaths with avoidable factors may be reduced, though an opposing trend is that the assessors may become more strict in their interpretation. Comparison with reports from previous years is therefore not necessarily absolute.

2.5.23. *Mental illness*

Norris [QRL 501] assessed the incidence of hospitalized mental illness in London in 1947–9, by collecting data from two observation units and three hospitals. This preceded the establishment of the Mental Health Enquiry [B 14]; the increasing use of this routine DHSS system has been complemented by a number of special surveys. Hare and Shaw [QRL 291] carried out a survey to ascertain the mental health of people living in a new housing estate and to examine the influence of social conditions. Two districts were studied, one a new housing estate on the periphery of Croydon and the other an older ward in the central area. A 10 per cent sample of addresses in the districts were taken and information collected on the health of all people at these addresses. The overall response was 1855 persons (97·7 per cent) for the new district and 1181 persons (94·6 per cent) for the old districts. The intention was to obtain information directly from every person over 16 and by proxy on every child. The interviewer used a structured questionnaire covering health, social circumstances and attitudes, and a personality test; a personality assessment was made by the interviewer. The survey was carried out by five medical and eight lay interviewers; duplicate interviewing was carried out for sixty-five new and fifty-eight old households (using a pair of interviewers who were both lay, both medical, or medical and lay). There were considerable differences in the records, particularly for the personality assessments.

During the interview the respondents were asked their general practitioners' names; the five doctors in the new estate were then invited to keep special records of consultations by the respondents. There were sixty practices involved in the old area and a sample of thirteen doctors with 89 per cent of the respondents on their lists were asked to co-operate; all agreed. Special precautions were taken to ensure confidentiality. The general method of recording followed that used by Chave and Taylor [B 98], but there does not appear to have been any standardization of diagnostic criteria. The hospital records of Croydon Hospitals, the Maudsley, and Kings College were examined for details of psychiatric in- and out-patients from addresses in the two districts; the number of persons attending the child-guidance clinic was also identified.

An important confounding issue is whether people are rehoused because of their state of health; the research team examined the number of recommendations coming to the MOH and the proportion that were accepted. They concluded that this was a negligible factor.

Jones and Miles [QRL 359] studied the psychiatric burden in the community using a variety of approaches, as a guide to the needs for mental health services in the largely rural area of Anglesey. This study is interesting from the method point of view—though the findings are not automatically applicable in other areas with different population characteristics. The need for care was identified from three different sources:

1. Scrutiny of the records of the local psychiatric hospital from 1951 to 1960 inclusive, for discharged patients, and the local health authority records were examined for mentally subnormal.

2. Home visits in 1961 to the families of all those patients in long-stay care in the psychiatric hospitals on 1 January 1961 and the families of the mentally subnormal under supervision or in residential care.

3. A prevalence survey using the general practitioners to identify community cases who have not been in contact with the psychiatric services.

Very few Anglesey patients apparently received psychiatric attention other than in the North Wales Hospital, Denbigh; attempts were made to trace patients in other hospitals. Care was taken to identify those patients who were normally resident in Anglesey and separate off those who were temporarily domiciled in Anglesey.

After testing out three different approaches it was decided to ask the GP to go through all his records and indicate those cases he considered 'psychiatric'; it was considered that the doctors enjoyed it and found it a stimulating experience. It was explained that they should identify patients with mental subnormality or severe disturbances and also those with milder conditions where the doctor regarded them as outside the limits of normality. It was usually found that minor transient conditions of anxiety and depression were not included—they were thought to be as 'normal' as headcolds. The Anglesey EC provided the age and sex composition of every practice in Anglesey which were combined to give the denominator for calculating rates.

An attempt was made to check the validity of the GP prevalence study, by matching the patients so identified with the list of patients who had been in the Denbigh Hospital and had been discharged. The doctors identified a considerably higher proportion of those currently ill (85 per cent), compared with only 36 per cent of those currently well. Those patients who had been discharged from hospital out-patients were not picked up as well by the GP survey as the ex-in-patients—it was not clear whether this was due to the fact that hospital admission is a stimulus to the GP's memory, or an indication of severity of the disease.

The above three studies have used data on in-patients in psychiatric hospitals; Culpan *et al.* [QRL 174] screened various out-patient clinics at an acute hospital. They showed there was an appreciable prevalence of psychiatric disorders that had not been identified. Two of the above studies also relied upon GPs to identify directly their patients with psychiatric morbidity; Kessel [QRL 369] discussed the difficulties of this approach, when reporting a study in a single London practice. Johnstone and Goldberg [QRL 356] have indicated how routine screening of all persons attending a surgery can identify 'hidden psychiatric disorders'. A much more extensive study was carried out by Sheppard *et al.* [QRL 610], *Psychiatric Illness in General Practice*. The aim of this investigation was to obtain reliable information on the amount and nature of psychiatric morbidity encountered in general practice and to study the factors which influence the GP in identifying and treating psychiatric illness. The study was regarded as being exploratory in design and it examined the methodological and theoretical issues involved in morbidity surveys in general practice. Some of the conclusions of this work are highly relevant to the earlier section on morbidity statistics from general practice (2.3.2)—in particular the confirmation of the difficulty of comparing results from general studies which stem from differences in the methods and definitions used.

Practices for the main survey were found by approaching a large number within the area covered by the London EC, which differed in size, geographical area and socio-economic pattern. The distribution of the practices which then volunteered was plotted, and doctors in areas where additional practices were needed approached consecutively until an appropriate number of volunteers in each area had been found. The practices finally selected were thought to constitute a fairly representative group of GPs.

Having identified the practices, it was decided to take a one-in-eight sample of adults (i.e. persons over 15 years) in the practice populations. The basic recording instrument was a card inserted into the NHS envelopes of the selected patients. Doctors recorded details of each consultation made by the sample patient during the year; home visits were not recorded, as it was impossible to ensure uniformity in recording due to differences in the ways doctors normally recorded (or failed to record) them. It was felt that this would not be a great loss as most psychiatric cases are referred to the doctors' surgery for subsequent consultations; acute psychotic patients and attempted suicides, who are frequently admitted directly to hospital following a home visit, may be under-represented. One probable source of inaccuracy was 'non-medical and prophylactic' consultations, as it proved difficult to persuade doctors that miscellaneous items such as signing passport photographs should be recorded. At the end of the year, the research team checked the cards for completeness and in addition a set proportion were checked against NHS records. There were variations in recording standards in different practices; four practices were judged to be inadequate and they were excluded from the survey. The final sample included forty-six practices and eighty doctors.

The London EC checked the registrations of members of the sample who did not demonstrate their presence by consulting during the year and over 1000 of these were found to have left the practices. The population at risk, the basis for the calculation of rates, was taken as all patients in the sample who remained on the doctors' lists throughout the year—14,697. The majority of the analyses concern the 9000 members of the sample who consulted their doctors at least once during the year, 61 per cent of those at risk.

The factors influencing the identification and diagnosis of psychiatric disorder by individual doctors was a major interest of the research. To provide some information on the attitudes of different doctors, they were asked to complete a questionnaire which was designed to measure their attitudes towards psychiatry. The questionnaire contained items which discriminated between doctors with a known interest in psychiatry and those with stronger leaning towards organic branches of medicine.

To provide an independent estimate of psychiatric prevalence, particularly in regard to variance between practices, doctors were asked to encourage their patients to complete the CMI. (This standard instrument has been described by Brodman and his colleagues [B 67].) Eighteen practices agreed to take part in this and in fourteen there was a high enough rate of return (average 81 per cent) to justify inclusion in the analysis. Altogether 2245 patients, who consulted their doctors during the survey, returned the questionnaire; the rate of return was lower for elderly persons than for other age groups.

Three substudies were planned to provide additional information and throw light on some of the issues raised. First, to provide a check on practitioners' clinical assessments, psychiatric interviews were conducted with patients identified as chronic psychiatric cases in ten practices. A hundred interviews were obtained out of a possible 167 and, in the vast majority of cases, the practitioners' diagnoses were confirmed. However, there was only a low correlation between doctors' assessments and the analysis of the CMI responses; it is suggested that this is due to the low reliability of the CMI as a screening instrument in general practice surveys.

The second study was aimed at eliminating the possibility that a large amount of psychiatric illness is undetected by GPs because patients do not consult them. This took place in one practice where there were exceptionally good records stretching back over a period of time. The records for the period 1949–58 were examined in one practice and a sample of non-attenders drawn from patients who were registered with the practice throughout the 10 years. The sample consisted of all people who had not consulted for 2 years in 1958 and a small number had not consulted at all during the decade. Eighty-eight index cases were interviewed and eighty-eight controls drawn from those who consulted in 1958 and matched by age and sex. The findings suggested that non-attenders were not more psychiatrically disturbed than the controls.

The third study was designed to investigate the total illness of neurotic patients and their families and whether they tended to seek medical help over trivial complaints. The survey was carried out on families registered in one large practice known to have good records. The survey included thirty-two women diagnosed as neurotic during the survey and thirty-two controls who consulted during the survey but were not diagnosed as neurotic and who had never been so regarded by their doctors. The practice was situated in a middle-class residential area and the women did not constitute a representative sample of the general population; this severely limits the general applicability of the findings.

A special analysis has been published by the GRO [B 212]. The aim of this report was to provide tabulations showing the local variation in frequency of different diagnoses for patients admitted to mental hospitals. The sources of data were the routine returns for each patient admitted to psychiatric hospitals and units; this report provided a detailed analysis on place of residence, which had not been nor has been subsequently produced in such detail in the regular reports on the Mental Health Enquiry (MHE—see [B 14]). The address for each patient admitted to hospital in 1957 was coded to the local authority, distinguishing residents in county boroughs, administrative counties, and the metropolitan boroughs. The data also separated first and non-first admissions.

None of the above reports relate to studies of the general population. In Newcastle [QRL 366] and Swansea [QRL 528] samples of the elderly living at home have been interviewed by a psychiatrist to identify mental disorder, whilst a detailed study was recently carried out on a random sample of adult women in South London [QRL 100]. These are the nearest approaches to total population surveys identifying untreated psychiatric disturbance.

2.5.24. *Mental subnormality*

A recent DHSS report [B 148] on mentally handicapped children in care suggested that the situation was so complicated that an extensive enquiry would have been required in order to obtain up-to-date information on the placement of all children. Statistics have been collated from a variety of sources for six areas in the UK; one of the studies is described in detail, whilst brief mention is made of the others.

The prevalence of mental subnormality has been studied by Birch *et al.* [QRL 69]. The aim of this study was to determine the prevalence of mental subnormality in a defined age-range and to describe the children so identified in terms of the degree of their mental defect, the presence of other abnormalities, and the association or lack of this with various social, familial and health conditions. Since 1948 there have been excellent obstetric records available for pregnancies in Aberdeen. Because of standard practice for the recognition and designation of educationally subnormal children, it was felt that nearly all the affected children were identified. The study was carried out in 1962 and included all children born in 1952/4 inclusive, who had been identified as being mentally subnormal by the local authorities. There is discussion in the book about the possible selective effect of migration. In the period 1952–62 more children had left the city than had moved in with a higher loss in Social Classes I and II. The records available in Aberdeen were used to identify the background medical factors associated with mental subnormality. A detailed questionnaire on social and economic factors was administered to all the families of mentally subnormal children and to a one in five random sample of comparison families (91·5 per cent of those selected were successfully interviewed). Each of the ninety-seven mentally subnormal children was individually evaluated for intellectual level, neurological findings and psychiatric status. The data so collected enabled the background histories of the mentally subnormal children to be compared with the sample who were not known to be subnormal. In addition internal analysis was carried out on the data for the subnormal children to see if there was a relationship between severity of subnormality and other factors.

Other studies have been based on a variety of retrievable records to identify the prevalence of mental subnormality in the community. Goodman and Tizard [QRL 277] examined records of persons known to the local health authorities of London and Middlesex; Drillien and her colleagues [QRL 216, 215] followed up children born in 1950–6 resident in Edinburgh in 1960–2 with an IQ test score below 70; Scally and MacKay [QRL 593] derived estimates of those special-care patients in the community in Northern Ireland ascertained as mentally handicapped, together with those in residential care in hospitals and a hostel; Kushlick and Cox [QRL 381] measured the prevalence of mentally subnormal adolescents in Wessex in 1963, known to several agencies; Innes and his colleagues [QRL 346] used the regional psychiatric-care register in North-east Scotland to estimate the prevalence of mental subnormality in that region in 1966, whilst Younie [QRL 727] used the registers of the seven local authorities in the same region of Scotland.

Wing [QRL 720] has presented statistics for Camberwell, arguing that though the rates are less stable due to the restricted population there is likely to be more thorough case-finding within a single authority.

2.5.25. *Nutrition*

A number of dietary surveys have been carried out on national or local population samples. These general surveys have concentrated on either end of the age scale—the young and elderly. As part of the investigation of aetiological factors in coronary heart disease dietary studies of middle-aged males have been carried out.

A large-scale survey of the nutritional condition of various subgroups in Britain was conducted between 1948 and 1951. Though the National Food Survey and studies on growth of school children continue to provide some background information, it was felt important in the 1960s that a programme of nutrition surveys was carried out on various sections of the community. This was to detect any retrogression in the diet of particular sections of the community, and ensure that the central government was in a position to make early predictions of the effect of changes of food policy, in economic circumstances, or in feeding habits. A pilot study was, therefore, mounted in the 1960s by the MoH [QRL 476]. This study was particularly aimed at gaining experience of the method to be used for further work, but at the same time the results stemming from the study were thought to be of sufficient interest to merit publication, though caution is required in interpreting the findings.

A random sample of children in Great Britain stratified by single years of age up to 5 was drawn from Welfare Milk Application records. Of the thousand children selected 275 were outside the scope of the survey (moved, away, died, not known at address, at school, still breast fed and other reasons). Of the remaining 725 children, 651 successful interviews were carried out; 556 mothers agreed to keep a diet record and were (under guidance) provided with weighing scales and a week's dietary record book. Each separate item of food given to the child was weighed and the amount left also weighed; 434 of them produced acceptable records; 341 children were medically examined and 314 received a dental examination. Some data were available on the family background; there was clear evidence that the response rate was lower in Social Classes IV and V, in families with four or more children, and in households where the mother did paid work—thus the poorest response was amongst those groups in which malnutrition was most likely to be present.

A more extensive survey was carried out in 1968–9 in thirty-nine areas of Great Britain. A similar technique was used and full dietary records were obtained for 1321 children out of an original sample of 2321. In addition to background information from an interview and the weighed dietary survey, the children had a dental examination and a medical [QRL 196]. Unquestionably, data were obtained that cannot be reached through the National Food Survey. One of the problems is that the response rate is about 66 per cent both for the weighed dietary survey and for the National Food Survey; it was suggested that localized studies in depth might influence civic pride and enthusiasm and provide a higher response rate. Local studies might also benefit by using fewer observers to carry out the clinical examination, whilst supplementary studies of biochemical findings, which cannot be directly related to the results from a broad survey, might be linked to in-depth local studies. There was also some doubt about the responsibility of the figures for individual intake of nutrients; this is due to inadequate supervision of interviewers in many widely scattered localities.

A survey restricted to study of vitamin D intakes of infants was reported by Bransby *et al.* [QRL 81]. The aim was to assess the total intake of vitamin D in the first year of life and the medical preparations consumed by children up to the age of 5. A two-stage sample identified 1623 mothers in England and Wales—only ten refused though data were not included for sixty-one children because feeding was atypical in the survey week whilst thirty-four children were over 5. The mothers were interviewed by health visitors either at home or in clinics during early 1960. Using a standard questionnaire the amounts of concentrated milk, infant foods, cereals, and vitamin D preparations taken in the week preceding interview were recorded.

Persons at the other extreme of the age range are also vulnerable to nutritional problems and a number of studies have been carried out on the diet of the elderly. A major survey of the health of the elderly had been carried out in Sheffield [QRL 321]; this had included a food survey reported by Bransby and Osborne [QRL 82]. In 1967 the Panel on Nutrition of the Elderly were concerned that the present evidence was too patchy and unrepresentative to enable a comprehensive picture to be obtained; they advocated that special studies should be carried out. A survey carried out in 1967–8 aimed to examine the dietary habits, health and social circumstances of the elderly (65 and over) in six areas living alone or with spouses, relatives or friends—but outside institutional accommodation [QRL 189].

In two areas the target was 100 records, i.e. twenty-five in each subgroup, whilst in the other four areas double that number were attempted. The sample was drawn through the registers of local ECs and the patients were approached by their GP in order to invite them to participate in the study. From an eligible sample of 1283, thirty-two were withdrawn by their GP; of the remainder 372 refused to participate (30 per cent). The response rate varied from area to area; the sample studied was deficient of females 65–74, with an excess of males 75 and over. The respondents were interviewed in their own home by the dietary investigator who carried out a general recall-type interview to identify the overall dietary pattern; this was supplemented by a record of food purchases and a written diary of food eaten during the succeeding week. A check on reliability of the dietary data was made by resurveying a sample of the respondents; this showed satisfactory agreement in the data. Each subject was asked to have a clinical examination at a hospital or clinic including an X-ray of the left hand; some subjects agreed only to medical examination at home. No attempt was made to standardize the clinicians' methods, though they had an opportunity to discuss this before the start of the survey. A range of haematological and biochemical investigations were made; in order to check on comparability some analyses were done of standard bloods and sera. The dietary investigators also enquired about the socio-economic circumstances of each subject. Full medical, dietary and social data were obtained from 90 per cent of the respondents; medical data were obtained from a further 6 per cent and dietary data from 4 per cent.

Three interrelated studies have been carried out for the King's Fund; the first of these (Exton-Smith and Stanton [QRL 232]) aimed to discover the levels of intake compatible with health in elderly women living alone. The recruitment of subjects for the study was a little strange in that in Hornsey lists of names and addresses were supplied by a Darby and Joan club, old people's welfare and the housing trust; in Islington the MOH provided a list of people who were thought to be malnourished. The intention was apparently to identify a well-nourished and poorly nourished group and compare their intakes and physical condition. Clinical assessments were made of the subjects and investigation of bone density, haemoglobin and blood levels of calcium, phosphorus and alkaline phosphatase. It is likely that the very people who are most poorly nourished could not participate in the study due to lack of co-operation or understanding associated with mental confusion and lethargy. A week's weighed diet survey was attempted, with peripatetic dieticians weighing larder stocks and purchases for those unable to weigh accurately. A few meals were eaten away from home and the investigators obtained descriptions of food consumed. Where club meals and meals on wheels were eaten a record of these was taken and a weighed survey of a sample of these meals was carried out. A random selection of these meals was analysed chemically.

The first survey showed that there was a remarkable decline in dietary intake for those in their eighth decade. Initially it was not possible to identify the reasons for this and a follow-up study was carried out in 1969 (Stanton and Exton-Smith [QRL 627]). Only twenty-seven (45 per cent) were still living alone in the same district and seven (12 per cent) in residential care; sixteen of the subjects agreed to a second week's weighed survey and six more gave detailed diet histories. A non-standard weighed dietary survey, similar to the first study, was carried out and after the completion of the dietary survey, nineteen of the subjects had a clinical and radiological examination.

A further study (Exton-Smith *et al.* [QRL 233]) involved old people in a large practice in Camden and residents of two local authority homes in Hertfordshire. Ninety-four subjects were identified by health visitors or geriatric visitors in North London as being 'house bound', of whom fifty-four participated. The diet of these individuals was assessed by interview and a 'measured survey' similar to the two earlier studies. An active group was selected in a Camden practice by taking every tenth patient over retiring age; 73 out of 105 agreed. Twenty volunteers in two local authority residential homes for the elderly in Hertfordshire also participated. Meals were eaten in a communal dining room which made it possible to weigh the food served and amount left on the plate for each meal. Fifty-one of the housebound completed a 7-day record, one a 6, one a 5, and one a 4. Ninety-eight of the active had a 7-day record, one a 6, four a 5, and two a 4-day record. The residential records were all comparable for 7 days.

Comparable studies have been carried out on very small samples of subjects in Scotland by Durnin and his colleagues [B 171, 172]. Other studies have been carried out on a range of different diseases and their relation to diet. A particular example of this is cardio-vascular disease; an extensive review of this subject was carried out by the advisory panel of the Committee on Medical Aspects of Food Policy [B 150].

A general report was issued on national nutritional surveillance by the DHSS [B 147]; this concentrated upon pregnancy and childhood. This report provides no statistics but is a discussion of information already available and the various methods that can be used to monitor food policy. As an interim the subcommittee recommended that a number of studies should be undertaken to provide baseline information about the present nutritional status of various subgroups of the population. They recommended a number of measures to improve the routine statistics and suggested a number of special studies on pregnant women and children.

2.5.26. *Physique*

There has been a periodic survey of the heights and weights of London school children since 1904. There have been changes over the years and in 1959 representatives from the MoH, Ministry of Agriculture, Fisheries and Food, and Institute of Child Health participated in the planning of the survey (see Scott [QRL 597]). The sampling frame was designed to secure a complete cross-section of pupils of compulsory school age attending ordinary day schools, allowing for distribution by social class, religion, type of secondary education and representation of individual educational divisions. The children had their height measured by metric rods attached to the wall, with a right-angle movable block; weight was recorded for children in pants and vest on scales frequently adjusted to zero; calf circumferences were measured by a steel tape to the nearest millimetre with the child sitting at a table; skinfold was measured by Harpenden calipers to the nearest 0·1 mm. All the measurements were carried out by school health visitors, who had had appropriate training and were instructed in the method to minimize observer error. In addition to recording these data, the children were asked single questions about puberty—girls whether the menarche had occurred and boys whether their voice had broken. Children in junior schools and secondary schools were also asked how many brothers and sisters had they at home and at school. Further studies of the build of school children were not carried out by the LCC due to doubts about the validity of data collected from a large number of observers in varying conditions.

The Newcastle cohort (see Subsection 2.5.10.1) of children born in 1947 were measured at 3, 5, 9, 13, 14 and 15. In 1968 an attempt was made to contact those still resident in the Newcastle area (i.e. when they were nearly 22). Four hundred and forty-two of the original 1142 were traced, weighed and measured; it was not possible to determine the bias due to loss from the cohort [QRL 466] but comprehensive data on growth in the respondents are presented.

In the course of many other epidemiological studies data on physique have been obtained, for example, from: Aberdeen mothers by Thomson *et al.* [QRL 645]; school children by Colley [QRL 156]; and manual workers by Khosla and Lowe [QRL 371].

2.5.27. *Rehabilitation*

A British Medical Association committee (Tunbridge [QRL 662]) reviewed the data available on the categories of patients admitted to acute hospitals who were disabled and required rehabilitation; they also looked at the outcome of care (this issue is dealt with in Chapter 6). Since this time there has been a dearth of published statistics identifying need for rehabilitation. Ferguson and MacPhail [QRL 238] followed up 705 men who had been discharged from acute medical wards in four hospitals in the west of

Scotland, for 2 years after discharge. They identified the number of deaths, the frequency and duration of hospitalization, the proportion who had worked, and for those at work the suitability of their job. An assessment was made of the cause of breakdown in those whose disease relapsed; comments were made about the lack of after-care services and the inadequate liaison between hospital, general practice and official machinery for care of the disabled. Further work was carried out in Glasgow [QRL 177], Aberdeen [QRL 706] and Dundee [QRL 293]. Each of these studies followed samples of patients discharged from hospital, though the diagnostic groups and ages varied. In Dundee women were included; in Aberdeen follow-up was only for 1 year after discharge. A further intensive survey has been carried out recently in Aberdeen, with regular interviewing of 194 patients followed for a year after discharge from hospital (Blaxter [QRL 75]). An attempt was made to identify the need for and the availability and functioning of the health and welfare services.

A recent report from the Central Health Services Council for England and Wales has emphasized that there are virtually no relevant figures on rehabilitation, and that social security statistics on incapacity for work were of little value [B 94].

2.5.28. *Respiratory diseases*

The subsection on population studies contains some examples of surveys that have been carried out on tuberculosis, pneumoconiosis and chronic bronchitis (2.2.2.2). Population surveys may identify the prevalence of asthma, and this was one particular aspect of the Isle of Wight school children survey (see Subsection 2.5.10.5). A more restricted survey was carried out in Aberdeen [QRL 184]; a sample of 2511 school children was interviewed and those positive to screening questions were medically examined for the presence of asthma. The prevalence has been examined in relation to child and family characteristics.

Many other epidemiological studies have been reported which either deal solely with respiratory disease, or have quantified the incidence or prevalence of respiratory and other conditions. Bearing in mind the points raised at the beginning of this chapter on validity of data and representativeness of the sample studies no further comments are made here; a number of studies are indexed in the QRL. Tuberculosis, which is not confined to the respiratory tract, is briefly discussed in Subsection 2.5.33.

2.5.29. *Self-medication*

Examination of this issue provides an insight into a major component of 'total health care'; because of the lack of medical supervision, it raises some important questions about care. Dunnell and Cartwright [QRL 220] reported a study whose aim was three-fold: to look at the distribution and nature of medicine taking, the role of the medical profession, and the storage of medicines in people's homes. In general they explored the relationship between patients and doctors and the functioning of the health service—particularly with reference to self-treated symptoms. A random sample of electors 21 and over was contacted during March–July in fourteen constituencies in Britain in 1969, using a two-stage sampling process. Eventually 76 per cent were successfully interviewed—1412; no analysis is given of the non-respondents. A sample of 969 households (drawn at random from the total sample) was used to identify if any children under 15 were present; information was obtained about medicines kept in 71 per cent of these households. No information was collected regarding people 15–20—because it was felt that late teenagers' medicine-taking habits could not be obtained from their parents and yet these individuals would be difficult to contact because of mobility, etc. In addition a sample of general practitioners, caring for the adults in the survey, were contacted. Data were obtained through a postal questionnaire; 598 GPs were named but only 56 per cent responded (these tended to be younger, but DHSS data did not suggest that they were different in their prescribing habits).

The adults were interviewed using a standard questionnaire on drugs: taken in the last 24 hours and the previous 2 weeks, symptoms, attitudes to health and to the medical profession, and consultation with their GP. A similar questionnaire was given to mothers of selected children. All those who had been given a prescription in the 2-week period were asked to complete a diary about all medicines in the subsequent 2 weeks—diaries were completed for 73 per cent of the 399 who had had prescriptions. Housewives were asked about medicines in the household and a list made of all stored medicines; samples of tablets were taken to check on their identification.

This issue has also been studied as one facet of the health sector of the GHS (see 2.2.1.2) and in the local survey in Bermondsey/Southwark (see 2.2.2.3).

2.5.30. *Sexually transmitted diseases*

Woodcock [B 485] has recently discussed the value of present statistics on sexually transmitted diseases; he indicates three problems: (1) a proportion of patients are still treated by their GP and do not enter the hospital statistics; (2) repeat attendances after cure are labelled as new cases (and thus one cannot identify reinfection rates and the cumulative incidence in persons); and (3) patients frequently have multiple diagnoses at one attendance and there is variation in the ways in which different clinics handle these statistics.

In order to supplement the nationally collected statistics (CGRHS [B 14]) the British Co-operative Clinic Group was formed; venereologists treating over 95 per cent of the patients in Great Britain participate. Standard returns are submitted, for hospital-treated patients, on various topics to the honorary secretary, who has been responsible for analysing the data and producing articles for publication. The group take care to standardize terms and definitions and the reports have covered a range of topics in greater detail than the statistics in the DHSS publications (see [QRL 85–90] inclusive).

2.5.31. *Smoking*

It may at first sight seem strange to have a subsection devoted to smoking amongst a classification of medical problems. However, the chief aim of this chapter is to identify the determinants of health need and the indicators of such need. One of the major known aetiological factors responsible for a wide range of diseases is cigarette smoking;

any studies that demonstrate the distribution and variation in smoking or identify the group susceptible to health education are thus demonstrating a health need (or future need).

A number of projects have been carried out by the Government Social Survey division. The study of schoolboy smoking (Bynner [QRL 115]) was part of the programme of the research of the MoH, required for a background to an anti-smoking campaign. It was concerned with the motivations and external pressures that result in some children smoking—after careful consideration it was decided that the work should take place on school premises and that the information should be obtained by questionnaire which the children would complete anonymously (rather than interviewing them), and the data collection should be under the direct supervision of Government Social Survey trained interviewers. After considerable piloting a questionnaire was devised which consisted of two parts; the first included questions about leisure, attitudes to school, home and friends, personal characteristics, and smoking experience. The children were then divided up into those who smoked, had given up smoking, or had never smoked; each of these categories completed a different questionnaire with details where appropriate on smoking history, contact with other smokers, attitudes and knowledge of the risk of smoking, and general attitudes to smoking and towards other boys who smoked.

The sample of boys aged 11–15 in sixty schools was designed so that an analysis was possible by age group within type of school. Six types of school attended by the majority of boys in the country were included: mixed secondary modern, boys' secondary modern, mixed grammar, boys' grammar, mixed comprehensive, boys' comprehensive. Approximately equal numbers were included from each type of school by selecting ten schools at random from those of each type in England and Wales; from each school approximately the same number of boys were selected in each of the first four school years. The total sample obtained by the procedure was 5601; with appropriate weighting this was adjusted to the distribution of the type of school across the country (secondary modern were under-represented and comprehensive over-represented by the technique of sampling).

Losses occurred from the sample in various ways; in some schools heads asked parents' permission and some parents refused. In addition some boys were absent on the day of survey. This reduced the total sample from 6772 to 5601. The response was poorest in the mixed secondary modern schools (dropping to 68 per cent in the fourth year), whilst grammar and comprehensive schools had a consistently high response above 80 per cent. The overall response was 82 per cent for the six categories of school. There was slight over-representation of boys in urban areas.

An earlier survey (Bynner [QRL 114]) was designed to identify the attitudes that medical students hold towards smoking and their role as health educators, and the check whether they differed from the public in their smoking habits and attitudes, and what they learnt during their training.

The MoH commissioned another general survey to collect background information about smoking, as an aid to defining an anti-smoking campaign (McKennell and Thomas [QRL 432]). A two-stage stratified random sample was used, the primary units being wards or combinations of wards and parishes in the rural areas. These were stratified by standard region, and within region by conurbation, other urban and rural location; within these strata by the J-index (proportion of jurors in the population). Two samples were taken: one of the adult individuals and the other of addresses designed to produce a sample of persons aged 16–20, using the electoral register. There were 1418 adults eligible in the sample drawn, of whom 6·5 per cent refused and 4·4 per cent were non-contacts. All the smokers and ex-smokers were interviewed and half of the non-smokers. Out of the 7121 households, 1161 contained one adolescent or more; amongst these there were 93 per cent full and adequate contacts. All the smokers and ex-smokers were interviewed but only a third of the non-smokers.

The GHS [QRL 512, 513] collects data on smoking habits of respondents and has been discussed in Subsection 2.2.1.2.

The introduction to this section explained that this subsection was included as the distribution of smoking amongst subgroups of the population was linked to the health hazards to which smokers exposed themselves. Knowledge of variation in smoking patterns may thus provide an indicator of variation in health need. The evidence that links the fact of smoking with subsequent ill-health stems from a massive literature that is beyond the scope of this review. Some of the key UK papers are indexed in the QRL, as they provide an insight into the distribution of morbidity in the population and the enhanced levels of this in smokers.

2.5.32. *Terminal care*

Cartwright *et al.* [QRL 130] looked at the lives and care of a random sample of adults who had died (i.e. persons 15 and over). The aim of the study was to obtain a picture of the way society cared for a group of people in the last year of their life; many of the subjects were old or had been sick for some while. The study shows the way in which a multiplicity of services functioned or failed to function, looking at these services from an unusual but highly relevant angle. The study was carried out in twelve areas in England and Wales, each being registration districts chosen with a probability proportional to population after stratification by region and type of area. Half the sample was selected from deaths occurring 3 months previously and the other half 9 months previously. Forty deaths in each of the two periods were selected for the twelve areas—a total of 960 in all. Interviewers were selected and trained with care and were given a standard questionnaire with which to interview the respondents. The first person to be contacted was the informant (i.e. the person who informed the registrar of the death and provided details about the patient). If that person did not live in the study area, could not be contacted, refused, or was not fit to be interviewed, the address at which the deceased person had lived was visited and an attempt made to contact the most appropriate person to interview.

Questionnaires were completed for 785 persons—82 per cent of the deaths; some incomplete data were obtained for another 3 per cent. No suitable person was able or willing to help in the remaining 15 per cent; refusal may have biased the sample away from deaths that were particularly upsetting to the bereaved relatives, though information was also lost because no appropriate person lived in the study area. Interviews were more often completed for working-class than middle-class persons, whilst response was also slightly higher in the north than in the south. As would be expected, there was a deficiency of successful interviews when the person who died had no close relatives.

During the interview questions were asked about the health during the 12 months before death of the person who died, including the medical care given by hospitals and general practitioners. Information was obtained about: the household arrangements and changes in these because of ill-health or old age; equipment used and additional expenditure; help given by relatives, friends and others. The last section dealt with the impact on the respondent as well as the deceased person of the final year of care.

Eighty-one of the deceased people had been in hospital or an institution for over a year; the others were asked about their GP. Six hundred and eighty-nine respondents provided traceable names, which related to 411 doctors; 323 (79 per cent) filled in a postal questionnaire or were interviewed. The doctors were asked about difficulties in obtaining hospital admission for various people with terminal conditions, their relationship with hospital staff and district nurses, their views on the adequacy of local authority services and on terminal nursing. They were not questioned about specific patients in the sample.

The MoHs agreed to district nurses and health visitors being interviewed and 508 (95 per cent) of the district nurses identified were interviewed about their involvement with the dying and bereaved; seventy-five out of seventy-six health visitors in the study areas who were involved with the care of the terminally ill or bereaved were also interviewed. The initial sample prepared by the OPCS had a significant deficiency of deaths in persons 75 and over and an excess of deaths from cancer. This was reflected in the data collected at interview; there was also an excess of deaths in the home and corresponding deficiency of institutional deaths.

2.5.33. *Tuberculosis*

Mortality and notification of tuberculosis were discussed in the previous review [B 14]. Logan and Benjamin [QRL 406] produced a collation of tuberculosis statistics for England and Wales, 1938–55, with a detailed and interesting commentary. There is a clear discussion of the difference between the individual getting a simple primary focus with no extension of the disease and the progressive development which leads to notification. It is emphasized that about 10 per cent of the patients with disease may not be notified, whilst some of the notifications relate to primary cases that are under observation following pick-up, for example at X-ray. The influence of mass X-ray campaigns upon the deficiency in notification is discussed and it is suggested that coverage had improved in recent years.

Heasman [QRL 305] reviewed the functioning of Mass Miniature Radiography (MMR) in England and Wales. His report contains an analysis of the routine data submitted to the GRO over the 3-year period 1955–7, in an attempt to contribute to the general study of tuberculosis and other chest diseases. Apparently the material is based on a 10 per cent sample of all examinations—which is referred to as a quasi-random sample; no detail of this is given. Other data are submitted for abnormalities which enables an examination to be made of the 'pick-up' rate and the source and characteristics of the individuals having positive X-rays. The introduction is careful to point out that the survey yields information on the prevalence of disease amongst those examined, but not its incidence. It can give an indication of the number of cases already in existence and not previously diagnosed but not the number of new cases appearing in a defined period. An important issue is that those coming for mass radiography are a biased sample of the total population; this is partly related to the category of examinee. These include: hospital patients, contacts, persons referred by their GP; antenatal patients; hospital staff; forces' recruits; residents in institutions; volunteers from factory surveys or from the general public. The prevalence of chest disease varied greatly between these categories which makes extrapolation to the general population difficult.

Carstairs and Howie [QRL 124] have produced a comparable, but briefer, report on the MMR service in Scotland. Again this was derived from an *ad hoc* analysis of the routine returns submitted by the units throughout the country. (During the enquiry it was found that two small static units had never made any returns!)

CHAPTER 3

UNMET DEMAND

A definition of need was provided in the previous chapter (Section 2.1). Once an individual (and/or his family) has identified a health-care need various lines of action can be followed. In certain circumstances a deliberate choice can be made to take no action. Some patients, particularly for minor complaints, will habitually resort to self-medication: self-care and self-medication have been discussed in the previous chapter (Subsection 2.5.29). In other circumstances the general practitioner will be contacted; this may involve a request for home visit or by attendance at surgery. Occasionally a family doctor cannot be contacted in an emergency (or he declines to visit) or no attempt will be made to contact the general practitioner; the patient may immediately go or be taken to the local Accident and Emergency (A & E) Department. Some patients seek help from 'paramedical' staff and a few may directly approach chiropractors, herbalists, faith healers, etc. What is not easy to determine is the sequence of events that can occur when some bottleneck or obstruction to contact of the first choice of care leads to reconsideration and approach of a second choice. When the initial 'portal' for care has been identified (whether it is first or second choice) various statistics on queues for care can be accumulated. In general, once a patient has requested 'care' from the health service he may: (1) not receive the care requested, but take no action; (2) organize self, private or unorthodox care; (3) enter a queue or series of queues for appropriate care—and statistics covering this are dealt with in subsequent sections in this chapter; (4) receive an inappropriate level of care or care not of the standard expected (this is dealt with in Chapter 6, Subsection 6.2.4.3).

From the initial contact in primary medical care the total pathways to complete care can be complex. These may involve referral to ancillary staff in the community health-care team; care from the staff in the Department of Social Services or from other welfare agencies; consultant opinion on domiciliary visit; referral for direct access investigation at hospital; ambulatory medical care at hospital out-patients which may involve investigation and/or treatment; certain categories of patient (the mentally ill, the elderly) may receive treatment over a long period of time by regular attendance at a day centre or day hospital; admission to hospital, whether this is for acute, chronic, maternity or psychiatric care; following in-patient care, a range of activities may occur including recurring spells of in-patient care or visits to out-patients. Through each referral 'node' there may be delay to the next point of care. Some of these queues for care may be fairly easy to identify and in certain circumstances regular statistics of such queues are available; for many aspects of this problem no routine statistics are available and various special studies have been mounted to provide an indication of the extent of this problem.

Once a queue for care occurs there may be an important stifling of demand; for example, the avenue to out-patient appointment is via a doctor's referral letter. The

99

hard knowledge of the present time lag between referral and date of next appointment may influence the family doctor in whether he recommends out-patient care. Thus the actual number of patients waiting for such care may underestimate the number that would be referred should further facilities be available. This issue has already been discussed (Section 2.1.2), but it is re-emphasized here because of the impact it can have on any statistics of 'queues'. As a specific example Wolff [B 478] has drawn attention to the very limited facilities that are available for psychotherapy and the way in which this has stifled demand. Sainsbury [B 401] described a rather different phenomenon, when he showed that provision of additional specialist facilities for psychiatric care did not result in patients with less severe illness attending but led to referral of a rather different group of patients who had previously been neglected. Another issue linked to demand and queues for care is the influence of the patients' views of what may be expected from the health service and the variation in the general practitioners' reliance upon hospital care for his patients. These issues have already been touched upon (Section 2.1.2), but they overlap with the points raised in this chapter. Some patients may opt by preference or as a result of delays for private care.

The factors that result in a patient initiating contact with the NHS are complex; for a given specific stimulus there will be variations from person to person in their response and for any individual patient variation from one point in time to another. Brotherston [B 70] has pointed out that public expectation is a major factor in determining demand. He suggested that public expectation depends on confidence in modern medicine, advancing levels of education, rising standards of life, diminishing tolerance of pain and disability. This can result in inappropriate (under or over) demand for care; the NHS may respond by delay, failure to provide appropriate care, or provision of inappropriate and excess care. Ashford [B 29] has suggested that very small changes in the willingness of patients to seek care can result in a very substantial change in the demand for care. This issue is dealt with further in Chapter 6 (Subsection 6.2.3). It must be emphasized that the quantification of queues for care can provide an unbalanced or misleading picture of the actual functioning of the service; as with any set of statistics the data have to be interpreted with caution.

The following sections deal with queues for (1) primary medical care, (2) out-patient and (3) in-patient care: statistics on general aspects are dealt with before specific problems. It must be remembered that there is overlap between the concepts of unmet demand and evaluation of health care. Some studies are discussed in Chapter 6 or indexed under that division of the QRL rather than being covered in this chapter, and vice versa.

3.1. Primary medical care

The paucity of routine data from primary medical care has been discussed in the previous chapter (Subsection 2.3.2); a few studies have been carried out on the difficulty patients encounter in seeing their general practitioner. Cartwright's study of general practice [QRL 127] (see Chapter 5, Subsection 5.1.1 for description) obtained data on waiting time at the surgery and factors associated with variation in waiting time. A major study on appointment systems [QRL 64] looked at their impact in waiting times at the surgery; family doctors commented that these systems even the flow of work and reduce the number of non-essential consultations—presumably this must result in some patients waiting several days or failing to obtain an appointment—when in the past they would have gone on the day of their choice but added to the queue in the waiting room.

A noticeable feature of general practice over the past 20 years has been the decreasing proportion of home visits to surgery consultations; this again must mean that patients are being persuaded to attend surgery or not contact the doctor for ailments which in the past would have generated a request for a home visit.

It is not clear how the frequency of home visits is being influenced by reduction in the number of repeat visits for persons with chronic illness or the transfer of care of such patients to ancillary staff. A particular aspect is the emergency 'night' call; a few surveys have looked at the frequency and factors associated with night calls [QRL 99] and at the impact of deputizing services upon the frequency and management of such calls [QRL 712; B 470–472].

Another important issue, but one that is difficult to study, is the lag that occurs between attendance of a patient at their general practitioner and referral to hospital. The family doctor may not think this is required initially, and the majority of patients are unlikely to make an overt 'demand' for referral; direct access investigation or therapeutic trial may occur before the referral occurs. There are very few data to show whether direct-access investigation is a preliminary or alternative to hospital referral, though this issue is touched upon in Chapter 6 (Subsection 6.2.4.1). Cartwright [QRL 126] endeavoured to collect data on the length of time for which a patient had contacted his doctor for a particular condition before an out-patient appointment was initiated. A particular issue for which this is important is early pregnancy when the woman wishes to have an abortion; the doctor may try to dissuade the woman and delay can influence the ease of abortion. This is an example where data on differences between aspirations and actuality are indexed in the QRL for this chapter and Chapter 6, 'Evaluation'.

3.2. Accident and Emergency departments

The self-referral to hospital Accident and Emergency departments (A & E) has been frequently identified as one of the major problems facing such services. The direct transmission of the injured or acutely ill patient is an understandable aspect of the work of A & E departments; quite different is (1) the attendance for non-emergency medical problems because of inability to contact the GP, or (2) the referral by the GP of patients to circumvent a delay for an out-patient appointment, or to precipitate hospital admission. Morgan and his colleagues investigated a sample of patients attending the hospital A & E departments in the Newcastle area [QRL 486]. They studied the patients' pathways to care, and assessed the appropriateness and opinions of their use of the service. Brief reference is made in the QRL to a few other studies that have also collected limited data on use of A & E departments; Chapter 5 (Subsection 5.4.2) also comments on relevant studies.

3.3. Referral to out-patients

There are no published statistics from the DHSS which quantify the delay between referral and provision of an out-patient appointment, though this is an issue that is usually kept under review at hospital. Many hospitals will identify the average delay for 'urgent' and 'non-urgent' referrals by specialty and consultant within specialty. The published statistics have been obtained from special studies on out-patients such as those of Forsyth and Logan [QRL 243] and a series of reports published by the NPHT [QRL 44, 112, 140, 599]. Williams [QRL 713] recorded the views of sixty-eight doctors in South Wales of the delay at hospitals in their localities. The GHS (see Chapter 2, Subsection 2.2.1.2) has collected data in 1973 about delay prior to out-patient appointment, and also length of time on the waiting list. However, tabulations have not been published from these items.

Rather separate from the delay in obtaining an appointment is the actual wait that occurs in the out-patient department. For example, Barr [QRL 54] examined this in the Oxford Region; he collected data on the proportion of patients arriving early or late, and the subsequent delay until they were seen. This issue is also discussed in Chapter 5 (Subsection 5.4.3.2).

3.4. In-patient care

The previous review [B 14] discussed the available central government statistics on waiting lists for admission to hospital. This source of statistics has been complemented by a number of special studies, which have examined specific details of the functioning of waiting lists; many of these are 'operational research' studies, which are beyond the scope of the present review. Cocking [B 110] has discussed the need to monitor the size of the waiting list, but emphasized the fallacies inherent in the statistics called for by the DHSS. Luckman and Murray [B 291] clearly demonstrated the need to study casemix and associated length of spell in hospital when assessing waiting time from size of waiting lists.

Apart from admission from the waiting list a patient may enter hospital as an emergency; the proportion of such admissions varies from specialty to specialty and is influenced by a number of factors. Warren *et al*. [QRL 691] examined this issue by analysing statistics of patients in London referred to the Emergency Bed Service (i.e. those for whom the GP had not arranged emergency admission in a local hospital). In particular they examined the degree of 'delay' in admissions and factors associated with this.

3.5. Inappropriate care

One facet of unmet demand is that of inappropriate care; this can occur for any state of care once the patient (or his relative) has initiated contact with the health service. It has already been mentioned as a topic of importance and one that is not well documented, but creates major repercussions for the other patients awaiting care. For example, if an elderly female patient who requires nursing but no active treatment occupies an acute

bed in an orthopaedic ward, she can be considered as queueing for care in a rehabilitation unit (or perhaps community hospital, etc.); at the same time she is occupying a
bed and causing the admission waiting list to stagnate (or grow if additions occur at
out-patients).

This issue is discussed in greater detail in Chapter 6 (see Section 6.2.4).

3.6. Private care

Fraser *et al*. [QRL 248] showed that of 694 patients referred for specialist out-patient
opinions, 139 (20 per cent) of the NHS registered patients opted for a private specialist
consultation. The reasons for this were predominantly to avoid either delay until an
appointment or waiting in out-patients. Thus private practice can be considered as one
(tenuous) measure of unmet demand; individuals are seeking private care because they
feel that their expectations are not met through the conventional NHS channels.

Sutcliffe [B 429] has indicated the paucity of available data on the use of the private
sector. An indication of expenditure is available from the Family Expenditure Survey
[B 138]) whilst the routine returns on available beds and occupied beds to the DHSS
identify those categorized as private (see appropriate section in previous review [B 14]).
An extensive review of the private sector in this country indicated that there was no
accurate reporting of those engaged in private practice, the number of private patients,
or the income from private practice [B 320].

Cartwright [QRL 126] in her study of hospital care found 3 per cent of the respondents had been admitted as fee-paying patients. She discussed the reasons for this and
the distribution of fees paid. In her subsequent study [QRL 127] of general practice, she
tabulated the distribution of doctors by number of private patients; other data on
frequency of private consultations and the effect of private consultation on ease of
hospital admission were collected. The author drew attention to the bias in the estimates, due to a higher non-response rate amongst private patients.

In the study of handicapped in this country (Harris *et al*. [QRL 297]) material was
collected on the proportion of respondents who consulted a medically qualified
specialist in a private capacity. Data were also available on the contact with 'non-
medical' sources of help such as osteopaths.

CHAPTER 4

RESOURCES

'Distribution of NHS resources by need rather than demand proposed.' This caption in *The Times*, 29 September 1976, heralded the final report of the Resource Allocation Working Party for England set up by the Department of Health and Social Security in May 1975 to review the arrangements for distributing National Health Service capital and revenue to regional health authorities, area health authorities and districts respectively. In so doing, the Working Party made recommendations about 'a method of securing, as soon as practicable, a pattern of distribution responsive objectively, equitably and efficiently to relative need ...' (page 5, [B 154]). The basic *need* criteria identified by the Working Party for the formula to determine the resource allocation for each region were the absolute population, its structure in terms of age and sex, and the regional standardized mortality ratios. Also considered necessary were fertility ratios in the calculation of maternity services and marital status for mental illness in-patient services, while the crude population only was to be used for Family Practitioner Committee (FPC) administrative expenditure. One recommendation of significance was that the caseload measure should be dropped from the formula because it is an unsatisfactory indicator of need since the number of cases treated is dependent to a large extent on the availability of facilities to treat them.

The recommendations, although accepted in principle by the Secretary of State, have given rise to considerable misgivings as evidenced in various medical journals. Criticism has been expressed about the inadequacy of the need criteria for they fail to take sufficient account of population densities, areas of social deprivation and local morbidity and mortality statistics. Other anxieties have been voiced about first, the risks to future advances in medical practice because of the channelling of funds away from the south-east and in particular, the teaching hospitals and, secondly, the absence of machinery to monitor the utilization of these resources. Resource allocation is, of course, solely concerned with the distribution of financial resources which are used for the provision of real resources. In England it is the RHAs who hold the responsibility for determining how the allocated resources are deployed; likewise in Scotland the powers lie with the Health Boards, in Northern Ireland with the Health and Social Services Boards, and for Wales with the Welsh Office. So, whatever reservations there may be about the appropriateness of the need criteria, and the timeliness of their implementation in England, the recommendations of the Working Party do confirm the shift over the past years away from the entrenched practice of deploying resources where demand is evident to the more appropriate though less easily defined concept whereby resources endeavour to relieve the needs and unmet demands of communities (as illustrated in Chapters 2 and 3).

The Resource Allocation Working Party saw the supply of health facilities in England, as elsewhere, to be variable and very much influenced by history, and this applies particularly to hospital provisions. In 1948 the NHS centralized control of a variety of institutions; teaching and voluntary hospitals, local authority hospitals including mental, maternity, tuberculosis and isolation institutions, and the former Poor Law infirmaries. Furthermore, by this date, the majority of medical teaching centres were established and such centres are now believed to influence the geographical distribution of general medical practitioner services. This, therefore, was the context of the Working Party's statement that 'the methods used to distribute financial resources to the NHS have, since its inception, tended to reflect the inertia built into the system by history. They have tended to increment the historic basis for the supply of real resources (for example, facilities and manpower); and, by responding comparatively slowly and marginally to changes in demography and morbidity, have also tended to perpetuate the historic situation' (page 7, *ibid.*). These inequalities have normally been manifest at regional level, but regional figures are but aggregates of local provision and recent publications by, for example, Buxton and Klein [B 81] and Rickard [B 386] have drawn attention to the marked intra-regional variations in resource deployment at area and even district levels.

This chapter furnishes information about health service resources from *ad hoc* statistical sources. It is in three parts: facilities (ambulances, acute beds, buildings); manpower; and other resources (drugs). Financial resources lie outside the ambit of the review. Data on the utilization of the services provided by these resources are described in the subsequent chapter. There are instances when some statistics on facilities and staffing are incorporated in reports concerned primarily with usage patterns; these are indexed in the QRL accompanying Chapter 5. Many reports on manpower topics contain statistics about the attitudes of staff to their work. Entries for these data are normally to be found in the QRL to Chapter 6 on 'Evaluation of Medical Care'. A few manpower studies are indexed entirely in the Evaluation QRL and so they are identified in this chapter by an asterisk (e.g. [QRL 52*]). In addition, the earliest of the studies into the provision of hospital facilities have an asterisk for they are indexed only in the QRL to Chapter 2. Finally, it is emphasized that the sources described in the following sections supplement those published routinely, and which were reviewed in the earlier volume in this series, *Central Government Routine Health Statistics* [B 14].

Resource statistics for Northern Ireland appear in two routinely published sources—although the authorities responsible for the administration of the resources and the presentation of the reports were restructured at the time of Reorganization. On 30 September 1973 the General Health Services Board [B 352] was replaced by the Central Services Agency of the Northern Ireland Health and Social Services. Among the functions that were conferred on the Agency under Section 26 of the Health and Personal Social Services (Northern Ireland) Order, 1972, were: general practitioner services covering central payments, registers of patients and lists of both medical and dental practitioners, and vacancies; staff selection procedures for hospital medical and dental staff, and the co-ordination of appointments in training grades; control machinery for prescribing, and record keeping; legal services; supplies; and various other services such as general ophthalmic. Statistics relating to aspects of almost all of these functions were incorporated into the annual reports from 1974 [QRL 502]. Hospital statistics were published annually in the reports of the Northern Ireland Hospitals Authority [QRL 503] until September 1973 when, in the restructuring of the health and personal social services, the hospital and specialist services were amalgamated with the local health authority, port health, school health, local authority welfare, child care and general health services. These are now administered by four Health and Social Services Boards who will be preparing annual statistical reports. The earliest are [B 174] and [B 457]. It is the intention of the Department of Health and Social Services for Northern Ireland to publish reports annually for calendar years, but the initial volume will span the years 1974–5 (Walby, A. L., 1976, personal communication). There is a further commentary about these Northern Ireland sources and the statistics relating to the use made of the services in Chapter 5.6.6.

4.1. Facilities

4.1.1. *Ambulances*

With Reorganization in April 1974 the administration of ambulance services in England and Wales passed from the local health authorities to the NHS. In Scotland, though, they were already under the control of the Scottish Home and Health Department, while in Northern Ireland, the transfer of responsibility for the services from the Hospitals Authority to the Health and Personal Social Services took place in October 1973. Routine statistics from central government publications on the operation of ambulance services were detailed in [B 14]. Other routine statistics on the number of persons carried, cost per person carried and cost per vehicle mile of the ambulance service in county boroughs, London boroughs and county councils of England and Wales were produced annually until 1974 by the Institute of Municipal Treasurers and Accountants (IMTA) and the Society of County Treasurers (SCT) ([QRL 348] and Section 5.3). *Ad hoc* studies of ambulance services have usually been undertaken as operational research projects with the consequence that statistical evidence that has been collected on the use of local services has frequently formed the basis of planning models.

4.1.2. *Acute bed provisions*

For more than two decades since the inception of the NHS, hospital resource planning has been bedevilled by the concept of bed norms, these being standard rates of bed provision per population. A generation of hospital studies has demonstrated the weaknesses in this concept. Furthermore, changing conventions regarding patient management for many medical and even surgical conditions, and the current retrenchment in capital building programmes have also brought about the realization that much in-patient care can be substituted by day hospital or community-based support. (This has applied particularly in the areas of mental illness, mental handicap and geriatrics, see for example [B 142, 146, 151, 155].) Beds have traditionally been used as the unit of supply in hospital plans despite the fact that their usage rates are dependent upon the availability of manpower (hospital doctors, nurses, ancillary staff and community health and social services), the current medical knowledge in diagnosis and treatment, and other resources such as laboratory facilities, operating theatres, etc. Further, they are not an arithmetic planning measure: ten hospitals of forty beds are not the equivalent to one hospital of 400 beds; again, the reduction of forty beds from a 400-bed hospital would probably leave the operating costs little changed whereas the closure of a forty-bed hospital would reduce operating costs to zero.

In January 1948 a memorandum circulated to the newly established Regional Hospital Boards (RHB) outlined estimates of hospital facilities and medical staff considered to be the optimum future requirements of a developed service, *The Development of Consultant Services* [QRL 470*]. In preparing the estimates, the Ministry of Health (MoH) drew upon the findings of the Surveys of Hospitals undertaken in the early 1940s (see [QRL 469*] and Subsection 2.3.3). It was a repeated recommendation in the reports that the clinical responsibility for hospital patients other than those in general practitioner or cottage hospitals should rest with consultants. The overall conclusion was that the optimal bed provision per 1000 population in England and Wales should be 5–7 and 8 for Scotland. The consultant services document therefore envisaged hypothetical average hospital districts with a population of the order of 100,000 to 120,000. For each specialty, proposals were made regarding consultant staffing and beds; for example, in general surgery it was suggested that there should be a group of 180 surgical beds and associated out-patient clinics, and that the staff required would be the equivalent of three whole-time surgeons. The overall recommended rate of bed provision (excluding mental health/deficiency) was therefore about 8 per 1000 persons. It is important, however, to realize that there already existed in Britain a complex hospital infrastructure [B 1 and B 372], so that there were already in England and Wales at the end of 1948 seven beds (excluding mental facilities) per 1000 population.

It was against this background that a succession of hospital studies were financed primarily by the Nuffield Provincial Hospitals Trust (NPHT) to determine the 'needs' of communities. The earliest studies endeavoured to describe the *current use* of the existing facilities by the catchment populations. (These studies are indexed in the QRL accompanying Chapter 2.) Later the emphasis was much more towards estimating *manifest demand* for facilities as evidenced in waiting lists plus reports by family doctors and other agencies of community morbidity which was not reaching the hospital sector (unmet demand). Thus the two surveys in Stirlingshire and Ayrshire published in 1948 and 1950 respectively [QRL 504,* 505*] surveyed the use made by all residents of hospital facilities (both within and outside the defined areas) over 1 year. Assuming a bed occupancy rate of 85 per cent the estimated number of beds required was 5·0 per 1000 population. In the subsequent investigations of Norwich, Northampton (1950–1) [B 356 and QRL 506*] and later Reading [QRL 52*], the 'critical number' of beds needed by the local communities was estimated using a method developed by Bailey [B 32]. In brief, the critical number was the daily rate of beds required *if* all persons recommended for admission in a given year had been actually admitted and had experienced the average in-patient duration of all discharges and deaths over the review period. At an occupancy level of 85 per cent, the numbers of beds required in the three areas were found to be around 2 per 1000 population. However, since these areas were in the south of England, it was decided by the NPHT to further explore some of the assumptions underlying Bailey's method in geographically dissimilar areas, Barrow-in-Furness (Forsyth and Logan [QRL 243]) and Tees-side (Airth and Newell [QRL 11]). Each study tried to measure both the current use of, and manifest demand for, local hospital facilities.

Hospital admissions in the Barrow-in-Furness hospital group plus a range of groups peripheral to the peninsula were examined during 1957 to assess, first, whether the actual population served by the Barrow hospitals differed from the administrative population, and secondly, the amount of movement of Barrow residents to neighbouring hospitals—this was found to be minimal. The effective population served was determined as 116,000, 11 per cent higher than the administrative population of 106,000 persons. Effective populations for the eight largest specialties were also calculated. The 'critical number' of acute beds to serve this effective population was found to be 2·56 per 1000 persons. There were two additional research phases. Information relating to general practitioners' practice sizes and prescribing frequencies and costs were related to their hospital referral patterns and use of direct-access diagnostic facilities. In addition, four quarterly censuses of the wards were conducted by a medical adviser to assess the clinical 'necessity' of the admissions. (This evaluation technique is discussed in Subsection 6.2.4.3.) The conclusions drew attention to fundamental issues in the prediction of hospital-resource utilization, for example, the propensity for under-utilization of beds scattered in many small units. A clinical 'necessity' was not recognized in many of the admissions and this highlighted the importance of adequate and co-ordinated domiciliary services (both from GPs and LHAs) to reduce bed-occupancy rates for primarily social reasons.

Three hospital groups serving industrial populations in central Tees-side and the Hartlepools were chosen for the other northern investigation as the rate of population expansion in the area was comparatively rapid, so making it a likely claimant for hospital expansion [QRL 11]. The purpose of the enquiry was to examine the current demand for non-mental hospital care, against which would be matched the adequacy of the current provision. Twenty-eight hospitals ranging in size from 300 to 20 beds comprised the three groups and some in-patients were admitted from the survey population to another thirty-one peripheral hospitals during the study period. The fieldwork extended over 15 months 1957–8, and three main sources of data were used. The first were monthly hospital returns similar to SH3 forms returned to the MoH. Individual patient records were the second source and, thirdly, general information was supplied by medical and administrative officers in the hospitals, the local Medical Officers of Health (MOsH) and a sample of family doctors.

It was the claim of the authors, Airth and Newell, that the contribution of the report of this study was not so much the statistics (which would only be of value if used for comparative purposes with similar studies) but for the presentation of the statistical methods and the authors' assessments. The 'critical number' method devised by Bailey was found to be less satisfactory on a practical plane when applied to individual specialties. The non-existence of a conventional waiting list for infectious diseases and obstetrics created a problem; and the whole question of the validity of waiting lists as barometers of demand was thrown into relief. The inflexibility in bed allocations to specialties meant that bed occupancy rates had to be fixed at about 85 per cent. If bed 'sharing' were acceptable the occupancy rates could be higher and the estimates of requirements lower. A further problem was to be encountered when applying the 'critical number' method to hospitals or groups which did not serve geographically compact populations. The 'critical number' of *acute* beds required for the three Hospital Management Groups was found to be 3·61 beds per 1000 population (but in actuality, there were 4·07 acute beds per 1000 population in the Groups). However, the modified procedure to take account of the special features of obstetrics and infectious diseases suggested that the requirement more probably lay between 3·88 and 4·14 acute beds per 1000 population.

The difficulties of measuring the demand of communities for hospital services were still far from resolved at the conclusion of this series of NPHT enquiries. Yet the relationships between the apparent demand and the utilization of the resources were beginning to crystallize. That the demand for hospital beds will probably approximate the supply, or supply create its own demand, was possibly the most significant conclusion to be drawn. Airth and Newell had looked at the relationship of the supply and demand for beds in hospital regions of England and Wales in four specialties, and they found it to be almost linear. These northern studies had though produced evidence of 'unmet demand' which family doctors had to cope with—restrictive admission policies for geriatric and maternity cases were cited in the Tees-side area. The general problems of measuring unmet demand not just for hospital facilities but also for primary health care were discussed in 1964 by Logan [B 290]. About the same time, Brotherston reviewed the research that had been undertaken into hospital usage [B 69].

In 1962 the MoH announced in a command paper *A Hospital Plan for England and Wales* [B 324] a policy aimed at reducing the number of hospital beds over a 13-year period. The projected ratio was 3·3 *acute* beds per 1000 population whereas the ratio in England and Wales in 1960 stood at 3·9 with regional variations ranging from 5·6 in Liverpool to 3·0 for East Anglia. The Plan offered little guidance as to how reductions were to be accomplished. In the Liverpool Region, which had the greatest percentage target, there were anxieties about the feasibility of achieving it. So, in response to a request from a Joint Research Committee of the United Liverpool Hospitals and the Liverpool RHB, the Medical Care Research Unit at the University of Manchester examined existing statistical sources and deduced that the region was marked by a high level of bed provision and expenditure, and a low level of throughput. Two years later, in 1964, the Hospital Authorities combined with the MoH and the NPHT to sponsor a 4-year study 'into the dynamics of medical care on Merseyside' [QRL 403]. It was hoped that the enquiry would provide information about the relationship between social environment and demand for medical facilities. Thus they were testing 'the conventional assumption—critical for the planning of hospital resources generally—that bad social conditions automatically produce a greater volume of medical and hospital care' (page 19, *ibid*.).

The Liverpool hospital resources study broke new ground both in its organization and methodology. Part of the initial brief was to train a team which could provide a nucleus of a permanent intelligence unit for the hospital region. Accordingly the organizational structure of the research project embodied a spectrum of planning interests. A widely representative Working Party considered the implications and implementation of the research findings, while the research itself was carried out jointly by the Manchester Medical Care Research Unit and a specially created Operational Activities Unit of the Liverpool RHB. The methodology was determined by the adoption of a need/demand/use and resources/outcome model. Secondary analyses of existing data sources comprised a major portion of the material amassed. A socio-economic index of 'need' was compiled on the basis of seventy-two different factors which included drawing upon the 1966 10 per cent census reports, the Registrar General's reports, criminal statistics and surveys of income. This index applied to seventy-five county boroughs in England and Wales. Facilities for medical, nursing and social care provided by local authorities in the Liverpool Region and other regions in England and Wales were compared. In the 'demand' sector two approaches were used to separate effective demand from latent need. The demand for surgical operations in Liverpool was compared, condition by condition, with that in other regions. A sample of 428 persons in Warrington was interviewed to elicit evidence about any 'unmet' need or demand. Routinely collected hospital statistics provided most of the evidence on use and resources. Some special tabulations were obtained from central government departments and wherever possible the data for the Liverpool Region were compared with other hospital regions in England. In addition, consultants were asked about the allocation of hospital facilities and their clinical policy in the treatment of uncomplicated common conditions. Nursing-dependency profiles of patients with certain conditions were assembled using a modification of the method developed by Barr [B 40]. A survey was conducted of long-stay patients to assess their reasons for admission, continued hospital care and the problems associated with discharges (see Butler and Pearson, [QRL 109] and Sub-section 5.6.2). Further, comparisons were possible between Liverpool, Uppsala (Sweden) and New England (USA) as the Medical Care Research Unit was participating in an international study covering these and other countries [B 277]. For estimates of costs, annual national and regional costing returns were perused, and exercises carried out comparing the relationship between costs per week and costs per case in an attempt to find out which combinations of resource usage produced the best returns in financial terms. The 'outcome' component was the least developed of the model. Available statistics on mortality and morbidity had to suffice, and more specific studies were not carried out to measure either the 'subjective' element of satisfaction/dissatisfaction or the extent of dependency following medical treatment. The data assembling took 5 years, and this final report prepared by Logan, Ashley, Klein and Robson [QRL 403] was published in 1972.

The projected national target of acute bed provision set in the 1962 Hospital Plan was reached by 1967 (8 years early), partly because of the population growth in the southern regions, and because of the transference of certain acute beds to the newly expanding geriatric specialty. So a Revision to the Plan was issued in 1966 [B 326] in which the hospital development programmes for each region were detailed, account having been taken of the latest population projections and the needs of psychiatric and geriatric services.

On 1 April 1968 plans were announced by the MoH for two new district general hospitals to be built at Bury St. Edmunds in Suffolk, and at Frimley in Surrey [B 63]. They were similar in design ('best-buy' hospitals) and each was to contain 308 acute beds which represented 2 acute beds per 1000 people, and was a major shift from the planning norm of 3·3 acute beds laid down 6 years earlier in the Hospital Plan [B 324]. This, it was felt, would be adequate so long as admissions and discharges were administered efficiently, aftercare was closely integrated into the community services, simple surgical procedures were undertaken often on a day basis, and fuller use was made of out-patient investigatory facilities. The adequacy of the proposed provisions were, however, critically assessed via sources reflecting the demands of the two communities for hospital services. A research team from St. Thomas's Hospital Medical School measured demand for hospital services in the catchment area of the proposed Frimley Hospital by asking approximately 100 general practitioners to record over a 3-month period details of almost all categories of referred patients to hospital departments (emergency in-patients, out-patients, casualties and domiciliary visits) and to local authority agencies [B 106]. Wheeler in 1972 analysed routinely available statistics and concluded that the planned ratio of 2 acute beds per 1000 population for the hospital under construction at Bury St. Edmunds was higher than the level of 1·92 already operating in the West Suffolk area [B 458]. Drastic shortening of the average lengths of stay over the decade had permitted corresponding increases in admission rates in the local hospitals, the consequence, Wheeler felt, of modified patterns in clinical management. He thought that similar levels could be achieved on a national scale. This view was, however, challenged soon after by Ross who wished to know if the health and social services in the Bury St. Edmunds area were under special strain coping with, in particular, cases discharged early from hospital [B 395]. And still too little is understood about clinical management and the reasons why acute beds are occupied for seemingly inappropriate reasons (assuming that clinical need is the gauge of appropriateness, see Subsection 5.6.2).

One final note: a DHSS Health Circular, HC(76)29, issued in May 1976 contained planning guidelines for the RHAs, AHAs and the BGs which included recommended levels of provision (or 'norms') for various in-patient and day-patient services. The guideline for new hospitals in England treating acute in-patients is now 2·8 beds per 1000 population.

4.1.3. *Day hospitals*

Day hospitals usually serve geriatric or psychiatric patients, and in-patients may also attend on a daily basis. A geriatric day hospital will incorporate facilities for medical examinations and nursing treatments, physiotherapy and occupational therapy and possibly other activities including speech therapy, chiropody, dentistry and hair-dressing. Day hospitals are distinct from day centres: the latter provide social facilities and possibly chiropody, but none of the remedial health services. They are usually run by local authorities or voluntary bodies, and for this reason have not been included in this volume (see, however, Volume I in this series [B 133]).

The establishment of day hospitals in Britain did not commence until 1946 when an independent psychiatric institution, the Marlborough Day Hospital, was opened. The geriatric day movement began with out-patients attending the wards and rehabilitation departments in hospitals. It was not until 1958 that the first purpose-built geriatric day hospital was opened at Cowley Road Hospital, Oxford. It was designed to treat both physically and psychiatrically disabled patients but with emphasis on the latter. It was at this time in 1958–9 that Farndale commented on the day hospital movement in Great Britain [B 188]. In a somewhat confusing presentation, he depicted each of the forty-five psychiatric day hospitals/facilities, ten geriatric day hospitals/facilities, and ten other rehabilitation units and day centres that he had visited, preceded by general observations about costs, transport, drugs, catering, etc.

Ten years later, Brocklehurst assessed the provision of geriatric day units ([QRL 95] and Subsection 5.7.1). A document was sent to all 239 consultant geriatricians in Great Britain and Northern Ireland. Ninety-four per cent replied representing 196 hospital departments. Identified were ninety existing day hospitals, twenty-nine departments with a day hospital planned to be open by the end of 1970, and seventy-seven departments without a day hospital and none planned to open by the end of 1970. Plans for beyond 1970 were seemingly not requested. Presented were details of geriatric hospital beds per 1000 population served, assessment units in general hospitals, out-patient consultative clinics, and nearby social day centres (with transport available). Other data on facilities and staffing were also tabulated.

4.1.4. *General practitioner hospitals*

The problems of defining general practitioner hospitals (GP hospitals) were illustrated by Robinson when reporting on dual censuses carried out in these hospitals in the South East Metropolitan RHB [B 391]. Characteristics common to most appear to be smallness in size (usually fewer than fifty beds); existence prior to 1948; a separate structure and administration; the acceptance of acute non-infectious admissions rather than long-stay cases; an absence of resident junior medical staff and contacts with consultants on a visiting basis; and the right of some (if not all) local GPs to admit, treat and discharge their cases for the majority of occupied bed days in a year. If, however, the recommendations for the community hospitals outlined in the DHSS's Memorandum of 1974 [B 156] and the 1976 Consultative Document [B 153] are implemented, the geographical distribution and role of the existing GP hospitals could be considerably modified with geriatric patients and the elderly with severe dementia occupying up to two-thirds of community beds.

In a review of the literature relating to GP beds, Israel and Draper produced a table showing bed numbers by location in the United Kingdom for 1969 [QRL 351]. It had been compiled from data collected by the Royal College of General Practitioners (RCGP) in a postal survey to Senior Administrative Medical Officers (SAMO). Also in this paper was an analysis of GP hospital beds, both maternity and other medical, from statistics in the annual reports of the DHSS. From these data and evidence in published small studies, the authors argued the case in favour of GP beds (see also Subsection 5.6.4). GP maternity beds total about one-fifth of maternity beds in England and Wales although there are marked regional variations, the South Western RHA having a much higher proportion. There were two surveys of GP maternity units carried out in England and Wales during 1966 [QRL 318] and 1968 [QRL 199].

4.1.5. *Health centres*

The National Health Service Act, 1946 embodied the principle of health centres which were to be established by LHAs. The possible activities to be accommodated in these premises were general medical services provided by medical practitioners, general dental services by dental practitioners, pharmaceutical services, services which the then LHAs provided, and out-patient services. Few health centres were established in England during the 1950s and early 1960s (only seventeen between 1949 and 1963). But from the mid-1960s onwards the movement escalated until by the end of 1972 there were in the United Kingdom over 500 centres. (A bibliography prepared by Baker and Bevan indicated the range of publications specific to this topic [B 36].) Statistics on numbers of health centres, gross expenditure, income and net expenditure in the LHAs of England and Wales were published annually until 1974 by the IMTA and SCT ([QRL 348] and Section 5.3), while in the second volume of the Court Report there are tables giving details of health-centre provisions since 1964 [QRL 728].

Individual health centres in the United Kingdom are listed in two sources. From 1975 the *Hospitals and Health Services Year Book* [B 96] has identified the names and addresses of health centres in the health districts of England, Wales and Scotland and the health and social services districts of Northern Ireland. The *British Health Centres Directory 1973* [QRL 98] had the same coverage but as at April 1972. Included were centres under construction or centres which had received formal approval for building by the appropriate government department, plus centres which had departmental approval in principle. The entry for each health centre covered the number of general practitioners and their total NHS list size, and, where relevant, dental services, general ophthalmic and pharmaceutical services. Additionally, school health services and RHB out-patient specialties were listed. There were, however, anxieties about the comprehensiveness of this latter item for some MOsH (who with the SHHD and other Scottish agencies provided the data) may have included some school health activities. Further, there were instances where consultants had made arrangements with the family doctors to undertake out-patient sessions in the health centre but this had not been brought to the attention of the local MOH.

4.2. Medical and dental manpower

The manpower studies (medical and dental, nursing and professional and technical) described in Sections 4.2 to 4.4, demonstrate a diversity both in their origins and their sampling sources. Many reports are the products of research projects initiated to investigate a specific problem such as the deployment of state enrolled nurses in community nursing services. Sometimes the subject has been explored in considerable depth with multi-phased surveys being undertaken and the participants even keeping workload recordings—this occurred in a range of nursing studies. The funding of these exercises has frequently been provided by agencies external to the bodies carrying out the research. Slightly different are the studies which were commissioned to provide statistical evidence for review bodies (such as Royal Commissions, special committees appointed by the various Secretaries of State in Great Britain, and committees of the Central Health Services Council) set up with broad terms of reference to assess the roles, educational requirements, etc., of certain components of medical, nursing or professional and technical manpower. The surveys have been carried out either by central government departments (usually the Social Survey Division of the OPCS, the Statistics and Research Division of the DHSS, the Office of Manpower Economics, and in Scotland now, by the Information Services Division of the Common Services Agency for the Scottish Health Service) or by independent research agencies. Normally the statistical findings are appended to the report of the review body, although in such publications the survey methodology is often scantily described if at all.

The majority of the manpower surveys have drawn upon one of three types of sampling sources. Certain of the enquiries into undergraduate and graduate doctors and dentists relied upon the medical schools to provide identification of past and current students. More commonly used have been the registers of professionally qualified persons, the most accessible listings for names of doctors being *The Medical Register* [B 211] and *The Medical Directory* [B 104], both published annually. The register comprises the names, addresses and qualifications of medical practitioners registered fully or provisionally with the General Medical Council (GMC) on 1 January of each year. Also included are the date and place of registration. The directory is compiled mainly from the returns of the annual schedule sent to every person on the principal (full) list of the register kept by the GMC. Considerably more biographical material is incorporated in the directory but the entry of doctors' names is voluntary, as is the maintenance of reliable accompanying information. Another medical listing is the Doctor Index maintained by the DHSS. Both of these two types of source (that is educational records and registers) include persons who are retired or are temporarily not working. This is not a problem when the third sampling source is utilized—the identification by employing authorities of health workers engaged by them, and it was the procedure adopted in the majority of studies. The RHAs and AHA(T)s can now provide separate listings of staff from their computerized payrolls, while the FPCs maintain cards or lists of medical and dental practitioners.

In addition to the *ad hoc* manpower studies described in this chapter and the central government routine staffing statistics reviewed in [B 14], there are two other potential sources of information. The reports of professional organizations responsible for standards, education and discipline (for example, the Central Midwives Boards, the General Nursing Councils, the Council for the Education and Training of Health Visitors, the Royal colleges and faculties overseeing the various branches of medicine and the boards of the professions supplementary to medicine) often contain figures relating to membership and, in particular, to new registrations. The censuses are another rich source of statistical material. Amongst the publications from the 1971 Census of Great Britain were volumes on economic activity at both 100 per cent and 10 per cent sample levels, and qualified manpower tables based on a 10 per cent sample.

4.2.1. *Community physicians and community health doctors*

From 1909 it was compulsory for all local authorities in England and Wales to appoint a Medical Officer of Health. However, the type of appointment and range of duties at any point of time varied from post to post, the consequence of the nature of the local authority making the appointment and the type of population to be served. With reorganization in 1974, and the transfer of local health services to within the NHS, the post of MOH was dissolved, the nearest equivalent now being the District Community Physician (DCP) or, in some instances, the Area Medical Officer (AMO).

The most comprehensive survey of MOsH in England undertaken since 1948 was that by Warren and Cooper, who in 1965 dispatched questionnaires to the MOsH of each of the 1287 local authorities [QRL 689]. There were in all 555 posts but nine were vacant; the response rate was 97 per cent. Where an MOH had responsibility for more than one authority, completed pro formas were to be returned for each authority served. From the replies, Warren and Cooper were able to build up a profile of the incumbents as regards sex, age, qualifications and experience. Further, they provided a comprehensive review of the responsibilities borne by many appointees which could cover environmental health services, personal health and welfare services, general medical and hospital services and voluntary bodies.

Local government medical staff were the subject of a second enquiry conducted by Warren and Cooper [QRL 690]. MOsH in England outlined details of full-time medical staff and numbers of part-time sessional staff employed on 1 April 1967. Vacancies were listed. All of the forty-four counties, thirty-three London boroughs, the Greater London Council (GLC), and seventy-seven of the seventy-eight county boroughs replied. Supplementary information was obtained from *The Medical Directory* and *The Medical Register* [B 104, 211]. The paper provided an analysis of staffing numbers both full-time and part-time and the specialties of hospital staff employed part-time or sessionally. The relationship between establishment sizes and population served was also explored. From the records of the Scottish branch of the Society of Medical Officers of Health, Riddell for 1961 and Wilson for 1966 detailed age, sex and qualifications by level of establishment of medical staff in post [B 388 and QRL 716].

Six months after Reorganization, all the 154 DCPs then in post in multi-district areas in England were asked about their working conditions, responsibilities and aspirations; 130 responded (Donaldson [QRL 207]). However, data on personal and professional characteristics were not presented. Those doctors who had held administrative positions prior to Reorganization but subsequently were not appointed to consultant posts in the new service were transferred to the new AHAs and RHAs. Anxious to provide suitable vocational training courses, the Centre for Extension Training in Community Medicine at the London School of Hygiene and Tropical Medicine elicited from 296 'transferred officers' their future employment hopes [QRL 5].

4.2.2. *Consultants*

Major manpower studies specific to the consultant grade do not appear to have been undertaken. There have though been occasional surveys to assess their views on junior hospital doctor staffing requirements ([QRL 334], Subsection 4.2.5) and geographical mobility ([QRL 386 and B 74], Subsection 4.2.4).

4.2.3. *Dental practitioners*

Information provided by the Dental Estimates Boards of England and Wales and Scotland and from the General Health Services Board of Northern Ireland enabled Cook and Walker to demonstrate the geographical distribution of dental care in the United Kingdom for 1962–3, and England and Wales only for 1952 [QRL 161]. For each Executive Council the numbers of dentists working for the general dental service, and the monies paid to the Council for treatments given during the course of selected years, were converted into indices. These were first, the rate of dentists per 10,000 inhabitants and, secondly, the average gross payment received by each dentist for treatments given in the course of a selected year, and for England and Wales only, changes that had occurred between the two indices during the period 1952–62. The emerging patterns of imbalance were interpreted graphically, as well as in tabulations.

4.2.4. *General practitioners*

The geographical imbalance of general medical practitioners in the United Kingdom has, since 1948, stimulated the implementation of three major strategies: the Medical Practices Committee, the Initial Practices Allowance and the Designated Area Allowance. This latter allowance was introduced in 1966 when the *Seventh Report of the Review Body on Doctors' and Dentists' Remuneration* [B 496] fixed an incentive payment of £400 per annum, payable to doctors practising in areas which, for a continuous period of 3 years, had been designated as short of doctors. (The allowance has subsequently been considerably increased.) Butler and Knight reviewed the problems relating to the distribution of general practice manpower [B 78] and the implications of the designated areas policy [B 80].

In 1969 the DHSS financed a research project to examine the issues surrounding the Designated Area Allowance and it was undertaken in the University of Kent by Butler, Bevan and Taylor [QRL 108]. The fieldwork comprised a postal survey of unrestricted principals contracted to ECs in England. Wales and Scotland were excluded because of their small numbers of designated areas. The Doctor Index as at October 1968, held by the DHSS, provided the sample. The population was stratified by standard region and designated/non-designated practice areas. Slightly differing sampling fractions were applied; a systematic one-in-eight sampling fraction in the designated areas giving 816 doctors and a one-in-ten fraction in the non-designated areas providing 1215 doctors. The total sample was thought to be representative with respect to sex, age, classification of area, type of practice and list size. The researchers achieved a response rate of 85 per cent. There was virtually no difference in the response rates for doctors working in the two types of practice area, and it was concluded that the completed questionnaires represented a satisfactory cross-section of all doctors in the sample. The survey sought answers to general questions of why inequalities in the distribution of doctors arise in the first place, how they are maintained and possible avenues for change. Thus, views were enlisted on the choice of area doctors practised in, the satisfactions and dissatisfactions experienced, and the factors that would be important should migration to another area be considered. Supplementing this material were details about the professional and personal backgrounds of respondents. The authors challenged some of the underlying assumptions of the designated area allowance; that a maximum list size of 2500 was a valid figure for all parts of the country; and that list size was a reasonable indicator of workload. Was the medical practice area the most appropriate unit on which to base the administration of the allowance? And should eligibility for the allowance continue to be based on average list size for an area instead of individual or practice list sizes? Further opinions of doctors distilled from a content-analysis of two survey questions relating to choice of practice area were published in a separate paper [B 79].

The attachment of general practitioners (and consultants) to the region of their youth rather than to the region of their medical school (where they differed) had been explored $3\frac{1}{2}$ years earlier by Last [QRL 386]. A 10 per cent probability sample of general practitioners and consultants in England and Wales was sent a postal questionnaire: the response rates for the two groups were approximately 86 per cent.

Concentrating their attention on three regions only, Brown and Walker (funded by the NPHT) also looked at the distribution of medical manpower. In Hull and the East Riding of Yorkshire, Cardiff and part of the Vale of Glamorgan (excluding the mining valleys), and Southampton and the adjacent parts of East Hampshire, profiles were assembled of the medical population for 1935, 1945, 1955 and 1965 from medical directories, so covering the 'medical lifetime' of almost all doctors in practice. Superannuation records held by the DHSS of identified doctors who qualified between 1950 and 1959 were examined for further career particulars—the coverage was only 84 per cent for general practitioners and 70 per cent for consultants. The findings from these two data-collecting stages were reported in [B 74]. A further step was the interviewing of about 250 family doctors to learn of factors affecting their career decisions and aspirations—see [B 73, 75].

The previous medical experience of doctors entering general practice for the first time as unrestricted principals or as assistants was the subject of an enquiry undertaken by the DHSS [QRL 191]. It was observed in the report of the Royal Commission on Medical Education in 1968 that vocational training was not required as a preparation for entry into general practice. So a survey of the 864 doctors who were registered as unrestricted principals between 2 April 1968 and 1 April 1969 was undertaken to ascertain their post-registration experience in hospitals, LHAs, general practice, the armed forces, etc., and overseas. Likewise, all assistants employed at 1 April 1969, less those who had previously been principals or were assistants prior to 2 April 1968 (213 in all), were included in the survey. Questionnaires were received from 82 per cent of the unrestricted principals but only 67 per cent of the assistants. This was thought to be a consequence of the relatively short time they had remained in their posts and were, therefore, more difficult to locate. Country of birth, country of qualification and sex were found to have little or no effect on the response rate.

In another study of new principals (those who entered general practice in England and Wales in the 12 months from 2 July 1969), Webb and Williams [QRL 703] analysed their mobility over the following 2 to 3 years from material specially prepared by the Statistics and Research Division of the DHSS from EC records. This cohort of 859 doctors was the subject of a longitudinal study of prescribing habits, conducted by the Medical Sociology Research Centre at the University College of Swansea ([QRL 458] and Subsection 5.1.2.8).

4.2.5. *Junior hospital doctors and dentists*

A census conducted in 1960 ascertained the average lengths of time doctors entering the junior medical grades were spending in those grades. This information was obtained by the MoH and the Department of Health for Scotland for a joint working party looking at the medical staffing structure in the hospital service [QRL 479]. All the hospital authorities in Great Britain returned particulars about whole-time junior medical staff as at 31 March 1960. Included in the details returned for each doctor were country and year of qualification and date of first hospital employment in Great Britain, whether or not national service had been undertaken and when in relation to qualification, and their current employment situation. Vacant posts were also defined. It was found, however, that 12 per cent of British doctors who qualified in 1959 from medical schools in Great Britain were neither in the census nor in the numbers of doctors known to be holding national service commissions. The main explanation appeared to lie in the hypothesis that these doctors were in between hospital posts on the census date.

The Department of Social Medicine in the University of Edinburgh carried out an exhaustive research programme during the 1960s into the careers of medical graduates. The research workers most closely associated with the programme were Last, Martin, Stanley, Broadie and Brotherston. A subsample of the undergraduates surveyed in 1961(see Subsection 4.2.7) was resurveyed in 1966. Thus a 50 per cent random sample of all respondents in the 1961 survey of United Kingdom medical schools who were at that time in their second, fourth or sixth year, and who had subsequently registered by December 1965, was sent questionnaires. Eighty-six per cent of the 1737 graduates surveyed replied. This was considered to be adequate in view of the difficulties of tracing a mobile population some of whom would have different surnames because of marriage. Twenty per cent of the 202 non-respondents were later contacted by interviewers from a market research organization, and they were found to be more mobile and less co-operative than the respondents as a whole.

The purpose of the follow-up survey was to learn about the doctors' experiences since the completion of their undergraduate courses, their career choices, present employment situation, and their future plans. Supplementary data were provided by the medical schools about examination achievements. Analyses of the material amassed were published in a series of papers: academic record and subsequent career [QRL 388]; emigration and international mobility [B 282]; the career preferences of young British doctors [QRL 389]; and careers of young medical women [QRL 626]. Finally, 444 individuals in the second- or third-year strata of the 1961 survey, who were identified in 1966 as being 'apparently unsuccessful' for their names were not in *The Medical Register*, were followed up. Only 171 were definitely classifiable 'drop-outs' because of academic failures or for other reasons—see Last and Stanley [B 283]. Three years later yet another resurvey was undertaken, the participants being the 1966 respondents [QRL 387]. Postal questionnaires were despatched to 1496 doctors—after three communications over a 4-month period a response rate of 90 per cent was achieved. The reasons for conducting this enquiry (which was supported by the DHSS) were primarily to assess the effect of both emigration and unemployment of married women doctors on the medical workforce, and to further resolve questions about doctors' formulations of career choice.

The career preferences of doctors graduating from medical schools in England, Scotland and Wales in 1974 were sought by Parkhouse and McLaughlin [QRL 524]. Questionnaires were sent to all 2348 graduates during the first half of 1975 and an 86 per cent response rate was obtained. In the previous few years, Parkhouse with McLaughlin had followed up the careers of graduates from the medical schools in Manchester and Sheffield; [B 363, 364] are two of their most recent publications from this exercise. Another medical school from which cohorts of graduates have been subjected to a succession of surveys is Birmingham. Whitfield pursued the careers of doctors graduating in 1948–58 and 1959–63; the publications from the series are numerous and three of the later papers presented data on the current work [B 464] and emigration [B 463] of the second cohort, and the higher medical and surgical degrees awarded by the University between 1949 and 1966 [B 462]. The career attainments of the 362 doctors graduating from Scottish medical schools in 1962 were assessed in 1973 by McIntyre and Parry [QRL 428]. A range of studies into the careers of women medical graduates is detailed in Subsection 4.2.8.

A survey of junior hospital doctors' and dentists' hours of duty in Great Britain was carried out in 1975 at the behest of the Review Body on Doctors' and Dentists' Remuneration (chaired by Sir Ernest Woodroofe) [QRL 194]. All full-time and part-time junior hospital medical and dental staff including locums, though not honorary contract holders (about 20,300), were sent questionnaires but only 15·3 per cent of the 19,525 whole-time staff returned usable forms. This was a disappointment to the Committee. The analysis of the response rate suggested that it was highest from the doctors working longer duties. Additionally, the requirements of the questionnaire in terms of apportioning hours of duty on 'stand-by' or 'on-call' into working and non-working time proved difficult for many doctors. Nevertheless, the survey provided some much needed baseline information for the Review Body about the spread of working hours, the distribution of different types of duties, the periods in which duties were carried out and the relative hours of different grades and specialties and between residents and non-residents.

There have, however, been at least three local work studies of junior hospital doctors. In 1967–8 the Management Services (NHS) Branch of the then MoH analysed the time spent by eighty-five doctors in nine acute hospitals [B 141]. They were in three specialties: general medical, general surgical and accident and emergency. Observers were used, each doctor being accompanied during most of his working and duty time excluding meals and non-working on-calls periods, for 7 days. Recordings of activities were made every half minute. In another local study, this time at the Northampton General Hospital, measurements were made over 1 week of the total working hours, total hours on call, and the time spent on each major activity by thirty out of the forty junior hospital doctors [B 379]. The work undertaken by non-consultant medical staff outside normal working hours in a general hospital in Kirkcaldy was scrutinized by Walker, Miller and McLean on behalf of the SHHD [B 452]. For 15 January days in 1968, thirty doctors of various grades entered on diary schedules the tasks performed between 1700 hours and 0900 hours on weekdays and between 1230 hours on Saturday and 0900 hours the following Monday. Baseline summary data were also recorded about work performed during normal working hours.

Consultants' views about the adequacy of the present medical staffing situation in their own hospital and on the minimum staff seen necessary to deal with a model workload in the relevant specialty were sought in 1972. An unusual survey design was adopted by the Hospitals Consultants and Specialists Association (known prior to 1974 as the Regional Hospitals Consultants and Specialists Association) [QRL 334]. The administrators felt that because of the urgency of the enquiry, the theoretically preferable method of selecting a sample in advance and pursuing individuals concerned via reminders to achieve a maximum response rate would be too time consuming. Instead the method was reversed. Questionnaires were sent to approximately 8000 consultants from whom 2378 replies were received. These were enclosed in sealed envelopes marked on the outside with the hospital region, consultant's specialty and age. A 10 per cent sample of all consultants stratified by age, specialty and region was then selected from the completions. Thus a total of 877 questionnaires only were used in the analysis, and they were thought to be similar to the specialty distributions of the total consultants and all respondents. However, the total responses may have been biased, those 30 per cent replying being particularly sympathetic to the subject under review.

4.2.6. *Medical migration*

The 'brain drain' debate of the early 1960s stimulated a series of empirical enquiries throughout the decade into the migration of British doctors. Various data sources were relied upon although some were later shown to have shortcomings. For instance, the earliest estimates of emigrant doctors based on overseas sources such as immigration statistics and national medical directories were likely to have double counted some individuals with multiple registration or citizenship. Thus in 1962 Abel-Smith and Gales (while funded by the NPHT) tried to overcome this problem by creating career profiles of a sample of graduates trained as doctors in the United Kingdom and Eire [QRL 3]. The basic sampling frame was the 'home list' of the GMC. A one-in-twenty sample of persons registering between 1925 and 1959 was drawn giving 3590 names. Rather than dispatching questionnaires to all and risking the receipt of incomplete or inaccurate information, alternative sources were first searched: the GMC's files, NHS superannuation files, other ministry records, medical directories, the armed services' records, concurrent manpower studies, the British Medical Association's records, registers of other countries, etc. The final phase was the sending of questionnaires to the 581 doctors for whom there was an address outside the United Kingdom or Eire—two-thirds responded. Subsequently, Ash and Mitchell [B 27] and Gish [B 215] published estimates for the years 1962–7 using the MoH/BMA Doctor Index which, from 1962, was maintained in a much more comprehensive fashion. Gish later published a substantial overview of the migration debate which included material about the deployment of foreign-born persons who had graduated between 1948 and 1966 from British medical schools [QRL 267].

4.2.7. *Student doctors*

In 1966 the Royal Commission on Medical Education requested the Association for the Study of Medical Education and the National Foundation for Educational Research in England and Wales to conduct a survey of medical students with funds provided by the Treasury. The Royal Commission (chaired by Lord Todd) had been set up in the previous year primarily to review undergraduate and postgraduate medical education in Great Britain [QRL 581]. It was intended that the findings be such that they could be comparable with a 1961 survey (unpublished) administered by the Department of Social Medicine, University of Edinburgh, on behalf of the Association for the Study of Medical Education. The later survey (conducted in the autumn of 1966) applied to first-(pre-clinical) year medical students and final-year students who were taking final examinations for the first time in either October or December 1966, May 1967 or June 1967. All the medical schools in the United Kingdom allowed their students to participate, but dental schools were outside the terms of reference. (In the 1961 survey three medical schools withheld their co-operation.) Postal questionnaires were distributed within the medical schools; the response rates from the individual institutions ranged from 72 per cent to 100 per cent, but the overall rates for the two student years under review were 95 per cent, so providing details about 1806 final-year students and 2413 first-year students.

The analysis in the report was organized in three parts: students' backgrounds prior to entering medical school, scholastic achievements and financial and living arrangements whilst enrolled, and career plans and aspirations including possible emigration. The tables incorporated statistics collected about 1684 final-year students in the 1961 survey.

4.2.8. *Women doctors*

The proportion of women students admitted to undergraduate medical schools in England has of late been increasing at a rate of about 1 per cent per annum and it has been estimated that during the 1980s half of the places could be filled by women. However, career prospects of women once qualified are seen to be far less promising (Bewley and Bewley [B 49] and Arie [B 23]). A small number of surveys have attempted to assess the careers aspired for and/or pursued by female students and graduates. From the data collected in the 1966 graduates survey by the University of Edinburgh (refer to Subsection 4.2.5), Stanley and Last prepared an analysis of women respondents only [QRL 626].

The marital status, family size, medical work undertaken or reasons for not being in employment were the subjects of a survey of women doctors in the United Kingdom, carried out by the Medical Practitioners' Union over 12 months during 1962–3 and reported by Jefferys and Elliott [QRL 353]. Included were women who had not permanently retired from work on account of age; their names were gathered from *The Medical Directory* and the annual lists of new registrations maintained by the GMC. Forms were sent to 11,594 individuals and the response rate of 75 per cent was considered to be very satisfactory. The non-respondents were thought to be older women. Another postal survey, but on a regional basis, of medically qualified women was undertaken in 1964 by the Medical Women's Federation [B 284]. Replies came in from 7861 but they were asked no personal details, only questions about the amount of work undertaken or the type of work desired. The published results from this survey were compared with those of the Medical Practitioners' Union.

The career patterns of women graduating from individual medical schools have been pursued by some researchers. More notable presentations, because of the large cohorts followed up, are the examinations of women doctors who graduated from Sheffield University between 1933 and 1957 [B 454], the Royal Free Hospital in London between 1945 and 1964 [B 198], and the Middlesex Hospital Medical School between 1950 and 1967 [B 8].

4.3. Nursing and midwifery manpower

4.3.1. *All nurses and midwives*

A committee set up in June 1970 by the Secretary of State for Social Services was given the following terms of reference: 'To review the role of the nurse and the midwife in the hospital and the community and the education and training required for that role, so that the best use is made of available manpower to meet present needs and the needs of an integrated health service' [QRL 190, page 1]. This Committee on Nursing, chaired by Professor Asa Briggs, felt it necessary to commission a number of research surveys from other bodies. (This was in addition to the activities of a small research team attached to the Committee.) Thus the following surveys were carried out on the committee's behalf: opinions of nurses and midwives on the various aspects of their work, motivations in entering the profession and their likely career prospects, by Social and Community Planning Research (SCPR); qualified nurses and midwives not currently employed by the NHS as nurses and midwives, by the Social Survey Division of the OPCS; and opinions and experience of overseas nurses, by Political and Economic Planning (PEP), but under the auspices of the United Kingdom Council for Overseas Student Affairs. In the *Report of the Committee on Nursing* [QRL 190], the research designs of these surveys were detailed as well as certain findings. Independent reports were also published by the agencies.

The investigation undertaken by SCPR was multi-phased. First, postal questionnaires were sent to nurses and midwives employed in hospitals and in LHA services. The survey was confined to England and Wales. In constructing the hospital sample, 100 randomly selected hospital groups (after some stratification) provided lists of their nursing and midwifery staff, and a one-in-six systematic sample of individuals was selected. The sample ratio for the teaching hospitals was, however, one-in-twelve. Thus, 10,407 names were chosen. For local authority staff, forty-five authorities likewise supplied lists of nurses and midwives. Every second name was selected, the total sample being 2483. After piloting, two very similar questionnaires but with selected questions relevant only to the hospital or community participants were despatched. The final net response rates were 79 per cent for hospital nurses and midwives and 87 per cent for the community counterparts. Comparisons between the respondents and the population of nurses and midwives employed in Great Britain showed that the results were adequately representative of sex, working status, hospital type and grade with the exception of assistants/auxiliaries. The topics covered in the questionnaires were: personal characteristics and family background; training; past career; hours of work and levels of individual responsibility; satisfaction with nursing as a career plus factors affecting morale and views on future career prospects. (Tables from this material appear in [QRL 190].) However, as these issues could only be dealt with at a somewhat superficial level using this survey technique, it was felt necessary to supplement the data with personal interviews using a structured schedule. So during May and June 1971, 1232 interviews were conducted with hospital staff and 373 in the community, all with persons who had responded to the postal survey. Many issues about recruitment, present employment conditions and work and professional attitudes were covered, but the analyses were presented in an unpublished SCPR report [B 341].

The Social Survey Division of the OPCS used a unique source for the sample population needed in its survey of nurses and midwives currently withdrawn from the labour force [QRL 589]. The 1971 Census taken on the night of 25 April contained five relevant questions: one asked for qualifications obtained since the age of 18 years—a category included the majority of nursing qualifications; and four which together established the employment of individuals (for example, the type of work being done, and the number of hours worked). Thus it was possible to identify persons resident in

Great Britain, who had nursing qualifications but who were not at the time of the census employed as nurses by the NHS. (The adoption of this method of selecting a sample population created a considerable furore with questions about breach of confidentiality being raised in Parliament.) As questions about future career intentions were found during piloting to be inappropriate for women in older age groups, it was decided to use a subsample of eligible persons being those born since 1919. Anticipated problems in the definition of acceptable qualifications, and whether or not a nurse was in employment with the NHS, were not as troublesome as expected. The coding frame from the 1966 Census was used for the qualifications question (the 1971 coding frame not having been completely assembled). The nursing level categories applied were those used in the survey carried out by SCPR. From the 2384 census districts in Great Britain, 100 were selected and within each one six enumeration districts. So in 600 enumeration districts, 709 women appeared from their census schedules to be eligible. Of these 628 were interviewed by trained interviewers of the Social Survey Division during August/ September 1971. The number who proved to be ineligible and those eligible but who refused to be interviewed were twenty-four respectively. The topics covered in the full report were: who the ex-nurses are, their past and present employment situations, future intentions towards nursing, contacts with nursing since leaving the profession and some of the respondents' attitudes towards women working and their own return to nursing.

Student nurses and midwives from overseas, especially those from developing countries, were of concern to the United Kingdom Council for Overseas Student Affairs which, on behalf of the Committee of Nursing, approached PEP to conduct a survey [QRL 644]. The fieldwork was initiated by a series of in-depth interviews with nurses who had come to train in Britain from one of the developing countries. The material drew attention to certain problem areas experienced by such persons—the difficulties of hospital and course selection, and the 'settling-in' process after arrival in the country. Eligible persons for this survey were identified from the returns of the postal survey undertaken by SCPR (see above). Thus interviews were conducted with 259 midwives and nurses of whom 54 were from Eire and 205 from 'overseas'; that is, born in a developing country of a father also born in a developing country and who had arrived in Britain after the age of 16. (Nurses from South Africa, Israel, Australia, New Zealand, North America and Europe were excluded.) It was admitted that the data were more of a 'qualitative' than 'quantitative' nature because of the sampling procedures and small final sample, coupled with the leeway given to interviewers to substitute non-participants with alternative respondents and to assist in interpreting questions and answers where there were language difficulties.

Finally, attention is drawn to the bibliographies of nursing literature edited by Thompson. The two volumes span 1859 to 1970 [B 431, 432]. Another source is the monthly publication, *Nursing Bibliography*, by the RCN which contains sections on management, staffing and research.

4.3.2. *Community nurses of all types in attachment schemes*

Ad hoc surveys of community nursing resources commenced in the early 1960s and continued apace throughout the decade. These enquiries were stimulated by the move in many LHAs to 'attach' health visitors, home nurses or even midwives to specified general practitioners rather than have them work within geographical districts. It was a trend which commenced in an experimental way in the 1950s and was strengthened by the recommendations in a report of a joint working party (issued in 1961) of the College of General Practitioners and Royal College of Nursing (RCN) set up to examine the subject of collaboration between general practitioners and health visitors.

From time to time during the 'attachment movement' there were nation-wide surveys to assess the extent of attachment of certain categories of nurses. Baker approached the MOsH of all counties and county boroughs of England and asked whether in 1963 any health visitors under their control worked in 'direct collaboration' (the meaning of which was unclear) with a general practice [QRL 45]. Two years later the Social Medicine Unit at Guy's Hospital conducted a similar survey [B 21]. Again a postal questionnaire was sent to the MOsH of each LHA in England and this time Wales was also included. Information was required about attachment schemes, either existing or proposed, and about arrangements for regular meetings between general practitioners and health authority staff. Those authorities who replied indicating the operation of some such scheme were later contacted once more by a postal survey. Subsequently in 1969 this team administered a follow-up survey to MOsH to ascertain the position as at 1 January of that year [QRL 23].

A more intensive enquiry was undertaken in 1967 by Abel, in the Social Science Research Unit of the DHSS on behalf of the Minister of Health [QRL 1]. Apart from assessing the extent and types of attachment schemes in England and Wales (knowledge about which was already available), her objectives were to discern the implications of such schemes from the manpower, economic and organization viewpoints. Postal questionnaires and interviews were used to collect the data from first, the clerks of fifty LHAs selected according to location, population size and stage of development of services, and second, twenty staff including MOsH, Nursing Officers and Health Visitor Superintendents from five LHAs with varying attachment policies. The topics under discussion with this latter group covered the procedures for starting a scheme, the effects of LHA boundaries on attachment schemes, the location of premises as a base for attached staff, and communication difficulties. However, since so few persons were interviewed within each hierarchical tier, any material reported could only be regarded as impressionistic. In the report, Abel provided evidence for each of the main aims. The analyses showed a marked variability in the level of attachment (as to be predicted from earlier surveys). Moreover, a number of authorities were operating simultaneously several schemes of different types. Sometimes, the in-depth interviews showed up confusion in the exact connotations of terms applied to describe schemes by medical and nursing staff in the same authority. From the data, Abel was able to construct a classification of schemes by type (attachment, partial attachment, association with regular contact and co-operation). Some of these definitions have been applied in subsequent studies.

Various monitored local schemes involving attached home nurses and/or health visitors were reported by public health staff (medical and nursing), family doctors and independent research workers during the 1960s. An overview of the research and literature surrounding the issues of nurses working with general practitioners was prepared by Hawthorn on behalf of the DHSS in 1971 [B 238]. There were, however, three separate local attachment schemes which were examined and reported in considerable depth. The earliest, *Feeling the Pulse*, prepared by Hockey and published by the Queen's Institute of District Nursing in 1966, attempted to establish a contemporary picture of district nursing from the experiences of district nurses, general practitioners and superintendents of district nursing in six LHAs [QRL 322*]. The selected authorities were matched in pairs representing urban areas of industrial character, seaside retirement areas and predominantly agricultural rural areas. Interviews were conducted with the three categories of personnel identified above, and the nurses also completed workload forms for each day of two working weeks. In addition, a postal questionnaire was sent to district nursing administrators all over the country to gain their assessments of the administrative arrangements in the nursing services. The commentary drew attention to the seeming misuse of the skills of the 'unattached' professional nurse—a conclusion also reached in another study incorporating district nurses, *Care in the Balance* ([QRL 323] and Subsection 4.3.4). Two years later, Hockey with Buttimore evaluated seven more district nurse/general practice attachment schemes in LHAs spread over the country, but with specific reference to an experiment in North Wales [QRL 113*]. The study design resembled the previous exercise described by Hockey (in 1966), that is, a combination of workload recordings by the nurses and questionnaires completed by personnel involved in the schemes. The third exhaustive report of an attachment scheme was prepared by MacGregor, Heasman and Kuenssberg [QRL 427*]. They evaluated an experiment in a north Edinburgh practice whereby two local authority Queen's nurses joined a seven-partner practice accommodated in two premises. Workload data were reported by the doctors and the practice nurses for 4 weeks before the attachment, and by all participants for a similar period of time, 6 months after the new nursing system was established.

The integration of health visitors and home nurses with general practitioners into newly innovated 'teams' providing primary medical care was the subject of an enquiry by Gilmore, Bruce and Hunt, published in 1974 [QRL 265]. The Council for the Education and Training of Health Visitors hoped that the study would provide some basis for the assessment of the training needs of health visitors working in general practice teams, for their assumption was that 'attachment' did not automatically create a 'team', it simply provided an opportunity for the development of a holistic approach to the delivery of community health services. The research procedures to test this tenet were complex. Three experimental schemes were selected plus thirty-six 'control' teams. Many specifications relating to membership, induction courses, counselling services and practice records and accommodation were to be met in the selection of the experimental teams. But despite efforts by LHAs to identify newly created teams in England and Scotland, only one was found to fulfil all the stated criteria. Two other compromise teams had to be chosen—they were already established and therefore were not participants in a preparatory course or counselling programme. All three were based in health centres; two in Scottish towns and the third in a large English industrial city. The data collection for these schemes was multi-faceted: over periods of varying lengths, working activities were timed, home visits detailed and day-books maintained. Additionally, team members were asked their views. The criteria used for selecting the 'control' teams were that the nursing staff were attached and had been working together with the GPs for at least 6 months before the commencement of the survey and so had established team relationships, and that all members should have permanent office accommodation in the same premises. The aims of this phase of the study were to compile a portfolio about each team—composition and size of populations served, clinic and group activities undertaken, methods of communication used and the role perceptions and discrepancies recognized by the members. The thirty-six study extension or 'control' teams were randomly chosen from eighty-two teams in England and Scotland thought to fit the required criteria by MOsH via questionnaires. Nineteen were in England and ten were accommodated in health centres. The most widely applied instruments were the questionnaires completed by 150 general practitioners, seventy health visitors and fifty-eight district nurses.

An attempt to cost domiciliary nursing care using the experience of two general practices with attached nursing teams was made by Rickard [B 385]. The costs (1972 prices) of both employing and supporting a district nurse and an auxiliary nurse were assessed from the accounts of the administering health departments. The nurses in each practice maintained work diaries for 2 weeks, so providing estimates of a year's items of service which were transformed into unit costs. Using a sample of seventy-five patients from each practice, the types of care delivered by the nurses were categorized and weekly estimates of costs constructed. Although this exercise was not a fully conducted cost-benefit analysis, and applied to the experience in two practices only, it was a new contribution to the general debates on attached nursing staff and community versus hospital nursing care. Finally, it should be noted that the published routine statistics on all community nursing personnel in England and Wales detailed in [B 14] were supplemented until 1974 by data provided by the IMTA and SCT [QRL 348]. The range of these latter statistics is outlined in Section 5.3.

4.3.3. Health visitors

There seems to have been only one early national survey specific to health visitors. An assessment of health-visiting resources (including tuberculosis visitors) as at 31 December 1953 was carried out on behalf of a joint working party representing the Ministries of Health and Education and the Department of Health in Scotland, and chaired by Sir Wilson Jameson [B 327]. Almost all employing authorities in England, Wales and Scotland provided information about the present numbers of qualified and unqualified staff engaged in the work, their age distribution, the proportion of staff time absorbed by various parts of the service and the ways in which various duties were grouped. An innovation was the keeping of diaries by health visitors during the first 5 days of one ordinary week. In all, 4800 visits in six areas were covered with the timing, objectives and contents being detailed. Numerous statistical tables were included in the report (which was reprinted in 1974).

A substantial descriptive analysis of the work content of health visiting in an English county (Berkshire), with supplementary information about the participants and their perceived relationships with other health and welfare services, was prepared by Clark [QRL 144]. The study design consisted first of a 'visit schedule' or record form completed by the health visitor for each visit made during 1 week (2055 in all), and secondly, a postal questionnaire and interview for which the health visitors were the subjects. Almost all of the eighty-two health visitors including part-time employees engaged by the Berkshire County Council at 1 May 1969 participated, and the great majority were in complete attachment schemes. From data collected via the visit schedules, Clark was not only able to determine the frequency that twenty-six different agencies initiated contacts between health visitors and 'clients', but the reasons, duration of the visits and outcomes were also discernible. The health visitors provided a 'content analysis' of the verbal topics covered in each visit: assessments were made immediately on completion of the visits as to who initiated the topics and the level of involvement of the health visitors themselves.

Diary sheets were completed over a 2-week period in the autumn of 1969 by 215 health visitors working in London [QRL 446]. The study, administered by the Intelligence Unit of the GLC, was carried out at the request of the Council for the Training of Health Visitors and the Association of London Borough Medical Officers of Health. Thus the objectives were oriented towards both the training needs of health visitors and their administration regarding efficient deployment. A one-in-five systematic sample of health visitors in all the London boroughs participated. On the diary sheets they indicated the time spent on various types of activities or visits, categories of people and topics covered. Office time, clinic work, travelling and meal breaks were covered—the total time for analysis exceeding one million minutes. Personal questionnaires were also completed. The comments in the report about the design of the diary sheets and the varying completion patterns adopted by the participants could be beneficial to others wishing to duplicate the diary method.

No research appeared to have been done into the use of health visitors' time for the teaching of health education to selected groups within the population by the late 1960s, and it was this gap that Hobbs tried to fill [B 245]. The study was carried out in four rather different ways: a review was done of the history of health visitors' training, a postal survey of health visitor training centres was carried out, as was a postal survey of LHAs in England and Wales, and interviews were conducted with health visitors from five high and low scoring authorities identified in the postal survey. The enquiry to the LHAs aimed to map out the range and amount of group teaching carried out by health visitors locally and to obtain the opinions of MOsH on the factors they considered to be affecting the amount undertaken. However, the response from the 173 authorities was disappointing, being less than 50 per cent (77), and it was thought to be in part the result of the publicized rejection of support for the study by the Society of Medical Officers of Health. (Indeed it seems questionable whether the study should have been pursued.) Twenty-two MOsH supplied their annual report instead of completing the questionnaire.

4.3.4. *Home nurses*

In Scotland until 1966 the only detailed factual information available on the functioning of the home nursing service was in the annual returns giving staffing and some simple workload statistics prepared by local authorities. As a better basis was needed for discussions with local authorities by the SHHD on the development of these services, a separate enquiry was undertaken within the SHHD's Health Services Operational Research Unit [QRL 122]. The enquiry was oriented towards the medical workloads of home nurses, especially the characteristics of patients, treatment regimes and lengths of treatment. But the allocation of time during the working day on visits, travel and clerical duties was also of interest, as were attitudes of staff towards their work. The employment prospects for ancillary and part-time nurses were also assessed. (It is noteworthy that almost half of the home nurses in Scotland were employed on triple duties—midwifery and health visiting as well as home nursing.) A one-in-seven ratio of nurses in eleven local authorities (cities, burghs and counties) were involved in the fieldwork. There were three phases. For 2 weeks in mid-1964, they itemized on work schedules for all patient contacts, levels of mobility and outcome including hospitalization where relevant plus domestic arrangements of the patients, and for new patients referral details. Concurrently, these nurses kept diaries indicating the time spent on clinics, visiting and other professional activities, the range of treatments given, and the patients on their books who were not seen during the survey period. Lastly, attitudinal questionnaires were completed. The numbers of nurses participating in each phase were 180, 187 and 212 respectively. A considerable breadth of statistical material was presented in the report.

State Enrolled Nurses (SEN) and their role in LHA nursing services was the subject of an enquiry described by Hockey, on behalf of the Queen's Institute of District Nursing, the DHSS and the NPHT [QRL 325]. The demand for extended community nursing services to relieve hospital facilities overtaxed by the increasing proportions of geriatric and young chronic long-stay patients in the population means that skilled manpower resources must be optimally deployed. Thus the hypotheses underlying this study were 'that the nursing resources of the health service are not being fully utilized, first because too few SENs are employed in the community and secondly, because many who are so employed are not being used in a way which is commensurate with their training and experience' (*ibid.*, page 3). A major field study was mounted in forty-seven areas in the United Kingdom. Various sources of information were drawn upon. The MOsH outlined, via postal questionnaires, the employment policy in their areas and their general views on the deployment of SENs. Chief or Principal Nursing Officers in all authorities were interviewed. From ECs' lists, a random sample of fifteen GPs in each area was surveyed although this phase of the study coincided with the 1971 postal strike. However, there were no statistical interpretations of these data in the report for two reasons: first, the public health officers often mutually completed their documents with nursing administrators or delegated the responsibility, and secondly, the response from the family doctors was rather low despite the use of reminders. Other sources provided the bulk of the data. Interviews were carried out with 1240 persons of whom 528 were SENs, 471 State Registered Nurses (SRN) and 241 health visitors. To supplement this material, complex workload schedules covering a 7-day period in the spring of 1971 were completed by SENs and SRNs who had been interviewed. The completion rate was nearly 75 per cent. Detailed for each patient seen was an analysis of technical procedures carried out, basic care provided and other activities. The timing of differing professional tasks undertaken during the working days was recorded. But what was unique to the study were views expressed by the nurses about night visits and procedures which might be carried out by a district nurse—who did they think were the most suitable persons to carry out the tasks, SENs, SRNs, doctors, nursing auxiliaries, or other persons such as home helps, neighbours or relatives?

An earlier study described by Hockey, which was about relationships between hospital and domiciliary components of nursing care, *Care in the Balance* [QRL 323], incorporated a survey of district nurses. The study was concerned overall to test two hypotheses, namely that patients are discharged from hospital without the availability of full domiciliary facilities, and they are requested to attend hospital as out-patients for treatment which could be given in their own homes. Material was amassed during 1967 from interviews with discharged in-patients, out-patients on review, hospital staff, general practitioners, and questionnaires filled in by district nurses. These nurses numbered 469 and were staff from the LA areas in which most of the patients from the six hospitals under review were resident. In addition to the completing in the questionnaires details about their working arrangements and personal opinions, the nurses kept recordings of their work over 1 week, the intention here being to discover what kinds of patients the district nurses were caring for. Altogether 2261 visits were analysed. Hockey's findings in this study, as in others she has conducted (see [QRL 322, 325]), were that the available district nursing resources and expertise did not always seem to be used to the best advantage.

4.3.5. *Hospital nurses*

Nurses' and midwives' deployment of working time was examined by the Committee of Enquiry into the Pay and Related Conditions of Service of Nurses and Midwives, the chairman being the Earl of Halsbury [QRL 193]. (The Committee also covered the professions supplementary to medicine and speech therapists, this report being published separately [QRL 195].) Questionnaires were sent to a representative sample of hospitals in Great Britain with fifty or more staffed beds—as listed in the *Hospitals and Health Services Year Book* [B 96]. The sampling ratios were one-in-two for London teaching hospitals, and one-in-ten for the remainder. So in all, 211 hospitals and thirty-seven clinics were approached via district administrators and the rate of response was 93 per cent. The forms sought information about how nursing staff requirements in the evenings, at night and at the week-end differed from the day-time situation during a week in 1974. The use of agency or part-time staff to cover these periods and types of shift systems and other duty arrangements operating were also probed. The report included results of the separate survey organized by the DHSS, of hours of work and earnings of NHS nursing and midwifery staff in Great Britain, both hospital and community-based. The sources were the NHS regional computer centres' payrolls in June 1974. Eleven of the fifteen regions in England and Wales complied; likewise five of the twelve Scottish areas.

Senior nursing staff were the subject of a special statistical enquiry conducted by the MoH for a Committee chaired by Lord Salmon [QRL 480]. This Committee was instructed to advise on the senior nursing staff structure in the hospital service, the administrative functions of the respective grades and methods of preparing staff to occupy them. The fieldwork was carried out amongst the following NHS employees: all staff in hospitals in Great Britain in grades above midwifery sister, ward sister and charge nurse; midwifery sisters, ward sisters and charge nurses in one-third of non-teaching hospitals in England and Wales and of teaching and non-teaching hospitals in Scotland, and of all teaching hospitals in England and Wales. The survey took place in mid-1964. The questionnaires were distributed internally in the hospitals and the overall response rate was 85 per cent comprising 37,393 nurses in England and Wales and 4802 in Scotland. Statistics on the personal characteristics of differing grades of staff (country of birth, sex, age, marital status and whether employed full-time or part-time), nursing/general education qualifications, and career histories were presented in an appendix to the final report from the Committee.

4.3.6. *Midwives*

The midwifery service, both hospital and domiciliary, was scrutinized by a sub-committee of the Standing Maternity and Midwifery Advisory Committee reporting in 1970 to the Central Health Services Council. The terms of reference were broad: 'To consider the future of the domiciliary midwifery service and the question of bed needs for maternity patients and to make recommendations [page 1, QRL 199]. Therefore, the sub-committee, chaired by Sir John Peel, drew upon a spectrum of statistical sources and opinions. In the first instance, the MOsH of all LHAs in England and Wales were approached and of the 174 only seven did not co-operate fully. They were asked for employment details (number and grade, other duties, attachments, vacancies and resignations) of domiciliary midwifery staff in the authorities under their jurisdiction. Workload details during certain months in 1967, the training programmes operating, and the MOsH's own views about the employment of domiciliary midwives were also sought. The survey of the SAMOs to the RHBs covered aspects of hospital midwifery staffing such as employment numbers, vacancies, retirement and training, plus the employment of domiciliary midwives in hospitals, the availability of GP maternity beds and the organization and workload of obstetric flying squads. Incorporated was evidence received from boards of governors within the regions. The report also contained abstractions from the views of seventy-seven chairmen of LMCs about the future pattern of the midwifery service as a whole. Further, two papers were appended dealing with factors affecting the needs for maternity beds and the provision of delivery beds, which were prepared by the Statistics and Research Division of the DHSS.

4.3.7. *Nurses in general practice*

The only data routinely amassed (though not published) about nurses *employed* by family doctors are the returns submitted by the FPCs to the DHSS (for England). Between 1968 and 1974 there was a three-fold increase in the number of whole-time equivalent nurses employed in general practice, the total figure in 1974 being about 740. However, it could not be assumed that all were necessarily trained nurses. Further, there was no way of telling just how many individuals these figures represented in terms of part-time employees or the number of practices with such a commitment. Thus, general practices in England were surveyed in 1974 by the Medical Care Research Unit at the University of Newcastle to probe these questions, and even more nurses were found to be employed than was generally expected [QRL 557].

   An assessment of the role that a practice nurse could adopt in general practice and its effect on the doctor's work was made by members of the North-east Faculty of the RCGP [B 398]. In four practices employing nurses, chronostamps were used to punch the beginning and end of all surgery consultations with the doctors and nurses over two separate periods of 2 and 4 weeks in the winter of 1965–6. The activities within the consultations were then classified according to whether a doctor or practice nurse need carry them out. More recent papers have concentrated on describing the workload activities of practice nurses (either attached or employed directly by the doctors) in health centre/group practice treatment rooms [B 34, 159].

4.3.8. *Student nurses*

An experimental nurse-training programme was introduced in the Glasgow Royal Infirmary in 1956 with a principal objective to reduce the period of student nurse training for the Final State Examination of the General Nursing Council from 3 years to 2 years. Evaluation of the programme during the late 1950s was undertaken by an assessment committee chaired by Professor J. H. F. Brotherston, and set up by the Secretary of State for Scotland in conjunction with the NPHT. One of the purposes of the evaluation was the assessment of the possibilities of extending the system to other hospitals. Thus the participants in the study consisted of seventy-five 'alternative' (experimental) students and 168 control students within the Glasgow Royal Infirmary, 187 control students at the Edinburgh Royal Infirmary (who, it was felt, would have similar abilities), plus a cohort of some 2000 student nurses training in fifty-two Scottish hospitals. The evaluation procedures and results were reported in depth [B 405].

4.4. Professional and technical manpower

An ambitious field study was undertaken in 1964–5 by Martin to collect statistical information about five professions: dietetics, occupational therapy, orthoptics, physio-therapy and radiography [QRL 451]. Several features are common to these professions. The staff are predominantly female, and they theoretically work under the direction of medically qualified persons. At the time of the survey, the entrance qualifications and training programmes, with the exception of dietetics, were similar. Also in 1964, each of the professions was in the process of becoming state registered, and an acute shortage of staff in all these occupations was alleged. With funding from the NPHT, Martin carried through a range of surveys in England and Wales: of all training schools in each profession; of samples of qualified members in each profession, the numbers involved ranging from 226 dietitians to 395 occupational therapists; of five RHBs in England; and finally of students in selected training schools for each of the professional groups. However, the book is essentially descriptive with only seventeen detailed tables.

Almost all of the 1225 professional and technical staff employed in the hospital service in Wales were asked about their employment expectations in the spring of 1963 [B 121]. The exercise directed by Crichton and Crawford from University College, Cardiff, provided the Welsh Hospital Board with data for the development of man-power programmes over the following decade.

The pay and related conditions of service of the professions supplementary to medicine and speech therapists were reviewed by a Committee of Enquiry led by the Earl of Halsbury [QRL 195]. (The committee jointly reviewed nurses and midwives but reported these findings separately [QRL 193], Subsection 4.3.5.) They were concerned with the situation of professions encompassed by the Professional and Technical Whitley Council 'A'—chiropodists, dietitians, occupational therapists, orthoptists, physiotherapists, radiographers, remedial gymnasts, and speech therapists' and helpers. As part of the enquiry, a survey was undertaken of hospital staffing (nurses and midwives as well as professions supplementary to medicine) for a week in August 1974. Using the listings in the *Hospitals and Health Services Year Book*, hospitals with fifty or more staffed available beds were sampled, the ratios being one-in-two of the London Teaching Hospitals, and for the rest one-in-ten. Additionally, one-in-ten of certain clinic types (for example, physiotherapy) were sampled. The response rate was unstated. Hospitals and clinics were asked to specify for each of the professions, and for helpers, the numbers on duty and on-call at different times of day or night on weekdays and week-ends. Included were sessional and part-time staff, but agency staff were separated out. A supplementary survey on earnings was administered by the DHSS drawing upon information from the NHS regional computer centres' payrolls. Full-time and part-time staff, but not agency employees in hospitals, training centres and community centres during June 1974, were covered. Data were obtained from twelve of the fifteen regions in England and Wales, and likewise from twelve of the fifteen Scottish areas.

Hospital pharmacy staffing in England, Wales and Scotland came under review by a working party set up in 1968 to advise on the efficient and economical organization of the hospital pharmaceutical service. The working party administered a questionnaire to hospitals which established the employment situation for hospital pharmacists, pharmaceutical students, pharmacy technicians and student technicians as at 31 August 1968, and summary tables appeared in the report [QRL 197].

The deployment of dietitians in the hospital service and community (England only) was assessed by Dawes during 1972–3 [QRL 183]. Questionnaires identified those LHAs, Hospital Management Committees and BGs who had an establishment for dietitians, and currently employed or had recently employed dietitians. Further, the MOsH were asked their opinions on the adequacy of dietetic services in their community, while part of the hospital document was completed by the group dietitian (or most senior appointment) and probed the content of the work undertaken, particularly that which involved giving dietary advice to patients outside hospitals, and to individuals and groups working in the community.

4.5. Other resources

4.5.1. *Prescribing costs*

Pricing bureaux at local or national levels provided the sources for district or regional analyses of general practitioners' overall prescribing patterns, these mostly being undertaken in the mid-1960s or earlier. A report published by the MoH statistics branch in 1964, *Recent N.H.S. Prescribing Trends* [QRL 471], presented prescribing statistics in Great Britain for the years 1961 and 1962. This exercise was facilitated by the revision at the beginning of 1961 in the system employed by the Ministry to amass information about drugs, dressings and appliances dispensed under the NHS pharmaceutical services. From a representative sample of one-in-twenty contractors (chemists, drug stores and appliance contractors) in England and Wales every tenth prescription form was submitted to the Ministry by the pricing bureaux. A comparable scheme operated in Scotland (from July 1961) but one-in-ten contractors were involved. For each prescription the contractor was identified including his location, the drug, the quantity dispensed and the net ingredient cost, and the data recorded on punch cards. This enabled the data on the actual prescription to be related to the therapeutic group and the medicament class of the drug used. Tables were thus provided showing for each quarter of the 2 years under review estimates of prescriptions dispensed by therapeutic group, costs and indexes for England, Wales and Scotland. Regional breakdowns were also provided plus analyses according to practitioners' age group and practice organization. Using the same method, a follow-up volume was prepared, *National Health Service Prescribing 1963* [QRL 473], giving corresponding figures about Great Britain as a whole for 1962 and 1963, and more extensive regional analyses for 1963 only.

Northern Ireland's prescribing statistics are comprehensive, for, since 1966, the data from all prescription forms have been computerized. This has facilitated a range of enquiries by Wade and colleagues into the prescribing patterns of various drugs, see [B 447] and Subsection 5.1.2.8.

The method of identifying 'high-cost' doctors established in the early days of the original National Health Insurance scheme of 1911 has continued in a modified form until the present day. So at the time when the major analyses were assembled, the procedure was that the overall prescribing costs of each doctor were analysed by the pricing bureaux for one month in each year and three figures were calculated: the total cost per prescription, number of prescriptions per person on the doctor's NHS prescribing lists and the combined average total cost per person on the NHS prescribing lists. Those doctors identified as high-cost (an average cost per person 1·25 times the average for all doctors in the local EC area) were contacted by the local regional medical officer. Where doctors worked in partnerships and so were likely to issue prescriptions for a partner's patients, account was taken of the partnership as a whole. Benjamin and Ash [B 45] scrutinized prescriptions which had been issued by a sample of 3150 doctors in twenty-nine ECs in England and Wales, and dispensed between September 1958 and July 1959. As they wished only to observe variations between individual doctor's prescribing costs, and did not intend to make inter-area comparisons, it did not matter that no more than 1 month's costs were analysed. (There is, of course, seasonal variability in the composition of drugs prescribed by family doctors.)

In an endeavour to discover whether wider use of the British National Formulary (BNF) in Northern Ireland might result in economies in the cost of prescribing, Wade and McDevitt [B 449] analysed two sets of data. (The BNF is published and revised at 2-yearly intervals by the Joint Formulary Committee of the BMA and the Pharmaceutical Society of Great Britain, and it is circulated free to prescribing doctors. The Committee claims that BNF preparations can serve almost all the requirements of both hospital and general practice. BNF preparations are usually less costly to the NHS than proprietary preparations.) Examined were: all the prescriptions dispensed by a single urban pharmacy but from many practices during June 1965; and, for the same month, all prescriptions written by doctors in two similar practices but one having persistently 'high' prescribing costs, and the other, persistently lower than average for Northern Ireland. Each prescription was checked to see if the preparations were either listed in the most recent edition of the BNF, or could be substituted by a BNF preparation with identical or similar consequences, or was a proprietary preparation which could *not* be replaced with a BNF equivalent. The original and amended lists were then costed by the pricing bureaux. It was felt that marked savings would accrue to the NHS by the greater use of BNF preparations. But patients' acceptability of revised drug preparations and the 'costs' to chemists faced with reduced reimbursements from pricing bureaux were issues not considered.

The extent of the disparity in unit costs between drugs dispensed in hospital pharmacy departments and those dispensed via general practitioners' prescriptions was demonstrated by Opit and Farmer [B 361]. The hospital services negotiate with the manufacturers or suppliers, whereas in the community, FPCs pay pharmaceutical contractors on a standard fee-for-service basis including a professional fee, according to a drug tariff. The allowed ingredient costs and professional fees of 5000 scripts issued during December 1972 were recorded by the Birmingham pricing bureaux. Each item was then recosted according to a current price list in use in a large general hospital.

Evaluative comments about the manner in which the health service resources discussed in this chapter are deployed really lie outside the scope of this review. However, Chapter 6 is concerned with the various techniques used in evaluating the NHS, and it contains a subsection (6.2.5.4) on economics in which some analyses of parts of the service are cited. Davies's study, *Social Needs and Resources in Local Services* [B 132], is another volume of interest in terms of the analytic techniques used in determining indices of relative needs of communities and standards of provision, and for assessing their relationships. Lastly, attention is drawn to two documents on priorities in England and Scotland prepared by the DHSS and the SHHD respectively, and published in 1976. *Priorities for Health and Personal Social Services in England* [B 153] attempted for the first time 'to establish rational systematic priorities throughout the health and personal social services' because, it was argued, when resources are limited, growth in any particular services can only be afforded if counterbalancing economies are made elsewhere. Thus, in this document are guidelines as to the services which should be treated as priorities once the financial resources are allocated within the NHS, namely the services for the mentally handicapped, the mentally ill and those used mainly by the elderly and physically handicapped, and by children and their families. (There had already been White Papers issued outlining the strategies for the mentally ill [B 151] and the mentally handicapped [B 155].) The Scottish document, *The Health Service in Scotland. The Way Ahead* [B 494], also saw these services and preventive measures as priorities which would be offset by a lessening in the growth rate of the acute sector of the hospital service. It is, though, admitted by the DHSS that local priorities will be affected by a range of factors—demographic, social and practical—peculiar to individual areas, and so it may often happen that local plans will not correspond with the order of proposed national priorities. Furthermore, it is not intended to stifle worthwhile local innovations and individual initiatives operating within the resources available. However, for a priorities policy to be successfully implemented at a local level let alone nationally, there must be, as a prerequisite, a thorough awareness of the current situation regarding both the stock of real resources and the use to which they are being (or could be) put. Only then can informed rationalization decisions be made. Chapter 7 draws attention to certain gaps in statistical data about the supply, and deployment of real resources in the health service, while the next chapter covers statistics of an *ad hoc* kind on use of services.

CHAPTER 5

USE OF SERVICES

This chapter considers the items of service performed by utilizing resources (facilities, manpower and other real resources) for persons whose needs have been acknowledged by the health professionals as being appropriate demands. The discussion focuses upon the services provided by the National Health Service (NHS) but included are the activities of the local health and school health authorities prior to Reorganization in 1974 when these functions were integrated into the NHS.

Information about the use made of services can be collected in various ways. Usually the statistics available are merely quantitative; that is, they provide counts of activities performed, persons treated, beds filled, etc. A qualitative element about the adequacy of the services is rarely present for such assessments are much more difficult to make within the constraints of the current conventions for data accumulation. Statistics on use may be amassed routinely or on an *ad hoc* basis. Some services appear to be more easily monitored routinely than others, but this is in part a function of the manner in which they are organized. In each hospital records department there are personnel responsible for the completion of the forms for the hospital in-patient enquiry, the mental health enquiry and the hospital activity analysis. The units of work returned from hospital pathology laboratories and radiology departments are taken into account in the allocation of resources to the individual laboratories and departments. The submissions of NHS items of service performed by general dental practitioners to the Dental Estimates Boards are also comprehensive for they too are required for financial reimbursement. On the other hand, the comparative scarcity of information about the workload activities of the 22,000 general medical practitioners in the United Kingdom is a consequence of their being independent contractors within the NHS and paid according to the size and composition of their lists of patients and the organization of their practices, rather than according to the work performed. (There is, however, a certain amount of information accumulated, although it is not readily accessible, about activities such as prescribing and certification, and claims for various services performed—see Subsection 5.1.2.)

There are many other routine returns accounting for activities performed in all parts of the NHS which are submitted annually to central government (the Department of Health and Social Security, the Welsh Office, the Scottish Home and Health Department and the Northern Ireland Health and Social Services). The accumulated statistics which are published regularly were reviewed in a previous volume in this series, *Central Government Routine Health Statistics* [B 14]. However, there are limitations for planning purposes in the nature of some of the material collected, for example, there are forms which now need revisions in their design and instructions regarding completion. Moreover, very few statutory requirements exist for the submission of workload returns and so there is cause for doubt about the comprehensiveness of certain statistics. It is

135

these limitations coupled with the known gaps in the routine information, especially from general practice, which have prompted the setting up of a range of *ad hoc* studies.

Ad hoc statistics about the use made of services have been derived from three types of sources. The first consists of special workload recordings made over defined periods of time either by the health workers themselves (doctors, nurses, etc.) or by personnel specially engaged. With careful monitoring for accuracy and comprehensiveness, data of this kind can be invaluable, for their content can be tailored to specific questions about the service under review. But a high degree of motivation on behalf of the participants is required. The second potential source is less satisfactory but is, nevertheless, of value. It consists of estimates by the health workers delivering the services, of the activities performed and to whom. These reports are collected via postal or interview surveys and, usually, supplementary information about the organization of the services and the attitudes of the health workers is sought. The recipients of the services, the patients, comprise the third possible source, for they too can provide estimates of the contacts they have had with health services of all kinds as well as offering their views about the effectiveness of the care. There must, of course, be reservations about the reliability of survey estimates made by both health workers and individuals because of the problem of memory recall; however, skilful questioning techniques can minimize inconsistencies.

For most persons, their NHS medical care is initiated when they present themselves to their dental or general practitioner and associated staff. (There is the possibility of self-referral to accident and emergency departments which is suggestive of unmet demand—see Chapter 3.) From that point onwards, the patient is dependent upon the health professional's discretion to manage or discharge the episode, or to transfer the responsibility to another professional either in the community or in the hospital sector. Thus this chapter is sectionalized according to the services through which a patient can progress; from general or dental practitioner services to either other community services or the hospital services (namely accident and emergency, out-patient, diagnostic and pharmaceutical, in-patient and day patient, and rehabilitation). Within each subsection, individuals' assessments of their use of the service precede studies with a workload-recording content, while relevant attitudinal surveys of health workers close the subsection. The chapter also incorporates references to special analyses of unpublished statistical material which have been collected routinely, and there are references to non-central government and Northern Ireland statistical reports published regularly.

It has been necessary to impose constraints upon the number of studies entered in the QRL on Use of Services. So in general, surveys of single or very few general practices/practitioners have been omitted, likewise individual hospital studies. In addition, some early national or regional surveys which have later been repeated have also been excluded from the QRL. But a few studies in these categories contain material relevant to other chapters and their accompanying QRLs. So, whenever there is a reference to any of such studies in the following text, it is identified by an asterisk (e.g. [QRL 96*]). A further point—there are studies reviewed in this chapter which incorporate in their methods surveys of patients. However, data indicating patients' 'satisfactions' about aspects of the health services are indexed in the QRL on Evaluation of Medical Care. And again, the attitudes of doctors and nurses towards their work are normally indexed in the Evaluation QRL.

5.1. General practitioner services

5.1.1. *Assessments by individuals of their contacts with general practitioner services*

The *General Household Survey* for 1971 [QRL 510], 1972 [QRL 512] and 1973 [QRL 513] contain extensive tabulations regarding individuals' usage of general practitioner services over reference periods of 2 weeks, 1 month and 1 year. In all 3 years more than 11,000 private households co-operated, interviews being undertaken with every member over 15 years of age. The survey design is detailed in Subsection 2.2.1.2. The question specific to doctor contacts in the 1972 survey was: 'During the 2 weeks ending last Sunday, apart from visits to a hospital, did you (or any of your children under 15) talk to a doctor for any reason at all?' [page 370, QRL 510]. The interviewers then probed as to the site of the consultations (telephone, home, surgery, elsewhere, and health centre in 1973 only), the status of the doctor (general practitioner, specialist or other), and the illness/disability presented by the patient. The question in the earlier survey was slightly more ambiguous in the wording of the reference period for it read, 'Last week or the week before ...', while in the 1973 schedule the age of children was raised to 'under 16'. In the second report, the GHS consultation rates (excluding telephone contacts) per 100 persons in 1971 were compared with the patient contact rates recorded by doctors during 1970–1 in the second National Morbidity Study [QRL 511]. The GHS rates were higher in each age group for both sexes with the exception of the 5–14 years where there was a remarkable similarity. The reported contacts by the elderly, particularly respondents aged 75 years or more, were greatly in excess of the doctor-recorded rates. No truly satisfactory explanation for this situation is apparent. Amongst the reasons offered by the authors of the GHS report was the suggestion that the self-selected participants in the morbidity study may have been 'atypical' in having rather efficiently organized practices. Thus, part of their workloads might have been borne by ancillary staff.

Prior to the publication of the GHS Introductory Report in 1973 the only national study of patients' perceived frequency of contacts with family doctor services, and their attitudes, was the 1964 survey carried out by Cartwright in the then Institute of Community Studies, *Patients and their Doctors* [QRL 127]. The main purposes were, first, to describe the care given by the general practitioner service and, secondly, to discover the attitudes of both patients and doctors to this care. Twelve study areas were chosen from all the 547 parliamentary constituencies in England and Wales which had been stratified on a number of criteria. From each of these twelve areas 144 people were selected at random from the electoral register. This gave a sample of 1728 'patients', of whom 1397 were successfully interviewed in their homes. They were asked for the name of their doctor and all except twenty-seven provided the information; 552 doctors were mentioned and to each a questionnaire was sent. The method of sample selection did mean that the chance of a doctor being asked to participate in the enquiry was related to the number of patients who considered him to be their doctor. However, validation against national statistics on doctors' list sizes showed the bias to be relatively small. After two reminders, 76 per cent (422 doctors) had complied. The non-respondents tended to have qualified less recently were less likely to be members of the then College of General Practitioners, and more frequently had licentiate qualifications only and more frequently worked on their own or in a small partnership of two or three, than those doctors who participated. In the patient interviews, respondents recalled the frequency of their contacts with general practitioner services in the previous 12 months as well as being given the opportunity to express their attitudes towards medical care. Additional questions were asked of mothers of children under 15, persons who had been to hospital as out-patients in the previous 12 months, people aged 65 and over, and persons who had consulted a GP in the previous 2 weeks.

Persons living in Bermondsey and Southwark, and Liverpool have also been asked about their uptake of a spectrum of health services (primary medical and dental services, hospitals, chemists, opticians, etc.). The former study involved 2153 adults during 1962–3—see [QRL 669] and Subsection 2.2.2.3. The latter survey took place in 1968–9, Liverpool being one of twelve study areas in seven countries. Households numbering 1012 were sampled and 2881 persons interviewed. To ensure comparability in the data from the study areas, the survey procedures were rigorously monitored by the research consortium, the World Health Organization/International Collaborative Study of Medical Care Utilization. However, most of the statistical findings in the substantial report were presented graphically [B 277].

Sometimes, nationally based studies of specific population groups have included questions asking about respondents' use of general medical services. *Handicapped and Impaired in Great Britain* [QRL 297] and *Life before Death* [QRL 130] which assembled retrospectively the medical experiences of 785 deceased persons are two such examples. The research method of the former study is described in Subsection 2.5.21 and that of the latter in Subsection 2.5.32. Similarly, persons who had been off sick from work for periods of 1, 3, 6 and 12 months respectively were asked about their contacts with health services. This study, *Prolonged Sickness and the Return to Work* [QRL 450], was carried out by the Social Survey Division of the Office of Population Censuses and Surveys on behalf of the DHSS in 1972–3. The sponsoring body was concerned to identify factors associated with increasing lengths of illness and the prospects of individuals returning to work after illness. Local national insurance office records were sampled and, in all, 4531 persons were interviewed.

5.1.2. *General practitioner workload and attitudinal studies*

It was observed in Volume II of this series that 'there is no routine information currently available on the workload carried by general practice' [B 14, page 64]. This situation continues to exist. General practitioners can complete returns claiming fees for certain items of service, although this is at their discretion, and there are no consolidated statistics generally available. General medical services for which payment is possible include vaccinations and immunizations, cervical cytology tests, maternity medical services, night visits (made between the hours of 11 p.m. and 7 a.m. but excluding the provisions of maternity care) and the treatment of temporary residents, emergency cases and patients with dental haemorrhage. Fees are also available for the administration of general anaesthetics other than in connection with hospital or specialist services, maternity medical services or in association with a trainee GP. All of these claims for payment are directed to the Family Practitioner Committee, which in certain circumstances, for example for vaccination and immunization claims, pass the appropriate documentation to the Area Health Authority. Additionally, family doctors receive a small payment for each reported case of certain infectious diseases, but there is reason to believe that considerable under-notification of the commoner infectious diseases exists ([B 237]).

There are two items of service about which data are amassed centrally. All prescription forms completed by GPs and presented for dispensing are sent to the Central Pricing Bureau in Newcastle upon Tyne, while medical certificates signed for national insurance purposes are processed annually in the Central Office of the DHSS, also based in Newcastle upon Tyne. But statistics indicating workload patterns are not derived from either data sources. Hospital records departments are further sites where data are deposited. Almost all cases referred by family doctors for specialist advice (as out-patients or emergency in-patient admissions) or for investigation in hospital departments will be documented by, for example, referral/discharge letters, hospital laboratory and radiology forms, etc. Yet such data are rarely systematized to provide indicators of the variability in the use of such services by general practitioners.

Family doctors are 'obliged' to keep notes of the medical histories of patients on their lists. Traditionally these have been kept on continuation cards inserted in envelopes in which have also been stored hospital and other communications, supplied by Executive Councils (now the FPCs). Recently, though, forms of an A4 size have become available. Problem-orientated record keeping is an even more recent innovation and there have been occasional experiments in computer-assisted medical records. A survey endeavouring to find out how 201 Scottish doctors kept their records, and their opinions about the type of records they maintained, was undertaken by Cormack in 1969 [QRL 165] and it was followed-up by Richardson and Berkeley in 1975 [QRL 570]. There is virtually no monitoring of the comprehensiveness and accuracy of the data relating to both patient identification and medical histories, in individual records, a problem exemplified by Dawes [B 135] in an examination of the medical records of eight practices (see also Subsection 2.3.2). This is a situation about which concern must be felt in the light of the expansion of the practice team concept with doctors, nurses, health visitors and even social workers jointly managing the care of patients. Farmer, Knox, Cross and Crombie [B 187] compared the files of four general practitioners and an EC to assess the feasibility of transferring EC lists to a computer filing system. The very high level of incongruencies detected, especially regarding civil state, were due, the authors felt, to the delayed updating of mutable information.

The unreliability in the numbers of medical records held is another problem of particular relevance if rates of items of service on behalf of a doctor's practice population are to be calculated. The mobility of patients caused by migration into or from a district, death or transference of registration means that a doctor's records will rarely match the actual number of persons who consider themselves to be his patients. Even more significantly, they are unlikely to correspond with the FPC Index which is the most complete population file within the NHS. Its principal use is the calculation of payments to GPs. The time lag in the transference of medical records between doctors and the FPC provides part of the explanation for the discrepancy between files. (Studies estimating rates of discrepancies are cited in Subsection 2.3.2.) Age/sex registers, disease indexes and family registers are supplementary record systems set up in practices to facilitate closer monitoring of patient 'profiles'. Many papers describing the methods of compilation of registers and the uses to which they have been put in individual practices (especially for research investigations) have been published in the

Journal of the Royal College of General Practitioners. The General Practice Research Unit of the Royal College of General Practitioners offers an advisory service to doctors planning research systems.

As the information on current medical records (excluding the patient identification data) is only accessible in GPs' surgeries, compilation of routine workload statistics from this source has not been a realistic proposition (that is, setting aside the problem of confidentiality). Thus the knowledge that does exist about GPs' workloads has been amassed from *ad hoc* studies undertaken by family doctors detailing their own work patterns, or by independent researchers co-operating closely with general practitioners.

5.1.2.1. *All-inclusive studies*. The most comprehensive recent workload study is the second NMS which was sponsored jointly by the RCGP, OPCS and DHSS [QRL 511]. This survey was intended primarily to record morbidity data in general practice which would be comparable with the results of a comprehensive study involving more than 100 practices, carried out 15 years earlier [QRL 408*]. The opportunity was also taken to collect information about patients' consulting patterns (home visits and attendances at practice premises) and the use made by family doctors of facilities outside their practices (hospital and local authority services). The method of this study has already been described (see Subsection 2.3.2.2); it suffices to recall here that 115 general practitioners in fifty-three practices in England and Wales recorded details of all direct consultations over a period of 12 months, during 1970–1. The items of a workload nature recorded at each face-to-face contact between doctor and patient were the site of the consultation (in the practice premises, other premises such as an institution, or in the patient's home) and, where relevant, the type of referral made. However, the only tabulated data on place of consultation were home visits as a percentage of all consultations for selected diagnoses by sex and age. Another table indicated the frequency of patients attending for reasons other than illness, for example various prophylactic procedures, normal pregnancy and prenatal care, and health education.

An understanding of the uniqueness of the research method applied in the 1970–1 NMS is necessary if, for workload purposes, the results are compared with other smaller studies. At each consultation, multiple diagnoses could be recorded and for each diagnosis the place of consultation and referral action would be entered on the record card. It was calculated that there was more than one diagnosis recorded in about 8·7 per cent of all face-to-face contacts. (The proportion of participating doctors who chose to record multiple diagnoses was not presented in the report.) The overall total consultation rate (face-to-face contacts) in this category was 3·0 per person per year but, when adjusted to take account of the inflation factor of 8·7 per cent, the rate became 2·75. Unless the incidence of multiple diagnosis recording was distributed evenly between all consultation sites, then it is possible that the data about home visits are not truly representative of the total face-to-face patient/doctor contacts which took place in the home. The referral data were thought to be under-recorded. In the validation process, which consisted of checking the details on the computer file of 100 patients per practice with the medical records held in the practices, a referral omission rate of 11·9 per cent was observed. For out-patient referrals only, the omission rate was 14·6 per cent.

Prior to the setting-up of the second NMS, two regionally based workload surveys of a very similar study design were conducted by GPs in south-west England and South Wales [QRL 726, 713]. Both of these studies have already been outlined in Subsection 2.3.2.3. Workload characteristics tabulated in the two reports included time spent other than with patients in the practice, procedures carried out in the practices and the use of other professional help, and referral rates to other agencies. Patient contact rates were calculated against the doctors' list sizes unlike in the second NMS when age/sex registers were created. These two studies have provided a useful guide to the variability of general practitioners' workloads in geographical areas with populations displaying distinctive occupational characteristics. A further 'use of services' study also reviewed in Subsection 2.3.2.3 was that undertaken in the City of Exeter by Ashford and Pearson [QRL 37]. The participating GPs entered on manuscript record cards inserted in their patients' NHS envelopes, the date and place of consultation, diagnosis or principal symptom, certification and referral.

Workload analyses for practitioners in north-east Scotland were provided in another study involving multiple recorders, 'A study of general-practitioner consultations in North-east Scotland' [QRL 572]. Sponsorship for the study was provided by the Department of General Practice in Aberdeen University and the Research Committee of the North-east Scotland Faculty of the RCGP. All of the 253 mainland principals in the north-east region were invited to participate; 163 accepted, but comprehensive recordings were returned by only 142 doctors. These doctors recorded nine items of information about every consultation (direct and indirect) on one day a fortnight during the period May 1969 to April 1970. The doctors also completed questionnaires seeking information about their professional experience and practice organization. In the published results of this study, consultation rates per 1000 patients *per day* were tabulated for a range of variables such as list sizes, the number of years principals had been in practice, and location of practices, but it was not always clear if these rates referred to *all* consultations or to direct consultations only.

There have been a number of workload surveys carried out in individual practices by GPs, and data from many of the published reports were abstracted in the 1973 edition of *Present State and Future Needs of General Practice* [B 203]. The data in some of these reports were amassed from routine daybook entries over variable lengths of time (from less than 1 year to 21 years) while, in other studies, special workload recording programmes had been set up usually for periods of less than 1 year in duration. In only a few instances had consultation rates and other workload rates per 1000 population been calculated against age/sex registers. Of interest from a methodological standpoint are the reports by Morrell, Gage and Robinson of their monitoring of items of service performed in their practice over a 12-month period as they carried out various validation checks on the data recordings [B 336, 337 and QRL 487]. Another doctor and his practice team combined an evaluation study with a year's workload monitoring—about 340 persons were interviewed by independent researchers, the sample being weighted towards the more frequent 'user' groups (Marsh and Kaim-Caudle [QRL 447*, 364*] and Subsection 6.2.5.3).

A forerunner of a small number of national surveys of general practitioners' attitudes was conducted by Cartwright and Marshall and entitled 'General practice in 1963: its conditions, contents and satisfactions' [B 90]. One hundred and fifty-seven doctors in England and Wales were interviewed during the summer of 1963: they formed 81 per cent of a representative sample drawn from thirteen parliamentary constituencies.

Cartwright adapted the methodology considerably in her subsequent study *Patients and Their Doctors* [QRL 127]. Postal questionnaires were completed by 422 general practitioners in England and Wales but they were the family doctors identified by a sample of 'patients' (see Subsection 5.1.1 for a full discussion of the fieldwork which took place in 1964). Topics in the doctor questionnaire which were specifically related to workload activities included on-call duties, the proportion of surgery consultations felt to be trivial or unnecessary and procedures undertaken within the practice. Additionally, details of practice arrangements and access to hospital facilities were amassed as well as attitudes towards current general practice. A small number of interviews were carried out but the material was used for illustrative purposes only.

Two years later Mechanic endeavoured to build up a profile of doctors' satisfactions and dissatisfactions, attitudes towards aspects of medical care and the organization of general practice within the NHS at a time when there was considerable unrest amongst family doctors over terms of service and remuneration. So in April 1966 a random sample of GPs in England and Wales was sent questionnaires. The response for completions after a maximum of three reminders was 60 per cent (813 doctors). To those doctors whose replies were still outstanding, a fourth approach was made using a short questionnaire and the response rate for this was an additional 13 per cent. Thus, for many key items in the survey, the total response rate was 73 per cent (995 doctors). Tabulations relating to practice organization and workload including reported access to and use of various diagnostic procedures were published in two papers [B 316, B 317], while other data from the study were compared with findings from an American survey carried out some $4\frac{1}{2}$ years later [B 318].

The most recent specific survey intended to form an 'up-to-date picture of the characteristics of general practitioners' in Great Britain was carried out in 1969 by a working party of the British Medical Association Planning Unit. This study was reported by Irvine and Jefferys [QRL 349]. The Unit was particularly interested in the growing trend for principals to work together in group practice premises or health centres. At the time of the survey there were in Britain 437 principals practising from health centres under Section 21 of the National Health Service Act, 1946 or the equivalent Scottish Act. Group practice allowances were being received by 10,297 doctors (GPA doctors), while 11,903 were neither in health centres nor recipients of group practice allowances (non-GPA doctors). The statistical divisions of the DHSS and the SHHD assisted in the drawing of the sample which was weighted for England and Wales in favour of health centre practitioners to allow valid comparisons to be made between this group and the GPA and non-GPA doctors. (The sampling fraction was unstated.) The response rate for these three groups was 74 per cent for health centre practitioners, 84 per cent for GPA doctors and 69 per cent for non-GPA doctors, but in the presentation of the results there was a reweighting of numbers in each type of practice to conform to national proportions. In Scotland 180 doctors were sampled, the numbers drawn from each EC area being proportional to the total in that area. In the report, comparisons were drawn with the situation in 1963 as described by Cartwright and Marshall from an interview survey of 157 GPs (see above). Some aspects of the practice organization and hospital relationships of 1721 GPs in England in 1969 were tabulated in the appendix to *Family Doctors and Public Policy* [QRL 108]. As this survey was primarily concerned with measuring the effectiveness of the designated area allowance policy, the full review appears in Subsection 4.2.4.

General practice in Northern Ireland was investigated in 1970 by the Ministry of Health and Social Services for Northern Ireland [QRL 482]. The 1969 Green Paper on the Administrative Structure of the Health and Personal Social Services in Northern Ireland highlighted the urgency for factual information on the organization and structure of general practice, and the degree of involvement of family doctors in other branches of the existing tripartite health service. An earlier, though unpublished, survey in 1965–6 had touched on these issues. The object of the 1970 survey was to obtain factual information about them. Few data on attitudes towards general practice were collected. All but one principal (out of 751) in general practice in Northern Ireland were interviewed during the period October/November 1970 by one of eight medical officers of the Medical Referee Service.

In 1968, 89 per cent (123) of the family doctors with surgery premises in the London Borough of Camden were interviewed by members of the Social Research Unit at Bedford College [QRL 611]. The intentions were first, to describe and compare general practice in an Inner London borough with other areas of London and of Great Britain; secondly, to consider how these doctors worked, both within their surgeries and in their contacts with other services; and thirdly, to elicit attitudes towards health service provision. Use was made of questions from other recent surveys of general practice, so making it possible to present results comparable with those obtained in other areas. Finally, it should be noted that data reflecting GPs' dispositions towards their work appear in the QRL accompanying Chapter 6 on 'Evaluation of Medical Care'.

5.1.2.2. *Allocation of working time.* The use made by GPs of their working time has been the specific subject of two enquiries involving multi-practices. The most extensive in terms of the total number of participating doctors was carried out in 1965 by the Merseyside and North Wales Faculty of the CGP in collaboration with the Medical Care Research Unit, University of Manchester [QRL 224]. During one mid-winter week in February 1965, 134 volunteers of the 309 members and associates of the Faculty completed day sheets which itemized the starting and finishing times of surgery consulting sessions and the numbers of patients seen at each session. Likewise, the times of home-visiting rounds and the numbers of patients visited were recorded. Other sessions completed in hospitals, clinics or for medical boards, and periods of practice administration were also timed. Supplementary information about each participant was obtained from medical directories. The forerunner of this study was a pilot workload survey over 1 week (August 1964) which included time recordings, carried out by the CGP with 370 recorders in England and Wales [B 114]. Some comparative data were presented with the 1965 survey results.

The more recent multi-practice study, *Time Study of Consultations in General Practice* [QRL 103], attempted not so much to measure the distribution of time between various activities in the doctors' working days, but to create profiles of the actions performed and time taken *within* patient consultations both in the surgery and at home. A recorder observed 2113 consultations (1636 in surgeries and 477 in homes) carried out by twenty-two GPs over a period of about 1 year. These doctors were practising in Scotland, eight in the City of Aberdeen, eight in small country towns and six in rural or village situations, and half were over the age of 45 years. Six trainee assistants were also studied. The timing of other professional activities, such as practice administration, was discounted because of the problems of maintaining the goodwill of the doctors and observer fatigue. Cumulative timing to one-tenth of a minute was the method chosen with the observer recording the time when a particular activity ceased.

Two alternative methods of timing activities have been used in other general practice workload studies. Chronostamps were utilized by Bevan and Draper in their investigation into appointment systems in general practice (detailed in Subsection 5.1.2.3). Morrell and his colleagues [B 338] used them for two 1-week periods in the workload survey of their north Lambeth practice, and they were also applied in a study of four practices employing practice nurses [B 398]. A chronostamp consists of a rubber stamp in the shape of a clock face with the hands geared to a clock mechanism, so when stamped the current time is recorded. However, the method is unsuitable for activity measurements within consultations because the clock-face is calibrated at 5-minute intervals and the time can only be stamped once every minute. To overcome this problem the 'bleep' method, described by Floyd and Livesey [B 197], was used by five Croydon doctors and some of their attached staff. The system is simple—when an apparatus emits a signal or 'bleep', the subject enters his current activity on a record sheet.

5.1.2.3. *Appointment systems*. The introduction of appointment systems escalated in the 1960s: only a few hundred practices operated one in 1962 whereas approximately two-thirds of all practices surveyed by the BMA Planning Unit Working Party in 1969 indicated their use [QRL 349]. The impetus was the remuneration revisions of 1966 which enabled GPs to claim reimbursement for a substantial part of the cost of employing receptionists. In 1967 Cardew presented statistics on the use of the service set up about 1960 to provide GPs with appointment diaries and work sheets [B 85]. A number of doctors have, in the past decade, reported upon their own experiences with appointment systems usually in the *Journal of the Royal College of General Practitioners*, but see also Morrell and Kasap [B 338].

An evaluative multi-phased enquiry into appointment systems in general practice was financed by the Nuffield Provincial Hospitals Trust and the Nuffield Foundation ([QRL 64] and Section 3.1). The fieldwork was undertaken between mid-1963 and mid-1965 and was reported upon by Bevan and Draper who were then members of the Unit of Biometry at the University of Oxford. The primary object was to present findings which would enable doctors to take informed decisions about the applicability of appointment systems to their own practices—this was prior to the 1966 remuneration amendments. The survey design was in three parts: postal surveys among doctors; postal surveys and personal interviews among 'potential patients'; and detailed record collecting from a number of practices. In the doctor-survey component, the initial problem was to identify those practices where an appointment system was currently in use. Ten per cent of all practices were thought to be using them. From the stratified ECs of England, Wales and Scotland, one-in-two partnerships were selected except for the ECs in London, Middlesex and Glasgow where the sampling fraction was one-in-four. This sample was then subdivided. The senior partners of a very large proportion of the partnerships were sent a short preliminary questionnaire asking whether or not an appointment system was in use. About 200 practices were required; 342 replied in the affirmative and to each a detailed questionnaire was despatched. Completions were received from 229 practices whose appointment systems were in accord with the study's definition. The smaller section of the partnership sample was used for the selection of doctors (not partnerships) *not using* an appointment system. Of the 621 doctors contacted by questionnaire, 516 replied.

In assessing patients' views, two separate surveys were carried out. The British Market Research Bureau during the mid-1960s operated a nationwide continuous survey in which quota samples of 5000 adults were interviewed monthly. Questions on appointment systems were posed to half of one month's sample and 2140 completed interviews were obtained. The second survey was administered by the Unit of Biometry. Patients from four practices where appointment systems were operating and five where they were not were sampled. From each practice's records forty-five names were selected, thirty of whom were considered by the doctors as 'working class' and the remainder 'middle class'. In the third part of the study, eleven practices who were planning to introduce appointment systems made chronostamp recordings of patients' arrivals and consultation durations, both before and after the implementation of the schemes. Practices willing to co-operate came to the attention of the research team via personal contact and letters published in the *British Medical Journal* and *The Lancet*. In addition, the participating doctors, as well as doctors from other practices operating appointment systems, kept some weekly records of the time spent in surgery sessions and of consultation types categorized as patient-requested and doctor-requested. Needless to say, the complexity of the research method resulted in a wealth of material being amassed.

5.1.2.4. *Deputizing services*. General practitioner deputizing services were first established in 1956 in London. Companies independent of the NHS recruit doctors from various sources to answer the calls of subscribers. The BMA sponsors some, and statistics of use are published from time to time in supplements to the *British Medical Journal*. The overall situation in England and Wales in 1972 was reviewed by Williams and Knowelden [QRL 712]. They wished to learn of the rate at which deputizing services had spread and the number of doctors in ECs who used them in 1972. Further, they were interested in the controls applied by the ECs when approving deputizing arrangements. The collection of relevant material was facilitated by the requirements of the Statistics Division of the DHSS which, in 1972, required ECs to provide supplementary data on these topics, in addition to the routine returns. The analysis showed that almost half of the ECs in England and Wales had approved deputizing services. The deputizing services in the Sheffield and Nottingham areas were also scrutinized by Williams, Dixon and Knowelden, in the early 1970s [B 470, 471, 472].

5.1.2.5. *Family planning and abortion*. The interim report of a cohort study involving initially 46,000 women aged 15–44 years, of whom half were prescribed oral contraceptives by some 1400 GPs, was published in 1974 ([QRL 365*] and Subsection 2.3.2.3). The survey, launched by the RCGP in 1968, was concluded in 1976.

Family planning attitudinal surveys of GPs in England and Wales have been organized by Cartwright from the Institute for Social Studies in Medical Care (previously the Institute of Community Studies) on three occasions. The first in 1967 was supported by a US Public Health Service research grant, and it aimed at showing what GPs were doing about family planning and how they saw their role in this field [B 88]. In all, 1954 doctors sampled from the Ministry of Health's Doctor Index were sent questionnaires of whom 72 per cent responded. The attitudes of both doctors and parents to family planning services were collected by Cartwright in her second survey (which followed closely on the first) during 1967 and 1968 [QRL 128]. However, the GPs were those identified by the sampled parents as being their family doctor. This yielded 702 doctors, of whom 76 per cent were either interviewed or had completed a postal questionnaire in the earlier survey described above. (The parents' survey method is reviewed in Subsection 2.5.18.) These doctors were asked how they saw their role in family planning, their probable responses to certain problem situations and the sources of contraceptive information available and methods recommended to patients. Interviews were also carried out with 229 health visitors and seventy doctors at family planning clinics.

Abortion was incorporated into the topics covered in the third of these surveys prepared this time by Cartwright and Lucas as evidence to the Committee on the Working of the Abortion Act (the chairman being Mrs Justice Lane) [QRL 131, 385]. In selecting a sample of fifty-two registration districts, the total number of 506 in England and Wales were stratified according to population, region and type of family planning services provided. Using the lists of the local ECs as the basic sampling frame, sampling fractions were calculated, giving all doctors an overall chance of about one-in-twenty-three of being included in the study. The final selection of 900 doctors was considered to be a national sample—not just an aggregate of doctors giving services in the study areas. The administering of the postal survey coincided with the postal strike late in 1970, but even so the overall response rate amongst the eligible doctors was 68 per cent. Material from this study has been published in two places. 'General practitioners and contraception in 1970–71' [QRL 134] contains some data which are complementary to the first 1967 study described above, but the latter study paid more attention to the clinical side-effects of contraception. Sterilization, too, was a separate topic. In the second report from the study, 'General practitioners and abortion. Evidence to the Committee on the working of the Abortion Act' [QRL 133], doctors' estimates of abortion referrals and their attitudes were related with age, sex and religion of the respondents and with the local hospital region statistics on birth/abortion rates. It is noteworthy that this survey of GPs (which was sponsored by the DHSS) formed part of a larger enquiry into the functioning of birth-control services in England and Wales. The Institute for Social Studies in Medical Care also amassed views from: 272 women having abortions in institutions licensed for abortion ([QRL 131] and Subsection 2.5.1); 759 health visitors [QRL 672*]; 511 domiciliary midwives [QRL 673*]; 410 consultant general surgeons and urologists [QRL 674*]; 388 consultant psychiatrists [B 451]; 332 consultants in obstetrics and gynaecology [B 450]; as well as data from 342 family planning clinics [B 329, 330]. The Social Survey Division of the OPCS looked at the services from the point of view of married and unmarried women (see Bone [QRL 76] and Subsection 2.5.18). The second volume of the report from the Committee on the Working of the Abortion Act contains numerous tables of routinely collected but unpublished statistics about gynaecology services in Great Britain, as well as details from surveys of hospital gynaecology departments which were commissioned by the Committee [QRL 385].

There have been some more recent enquiries into aspects of family planning. For example, 152 family doctors practising in the Coventry EC were questioned about the type of family planning services they currently provided, their experiences with immigrant patients and their willingness to extend the service (Brennan and Opit [B 61]). Cartwright conducted further investigations into family size and family spacing in England and Wales. Parents of young babies were interviewed in 1973 [QRL 129], and then followed-up by postal questionnaires when the children were 2 years old [QRL 135*]. However, doctors were not surveyed in this study.

This subsection has provided little more than a cursory review of the breadth of enquiries into family planning services. However, a review devoted specifically to the topic is to be published in this series of Reviews of UK Statistical Sources.

5.1.2.6. *Home visiting and patient transportation systems*. The trends reported by self-selected practices suggest that the average number of home visits conducted daily has generally fallen over the last 20 years [B 203], but one study in north-east England revealed wide variations in the visiting patterns of family doctors. Marsh, McNay and Whewell [QRL 448] described a survey by 190 general practitioners (half being members or associates of the North-east England Faculty of the RCGP) from 94 practices, who volunteered to record details of visits carried out between Monday and Friday during two consecutive weeks November/December 1969. This fortnight was thought to be representative of moderate workloads without the distortion of holiday periods and epidemics. The standard questions completed for each visit ranged over patient identification data, diagnosis, type of visit (new or repeat) and the time and duration of visits. Unique, though, were the judgements the doctors had to make about the necessity of the visit, and the apparent ability of the patient to attend at the surgery rather than receive a visit at home, particularly if a minibus service were available. This methodological approach was also applied in an assessment of the necessity of home visits carried out by GPs practising from a health centre in Oxfordshire [B 48]. From the data, estimates were made of the time savable to the doctors if the patients who received 'unnecessary' visits could have been transported to the health centre.

During the 1960s some practices experimented with patient transportation systems. For example, in two urban practices cars were used to ferry patients to the surgery [B 196, 415]. The principal in a dispersed Yorkshire practice centralized his main surgery, closed four branch surgeries and arranged for an eleven-seater bus to transport patients to the surgery [B 421], while in east Cornwall a mobile surgery in a converted passenger coach was experimented with by a practice which previously staffed a main surgery and five branch surgeries [B 83]. The enthusiasm expressed by some of the doctors involved in these schemes about the apparent saving in their time, the more thorough examinations made of patients, the therapeutic effects on some of the elderly, and the changes in patients' attitudes towards attending the surgery encouraged the setting-up of a major evaluative study in 1968.

The DHSS and the SHHD financed five transport services in selected general practices and the effects of the services on the doctors' work and their relationships with their patients were monitored by the then Institute of Community Studies, and reported by Lance in 'Transport services in general practice' [QRL 384]. Four of the practices chosen had no previous experience with transport services; they were located in Greater

London, an industrial valley of Monmouthshire (two) and in a small country town, but with a wide rural hinterland in Ross-shire. The fifth practice in Greater London was already operating a car service [B 196]. Five methods of data collection were adopted. First, comprehensive patient registers were compiled with the co-operation of the local ECs. These were used for data recording, age/sex analyses of the practices and for sampling frames. Secondly, throughout the first 18 months of the project all practices recorded some details about each request for a doctor to visit, each patient using the transport service and all consultations. The drivers, too, kept logs of the uses made and the servicing of the vehicles (minibuses or, in one instance, a Land Rover, all able to seat ten to twelve persons). Similar, but less comprehensive data were amassed during the subsequent 12 months of the fieldwork. The third method adopted was diary-keeping by the doctors for 1 week prior and another week after the introduction of the services. They recorded the amount of time spent on professional activities, plus the times and distances involved in home visiting. Fourthly, samples of the potentially more frequent users of the services, the elderly (over 65 years) and mothers with young children, were questioned before and after the services began about their knowledge, preferences and use of the services. Finally, the study design incorporated control practices, three urban and one urban/rural, drawn from differing regions of England. In these practices the numbers and sites of consultations were recorded and, in one practice, the doctors kept professional diaries for the same 2 weeks as in the experimental practices. The entire fieldwork phase extended over $2\frac{1}{2}$ years, May 1968 until November 1970. The general issue of transport in general practice and the experiences, including costs, of a number of practices, have been reviewed by Bevan, Dowie and Kay [B 48] as a corollary to an investigation into the need for a transport scheme to serve an Oxfordshire health centre.

5.1.2.7. *Investigations*. Data about hospital investigations ordered by general practitioners can be collected at two points: in the surgeries or in the hospital departments where records from numerous family doctors are centralized. (Direct access for most types of tests is now widely available unlike the situation around 1963, Levitt [B 288].) Surgery recordings were presented in the second NMS as rates of investigations ordered by rural and urban divisions of the standard regions [QRL 511]. But there was no differentiation in the tabulations between pathology and radiology requests. Categorizations according to type of test (for example, haematology, bacteriology and X-ray) and purpose (diagnostic or screening) were applied to the recordings of eighteen self-selected doctors in Leicester [QRL 531]. For $11\frac{1}{2}$ weeks late in 1970 they detailed objective and subjective information about their investigations. (Referrals to out-patient departments were also surveyed in this study, see [QRL 248].)

Much more information exists via hospital records about the nature of investigatory workloads created by family doctors. National trends of total usage by GPs of pathology and radiology services are published annually [B 149]. Some of the hospital out-patient studies conducted in the early 1960s examined usage patterns of open access diagnostic departments—these are reviewed in Subsection 5.4.3.1. Radiological referral rates per practice in the Aberdeen area were calculated for 1973 by Mair and colleagues [QRL 444]. A one-in-ten sample of the records from 189 principals yielded the frequency that different procedures were requested, while all referrals in the months of January, June and December were used in the estimation of rates per 1000 patients for each practice.

The effects of the introduction in the mid-1960s of open-access policies on the X-ray departments of two London teaching hospitals were monitored by Cook (Middlesex Hospital [QRL 162]) and Anderson (Guy's Hospital [QRL 22]). Types of examinations ordered and results were included in the analyses of the radiology use of the Cardiff teaching hospital by doctors in a health centre over $3\frac{1}{2}$ years (Wallace *et al.* [B 453]).

An open-access pathology service was made available to GPs in the north-east region of Scotland over 50 years ago. Evidence of the growth in the number of bacteriology, haematology and biochemistry tests performed in The Laboratory, City Hospital, Aberdeen, on behalf of family doctors during selected years between 1959 and 1971 was offered by Porter and Brodie [QRL 547]. All other surveys of pathology department records which provided GP usage rates were undertaken in the early to mid-1960s and are, therefore, likely to under-represent current patterns. The most substantial was Rose and Abel-Smith's analysis of the use made by both family and hospital doctors of the laboratory services in an unnamed English county town in 1966 [QRL 577]. A comprehensive review of published research and arguments surrounding GPs' use of open access pathology services was prepared by Green [B 223].

Investigatory facilities independent of hospital departments are now being provided. The first 2 years of operation of a Cardiff GP X-ray unit which offered a restricted range of tests to 138 doctors were reviewed by Davis and Williams [B 134]. Certain Scottish health centres have been equipped with X-ray units by the SHHD, and two such schemes have been evaluated: Springwell House Health Centre by Howie [QRL 337*] and Woodside Health Centre by Barber *et al.* [B 39]. The Clydebank Health Centre's electrocardiography (ECG) service used by thirty-two GPs was surveyed by Fyfe and Maclean over 29 weeks of operation [B 205]. Details presented included reasons for and frequency of use and outcome regarding patient management resulting from the ECG readings. An alternative type of service, that of hospital-based ECGs directly available to general practitioners, was offered by the Middlesex Hospital. In the first 30 months of operation, starting mid-1965, 429 doctors referred patients [B 411]. Finally, in 1974 a brief reply-paid postcard survey by Bradford [B 58] of 1000 GPs chosen systematically from *The Medical Directory* (for Great Britain) [B 104] yielded a 75 per cent response rate, and one-quarter of the respondents were without ECG services.

5.1.2.8. *Prescribing*. Numerous investigations into the prescribing habits of general practitioners have been conducted in the past two decades. Yet much is still to be learnt about the factors influencing the individual doctor's prescribing rate including the role played by the patients. Various prescribing sources have been used often in combination: family doctors have made special recordings of their activities and in one instance medical records were examined; centralized records of the pricing bureaux have been analysed; and attitudinal material has been collected from both doctors and patients. In the following discussion, studies of overall prescribing patterns precede enquiries about specific drugs, while attitudinal surveys conclude the subsection. (Excluded are sources primarily concerned with prescribing costs. These are reviewed in Subsection 4.5.1.) However, spanning all these topic areas is a report from the Medical Sociology Research Centre of the University College of Swansea [QRL 458] about a multi-phased project into the prescribing behaviour of a cohort of 859 doctors, being all those who entered general practice in England and Wales as new principals between 2 July 1969 and 1 July 1970. These doctors have been the subjects of three postal surveys, although the results from the third, conducted in 1976, were not incorporated in the report. The earlier surveys in 1970–1 and 1972 probed the sources of prescribing knowledge relied upon by these doctors as well as collecting personal and practice details. Forty-five per cent of the cohort participated in both surveys. Another source utilized by the research team was a selection of prescriptions written by the cohort members for at least 1 month during one of the years after the cohort was formed. The Prescription Pricing Authority had supplied the prescriptions to the Unit for Research into Drug Usage in the Department of Pharmacy, Heriot–Watt University, where they were transformed into a computer-readable state before being transferred to the Swansea Research Centre for further analysis. The analyses in the report do though apply only to a sample of 116 cohort doctors' prescriptions for 1 month each, between June 1970 and November 1971. Contained within the report is a collection of papers by various authors covering many topics including: variabilities in doctors' overall pre-scribing patterns; the types of drugs prescribed for various patient age groups; ancillary staff and prescription writing; doctors' views on prescribing information; and a separate investigation into pharmaceutical advertising.

Two decades previously Martin explored some of the social aspects of prescribing [B 310]. He utilized the 1951 data made available by the pricing bureaux for ECs representing sixty-seven medium-sized county boroughs in England. Prescribing variables for each EC were correlated with variables representing practice charac-teristics (for example, age of principals, average list sizes, etc.) and demographic and geographical variables. Martin observed regional variations in prescribing fre-quencies—very high in Lancashire and low in the North-east, Midlands and Southern England. Also it was noticeable that the average total cost per prescription was closely related to the social conditions of the local areas. The investigations in 1961 by Lee and colleagues [QRL 363, 395, 396] found no new explanatory factors for the markedly different prescribing patterns in three unspecified towns in the north of England. Characteristics of practice organizations within the towns and the medical training of practitioners were cross-tabulated against selected prescribing variables.

Anxieties about the steady increase during the mid-1960s in the prescribing of psychotropic drugs, particularly of the tranquillizers and anti-depressant varieties, stimulated the setting-up of another research project based in the Medical Sociology Research Centre, Swansea, which was financed by the MoH/DHSS, and reported by Parish [QRL 522]. A retrospective analysis over a 12-month period of the medical records of general practitioners in a Midlands industrial city was undertaken to determine and interpret the prescribing patterns of drugs under the five psychotropic main headings in the drug analyses published annually by the DHSS—hypnotics (barbiturates); hypnotics (non-barbiturates); tranquillizers; stimulants and appetite suppressants; and anti-depressants. The study design depended upon relatively com-plete medical records to minimize sources of error. (Estimates of under-recorded data are difficult to make, especially as it cannot be assumed that the recording or non-recording of prescribing data are randomly scattered throughout the medical records.) Forty-eight doctors, who claimed to keep careful records, were included in the survey. They represented 37 per cent of all GPs in the city and their average NHS list size was 2758 patients per doctor. A systematic random sample of one-in-ten records gave a total of 13,259 patients, although it was biased towards persons 20–40 years. These patients' medical histories over the 12 months from 1 May 1967 were checked and details extracted about any of the drugs under review. A further stage in the study was the analysis of a one-in-ten sample of 83,585 prescriptions dispensed by the city pharmacists in February 1968. Of the 126 GPs who issued these prescriptions, thirty-five were included in the survey, so this exercise provided some comparisons between the prescribing habits of participating and non-participating doctors, as well as enabling the validation of certain data extracted from the medical records. A similar analysis of psychotropic drugs only, dispensed by city pharmacists in May 1969, was also under-taken. Apart from detailing the characteristics of patients receiving differing drug treatments, the results from the study emphasized inter- and intra-practice variations in the use of various therapeutic subgroups of drugs. The role of ancillary staff in the issuing of prescriptions was also reviewed.

The frequency that psychotropic drugs were prescribed for children under the age of 12 years in a Scottish general practice of five principals and 8290 patients was presented by Bain [B 33]. This specific review of psychotropic drugs was part of an overall analysis of a year's drug prescribing in the practice [B 35], facilitated by the computer-assisted medical records system (see [B 240]) and it highlighted inter-doctor variations.

Corticosteroid prescriptions (excluding those for preparations applied directly to the skin) were accounted for by members of the Wessex and North-east England faculties of the RCGP. The former survey involved 91 doctors who recorded over a 6-month period, July–December 1967, while in the north-east, 154 doctors from 76 practices collected data for the last 3 months of 1970 [QRL 616, 340].

There have been two enquiries regarding chloramphenicol. In the earlier one, the prescribing rates over 1 month only in 1961 of 182 doctors in three English towns were related to indices of education, consultants' assessments and personal interview assess-ments (Meade [QRL 455]). In Northern Ireland, Wade, with the assistance of the Pricing Bureau of the General Health Services Board, was able to retrieve all scripts issued in December 1962 after they had been processed for payment to pharmacists. The advantages of this method were that the quantities of chloramphenicol dispensed could be assessed, and both the prescribing doctors and the patients followed-up [B 446]. The computerized system of prescription processing, installed by the North-ern Ireland General Health Services Board in 1966, has permitted observation of the geographical variations in the dispensing of anti-diabetic drugs [QRL 667], thyroid preparations [B 447], an hypnotic medication [B 448] and chloramphenicol/amphetamines/bronchodilator aerosols [QRL 668].

Doctors' attitudes towards prescribing and the sources of information available to them have been assembled twice in national surveys. Although there was some overlap in the general context of questions asked, the conception of the studies and sample selection methods differed markedly. The earlier study was undertaken during October 1966 by the Government Social Survey at the request of the Committee of Enquiry into the Relationship of the Pharmaceutical Industry with the National Health Service, chaired by Lord Sainsbury [QRL 651]. The survey area was Great Britain and only principal GPs, although no more than one per practice, were eligible. To enable the fieldwork to be completed within the timetable laid down by the Committee of Enquiry, and taking account of the geographical spread of the survey area, a sampled population of about 500 doctors was considered appropriate. So a two-stage sample was applied; first, EC areas stratified according to type of county or borough, followed secondly, by principal GPs in these areas. The sample provided 529 eligible doctors of whom 463, or 88 per cent, agreed to co-operate. When the available characteristics of the non-co-operators were analysed, two independent effects were recognizable, an increase in refusals with age and a decrease in refusals with increasing size of partnership. However, their absence was thought to have had little effect on the results. The topics covered in the interview schedule ranged over sources of prescribing information especially for new products, and the doctor's rate of response in acting on this information. Specific named products were discussed. In addition, respondents were presented with six hypothetical illness situations and were required to name the preparations they were most likely to prescribe, as well as the estimated cost of the dispensed drug (within twenty-five key price ranges). Supplementary data (for example, dates of birth, list sizes and com-position, practice organization, and, in particular, details of prescribing from the latest Annual Review) were made available by the MoH.

The second attitudinal survey of family doctors' prescribing habits formed part of a general enquiry into relationships between patients and doctors with particular refer-ence to medicine-taking. The study was carried out by Dunnell and Cartwright from the Institute of Social Studies in Medical Care [QRL 220]. The first phase of the inves-tigation entailed interviewing between March and July 1969, samples of adults in households in fourteen parliamentary constituencies in Britain. (This phase is described in Subsection 2.5.29.) Of the 1412 adults who complied, 98 per cent were registered with a doctor under the NHS, many with the same doctor. These respondents identified in their interviews 598 GPs as being their 'own' doctor. The initial contact was made with these doctors soon after identification, when a letter was sent explaining the survey and asking for help at a subsequent date. However, it was not until 12 months or so later that questionnaires were despatched. Two reminders yielded a 56 per cent response rate. Comparisons between available information relating to both respondents and non-respondents showed that, apart from a tendency for respondents being younger, there was no evidence of any differences in their prescribing patterns. Many of the questions asked concerned patient self-medication. Policies regarding the issuing of repeat prescriptions were also explored.

Sources of information used by Liverpool GPs when choosing therapeutic actions have been the subject of three enquiries. In 1962 thirty-two to thirty-nine doctors participated in dual surveys by recording their therapeutic decisions for a wide range of diagnostic situations experienced over a week (Wilson *et al*. [B 474, 475]). The most recent concentrated on the adoption of new drugs, 140 doctors being interviewed during 1974 (Williamson [B 473]).

5.1.2.9. *Referrals*. Data on GP referral behaviour can be collected at two sites: in the surgery or at the patient-receiving end—the hospital or other agency. Practice-derived statistics, if accurately recorded, have the advantage of providing a comprehensive overview of referrals to *all* hospitals and other agencies and can be related to the doctor's total workload. In the analysis of hospital-based data, assumptions have to be made about the reliance of local GPs on the hospital's resources. Where there is no well-defined catchment area served by a district hospital, doctors may choose to refer patients to a range of hospitals. This may also apply within compact districts although on a more limited number of occasions, because doctors wish to refer patients to specialties not represented in the hospital or to consultants with unique skills. Referral rates are then of doubtful value if account cannot be taken of the propensity of doctors to refer in this way. Furthermore, if referral rates from differing geographical areas are being compared, account must be taken as to whether all the GPs had direct access to diagnostic facilities. Hospital referrals for consultant opinion are classifiable as in-patient (usually for an emergency admission), out-patient and domiciliary consultation. However, many published studies have chosen to group these categories.

Of the practice-based studies, the most comprehensive to date is the second NMS [QRL 511]—the method of which is detailed in Subsection 2.3.2.2. The 115 participating doctors recorded referrals defined as 'any action taken by the doctor on behalf of the patient to enlist support from outside the practice' (page 18). Six types of referral were recognized: in-patient referrals, being direct admissions to hospital; out-patient referrals for specialist opinion or service, including domiciliary consultations; referrals for investigations initiated by the GP; referrals to local authority services, excluding referrals to local authority staff seconded to the practice; outcome death where the doctor was called to view the body; and other referrals to opticians, chiropodists, dentists, etc. Multiple referrals at the same consultation were noted separately. In the published tables the numbers and referral rates per 1000 population for each type of referral were presented according to sex and age of patients, selected diagnoses and standard region subdivided into urban and rural components. This last breakdown demonstrated the wide variation in GP referral rates which had been observed in various early studies and summarized by Carstairs and Skrimshire [B 87]. Certain referral statistics were included in the overall analyses of the South Wales and south-west England workload studies [QRL 713, 726] and in the Exeter City survey [QRL 37].

Localized multi-practice surveys where doctors recorded workload data specific to referral decisions have been infrequently carried out. Thirty doctors practising in the counties of Berkshire, Buckinghamshire and Oxfordshire examined their referral habits over 13 weeks in 1960 [B 424] and 10 years later, eighteen doctors in Leicester did likewise over $11\frac{1}{2}$ weeks [QRL 248]—they also noted their diagnostic investigations [QRL 531]. For 13 weeks of 1969–70 approximately 100 doctors in the catchment area of the proposed Frimley Hospital recorded referrals to almost all agencies to enable estimates of the demand for health services in the area to be calculated [B 106].

Whenever GP referral material has been extracted from hospital records it has only been a component of a broader investigation into the activities in out-patient departments. In the subsequent reports, the results relating to referrals have been reduced to a single-summary table/graph or merely commented on. For this reason the methods of relevant studies are not detailed here but appear in the discussion on out-patient statistics in Subsection 5.4.3.1.

General practitioner referral patterns to psychiatric services have been examined in occasional local surveys. In their study of psychiatric illness in general practice, Shepherd and colleagues enlisted the co-operation of twenty-four doctors in twelve practices scattered over Greater London [QRL 610]. They agreed to record extra information including referral decisions about each consultation over a 12-month period for a one-in-eight sample of the practice population over 15 years of age. The date of the fieldwork was 1961–2. The study design which included an interview survey of seventy-five GPs is fully detailed in Subsection 2.5.23. The North-east Scottish

Psychiatric Case Register provided baseline data regarding 198 general practitioners' referrals over the period 1963 to 1970. These doctors, too, were approached by questionnaire and, where willing, were subsequently interviewed [B 390]. Some exercises have attempted to link referral decisions with other factors, such as treatment programmes prior to referral (as recalled by patients in Aberdeen, 1965–6) [B 206], and GPs' reasons for referral and anticipated outcomes, plus patients' expectations and performances were noted in Manchester [B 264], and in the Maudsley Hospital catchment area [B 269]. Nine years of referrals to local mental health services from six practices in a South Wales mining valley were scrutinized by Rawnsley and Loudon [B 376].

5.1.2.10. *Sickness certification*. It is usual for certificates claiming National Insurance Sickness Benefit payable in respect of days of incapacity for work forming part of 'periods of interruption of employment' to be signed by medical practitioners. National Insurance sickness benefits available in 1972 were indexed by Whitehead in Volume II of this series [B 459]. The routinely published annual figures [B 149] suggest that sickness certification for extensions of 'old' incapacity episodes, as well as new episodes, is an item of service performed very regularly by GPs. Yet statistical material relating to this activity in general practice is very scarce. No multi-practice studies concerned specifically with this topic are known to have been mounted and reported, although certification rates per 1000-patient contacts (by sex and age group) were published in one paper about the Exeter City 'use of health services' study ([QRL 37] and Subsection 2.3.2.3).

A small number of investigations have been undertaken in individual group practices, but extrapolating the findings into predictions of rates of certification for multi-practices distributed either regionally or nationally would be unwise on several accounts. The composition of the practice populations has often been atypical in terms of ethnic and occupational characteristics. They could, therefore, have been making exceptional demands (either high or low) for certification. Recording periods have infrequently lasted for 12 months; some analyses related just to winter months when sickness absences due to respiratory disorders are at a peak. Too little is known about doctors' compliance to patients' demands in this area, and there is still no way of assessing how representative these research-oriented doctors are of GPs with similar medical qualifications and social backgrounds. There was, however, one London group practice study which drew attention to the considerable magnitude of 'private' sickness certificates (that is forms other than National Insurance Med. 3) which are signed annually by family doctors [B 86].

5.2. Dental practitioner services

5.2.1. *Assessments by individuals of their contacts with dental services*

The three surveys carried out by the Social Survey Division of OPCS, on adult dental health in England and Wales in 1968 [QRL 282] and in Scotland 1972 [QRL 652], and children's dental health in England and Wales 1973 [QRL 650] incorporated questions on perceived usage of dental facilities. The methods employed in each of these surveys are detailed in Subsection 2.5.12. In the adult surveys, respondents were asked about their pattern of usage for checkups, and when they had last attended a dentist; within the last 6 months, 1 year or longer. The reasons which initiated the last visit were probed as well as details of the treatment course pursued but these latter data were only tabulated for England and Wales. The validation exercise in the Scottish survey of respondents' assessments of attendances within the past year, with the records held by the Scottish Dental Estimates Board, was inconclusive owing to numerous difficulties in matching names. One-third of the Scottish adults with some natural teeth claimed to have regular checkups while in England there were marked regional variations. However, there was no apparent definition applied to the term 'regular checkup'. Dental attendances were tabulated against dental health conditions, age and sex, and household social class in both reports.

In the children's dental health survey based on children of the then statutory school age, 5–15 years, all 3137 interviews were conducted with the mother of the child or adult responsible [QRL 650]. Information was sought about possible contacts with school dental clinics, NHS dentists, dentists in private practice, local authority clinics for the under-5-year-olds and dental hospitals. The mothers' own dental-attendance patterns were established. Thus the report related the reported child contacts with the various alternative sources of care, and with mothers' behaviour in this area, plus social class. In the dental examination stage of this study, 12,250 children were inspected.

There had been a methodological forerunner to these national studies, financed by the NPHT, and undertaken in 1963 by a newly created research unit at the London Hospital Medical College (see Bulman *et al*. [QRL 105]). The demand and need for care in Salisbury and Darlington, two areas with relatively high and low ratios of residents to dentists respectively, were measured by interviewing and then briefly examining dentally a random sample of 1156 adults of whom 724 co-operated fully, so giving a response rate in Darlington of 68 per cent and 56 per cent in Salisbury. Variations in perceived usage between the two towns and between social classes were demonstrated.

5.2.2. *Dental practitioner surveys and workload statistics*

There has not been an evident need for *ad hoc* surveys of workload activities of dental practitioners because all dental treatments carried out under the NHS are reported routinely to the Dental Estimates Board via the FPCs. Payment is then made to individual dentists for items of service performed. National aggregated data on courses of treatment and cases of emergency treatment, and the relevant costs, are published annually [B 149, 408, 456], while some statistics for Northern Ireland are in [QRL 502; B 174, 457]. However, as so little detailed information existed about the pattern of dental practice, a survey was mounted in 1972 by Silversin and his colleagues [QRL 612]. A random sample of 'relatively young' dentists, being those who had graduated between 1956 and 1970 from twelve of the sixteen British dental schools (see below), were selected from the British Dentists' Register. The sample was stratified by school and year of graduation, and included 42 per cent of the dentists in the United Kingdom who had qualified between the specified dates, and almost 12 per cent of all dentists.

Postal questionnaires were despatched with three reminder letters where necessary to 2040 dentists. Usable responses were received from 1663 (81·5 per cent). Dentists who worked solely for the local authority dental service, armed forces, university, hospital or industrial practice were asked to return the questionnaire unanswered; 475 did so. In addition, the study encompassed a private practitioner section—all the dentists with practices in the Harley/Wimpole Streets area of London were sent questionnaires and 103 replied. Size of practice and the deployment of dental surgery assistants and dental hygienists, time allocations to various treatments, and the proportions of practice populations under 12 years of age, and percentages of patients receiving treatment either under the NHS or privately, were tabulated.

A complementary publication from this survey by the same authors [QRL 613] concentrated on the pattern of use of dental surgery assistants by respondents. Effective utilization of dental assistants is now recognized as crucial if the dental profession is to meet the demand for care within the NHS. Since there was little evidence of the use being made of dental assistants (or even teaching in the subject in dental schools) this paper was intended to help fill the gap by providing both details of use and attitudes. A dental surgery assistant was in the paper understood to be a person who assists the dentist in his clinical work but does not carry out any independent procedures in the oral cavity. Although these are slim papers, they do provide some insights into the organization of dental practice amongst relatively young practitioners. The initial stage in the study had involved a familiarization of the curricula of twelve undergraduate dental schools in England, Scotland and Wales as at October 1971. At each school, the dean and heads of departments of pedodontics, operative dentistry, periodontology and prosthetics were interviewed. Some final-year students were also questioned. In the published overview [B 414] certain of the findings were compared with aspects of dental education in the United States.

Orthodontics is a well-established subject in undergraduate teaching curricula, and nearly four-fifths of orthodontic treatments are performed in dental surgeries (the remainder being carried out almost equally by the school dental service and the hospital and specialist service). Yet information about the numbers and distribution of dental practitioners carrying out such treatments was lacking until Sheiham and his colleagues analysed all the 1965 orthodontic forms for England and Wales held by the Dental Estimates Board at Eastbourne [QRL 607]. The figures related to practices rather than individual dentists. In Scotland, Haynes examined data provided by the Scottish Dental Estimates Board to assess the rate of discontinuation by patients of orthodontic treatments over the period 1964–71 [QRL 303].

Views about aspects of dental practice were collected from approximately 54 per cent of the dentists who graduated from the London Hospital Medical College between 1920 and the spring of 1968 when the survey took place (Flood Page *et al.* [B 195]). The survey's main purpose was to provide information which might be relevant in a review of the content of dental courses. But included were several questions based on ones used in the 1965–6 survey into the practice organization and well-being of South Wales dentists (Eccles and Powell [B 175]). The 'Old Londoners' paper offered comparative data with the South Wales study before considering ways for improving working relationships for practising dentists and within dental schools. Then in 1975 Craft and Sheiham surveyed dental practitioners in three northern and three southern towns in England to assess their attitudes to preventive dentistry and their use of dental hygienists [QRL 167]. (Note that sources about the geographical distribution of dental practitioners appear in Subsection 4.2.3.)

5.3. Community health services

The activities identified by the DHSS as community health services are health visiting, midwifery, home nursing, tuberculosis visiting; chiropody; family planning; the ambulance service; and the provision of health clinics and centres. Ante- and post-natal care, maternal dental care and vaccination and immunization programmes also come under this umbrella. Routine statistics for these health services, which were administered by local health authorities until Reorganization on 1 April 1974, were published annually and are described in an earlier volume of this series (see [B 14]). An additional source of Welsh statistics was published by the Welsh Office for the first time in 1974 [B 456], while data for certain areas of Northern Ireland were incorporated in [B 174, 457]—see Subsection 5.6.6. Furthermore, the National Health Service Reorganization Act of 1973 laid the responsibility for medical and dental inspection, and treatment of pupils at schools maintained by local education authorities on the Secretary of State for Social Services. Under the Act local education authorities have retained their duty for the ascertainment of children requiring special education, but the NHS provides necessary health staff to enable these functions to be carried out. Until Reorganization, routine statistics on school health services in England and Wales were published biennially in the reports of the Chief Medical Officer of the Department of Education and Science (DES) [B 136]. (These and other relevant routine statistics are also detailed in [B 14].) The final report reviewed the developments in the school health service over the years 1908–74 [B 137].

Until 1974 data on community health services were published annually by the then Institute of Municipal Treasurers and Accountants, but now the Chartered Institute of Public Finance and Accountancy and the Society of County Treasurers. The local health services series commenced in 1949–50, but following the implementation of the Social Services Act, 1970, the title was amended from *Local Health Services Statistics* to *Local Health and Social Services Statistics* [QRL 348]. They were an amalgam of returns made by London boroughs, county boroughs and counties of England and Wales, and the data applied to the year ending 31 March. Detailed for each local authority were the population, and expenditure met from rates and rate-support grants. The midwifery, health visiting and home nursing columns itemized cases and/or visits and costs. The ambulance column covered numbers of persons carried plus costs per person and vehicle mile. For chiropody and family planning, local authority workloads and costs where appropriate were separated out from those of voluntary organizations. The numbers of health centres opened or in the course of construction and the expenditure were also listed. In interpreting the data though, it is necessary to be familiar with the accompanying explanatory notes. For example, in the midwifery statistics, the figures on domiciliary cases included a weighting of hospital deliveries attended by domiciliary midwives after discharge from the hospital—four such confinements were equivalent to one confinement which was cared for completely in a domiciliary setting. The education series, *Education Statistics* [QRL 347], presented the net expenditures on the school health service per 1000 population by each local authority and the Inner London Education Authority.

Prior to Reorganization, Medical Officers of Health were obliged to prepare annual reports about the general state of the public's health in the LHAs under their administration. The contents usually combined a review of vital statistics for the area with workload statistics for the various components of the community health services. Since the great majority of MOsH had a dual role as Principal School Medical Officer for the local education authority, they frequently incorporated analyses of the school health workloads into a single report. The reports, which were variable both in substantive material and promptness in availability, were submitted to the Chief Medical Officers of the DHSS and DES where relevant, who, in turn, relied upon this material and the routinely submitted workload statistics when compiling their own annual and biennial reports [B 152, 136], respectively. (A complete series of MO'sH reports dating from 1945, plus many others from earlier years, is still held by the DHSS library.) Some reports contained descriptions of special projects such as cervical cytology screening programmes, but the findings were often subsequently presented in journals such as the *Medical Officer*, *Community Medicine* and *Public Health*, *London*, all of which have now ceased publication under these titles. The cytology screening programmes in Manchester [QRL 518* and B 403], Nottingham [QRL 526*], Herefordshire [B 273], and West Sussex [B 404] were just four schemes described in this way. (Screening is discussed in Subsection 2.3.1.)

Ad hoc surveys of community-based health services intended primarily to assess the nature of the workloads borne have been infrequent. But as workload data-collecting stages were integrated into a number of manpower studies of home nurses and health visitors, a considerable volume of statistics is available describing the work of community nursing services. However, the relevant major studies are reviewed in the previous chapter on Manpower, Subsections 4.3.2, 4.3.3 and 4.3.4. There is, though, a now dated, but of its kind a unique examination of the work of a comprehensive range of county social welfare agencies—*An Anatomy of Social Welfare Services* by Jefferys [B 262]. During 1960–1, 398 workers in Buckinghamshire were interviewed and, of these, 348 recorded domestic, social, housing and agency details about each contact seen over a period of 1 week (7696 in all). Represented were the National Assistance Board, Ministry of Labour, Ministry of Pensions and National Insurance, hospital almoners, social workers and psychiatric social workers, sections of the county education department, the children's department, probation service and women's constabulary, and the county health department including all nursing services, the home-help service, occupational therapy service, home teachers for the blind, almoners, social workers and welfare officers. Housing authority officials and members of various voluntary services also participated. However, very little statistical material was presented in the publication.

5.3.1. *Assessments by individuals of their use of community health services*

The GHS in all 3 years asked informants whether they or any of their children under 15–16 years had made use of a range of community health services during one specified month, and who had put the users in touch with the respective service [QRL 510, 512,

513]. In the original report the tabulations were: first, a list of fourteen community health services each correlated with source of referral; secondly, six domiciliary services presented as rates per 1000 population by age; and lastly, for persons aged 65 and over, their usage patterns of these six domiciliary services were related to gross weekly household income. The tables applied to respondents in England and Wales for a 1-month reference period. However, in the two subsequent reports relevant tabulations were omitted because of doubts about the validity of the data (Moss, L. 1975, personal communication). The GHS method is detailed in Subsection 2.2.1.2. Questions about individuals' contacts with community health services have appeared in a range of other surveys dealing with specific services or subgroups of the population. Major studies containing such material have been reviewed elsewhere in this volume: *Handicapped and Impaired in Great Britain* [QRL 297], Subsection 2.5.21; *Trouble with Feet* [QRL 146], Subsection 2.5.19; *Life before Death* [QRL 130], Subsection 2.5.32; *Family Planning Services in England and Wales* [QRL 76], Subsection 2.5.18; *Prolonged Sickness and the Return to Work* [QRL 450], Subsection 5.1.1; and *Children's Dental Health in England and Wales 1973* [QRL 650], Subsection 5.2.1.

Validation of reported contacts against records held by the various health agencies is notoriously difficult. Apart from the general problems about the accuracy of recall over a defined period, respondents, in particular the aged, often confuse the identity of the domiciliary visitor. Further, the policy of recording cases only by some services prevents identification of actual contacts made with patients (for example, a health visitor's records may show the total number of cases attended in a year, but not the frequency of visiting to each one which could range from an occasional contact with many patients to very regular visits to some). There is a review of the problem of reliability in the commentary accompanying the relevant tables in the Introductory Report of the GHS [QRL 510].

5.3.2. *Referrals by doctors*

Referrals of patients to the then local authority services were recorded by general practitioners participating in the second NMS ([QRL 511], Subsection 5.1.2.9). Excluded from the recordings were referrals to local authority staff seconded to the doctor's own practice. Unfortunately, there was no differentiation between the types of services called upon. Therefore, in the relevant table only the overall referral rate per 1000 practice population is presented by standard region subdivided into urban and rural components. Individual GPs' referral patterns for home and surgery nursing care in the City of Aberdeen were demonstrated by Richardson [B 384] to be substantially different, the identifiable influencing factors being experience, practice size and age composition, nurse attachment and the doctor's own perceptions of nursing need and nursing skill. Records held by the Aberdeen District Nursing Association showing referrals by each doctor for home nursing care, and records kept in practices with attached nurses giving numbers of new patients referred for nursing attention in surgery premises, were analysed for two 3-month periods in 1972 and 1973.

The effectiveness of sources of information offered to GPs about statutory and voluntary health and welfare services in the mid-1960s were assessed by the

Department of Public Health at the London School of Hygiene and Tropical Medicine, and reported by Anderson and Warren (1966 [B 22] and 1967 [QRL 24]). The project was in two parts. Interviews were conducted in the first stage with GPs (52), MOsH, Hospital Management Committee secretaries, and clerks to ECs in three conurbations including London, three towns and four rural areas in England and Wales. The doctors were asked about their knowledge and use of twenty-three services while the other participants provided details of the information distributed about these services by the relevant authorities. The revelation that so many methods of disseminating information existed, coupled with the wide disparity of knowledge displayed by the doctors even in areas where booklets were supposed to have been circulated, stimulated the setting up of the subsequent stage in the project. The MOsH for thirty-eigh^t LHAs (thirteen counties and twenty-five county boroughs) outlined in postal questionnaires their authorities' methods and frequencies of distributing information. The earlier findings were confirmed—in certain areas, information was only available on request. So a pair of counties displaying contrasting policies were selected for intensive examination. Interviews were carried out with samples of GPs in the two areas, 110 and 95 respectively, and the questioning focused on the five services thought then to be most likely in frequent use: home helps, meals on wheels, mental welfare officers, loan equipment for the disabled, and health visitors. The general problem of how best to disseminate information was highlighted for there was no evidence to suggest that doctors who had been sent a booklet made more recent use of the services than those without such a provision—indeed, many who were recipients of a booklet complained that they had never received any information about services which were described within it. In a converse scheme, a gazetteer of the arrangements of fifty-five general practices was distributed in 1972 to hospital, health authority and social services staff in the Aylesbury area. Later the scheme was evaluated [B 380].

5.3.3. *School children*

Ad hoc surveys of school health workloads have been mainly directed towards the periodic examination system, whereby children are medically examined at intervals throughout their school life. Attention was focused on the need for such a policy in the reports of the Royal Commission on Physical Training in Scotland, and the Inter-Departmental Committee on Physical Deterioration published in 1903 and 1904 respectively, and the principles were subsequently established in the 1907 Education Act. Thus, children were to be examined on entering school at the age of 5 years, again at 7 years and/or 10–11 years, and just before reaching the school-leaving age. Until the early 1950s it was the practice for every child of relevant age to be inspected individually during each periodic examination phase. However, the overall improvement in child health as evidenced from the diminution in the rate of defects detected in the school screenings made the continuation of such a thorough policy unnecessary. Local education authorities were therefore encouraged by the then Department of Education to introduce selective systems although Lee, in the late 1950s, challenged the effectiveness of the school examination system for detecting disorders which would later render boys aged 18 years as unfit on medical grounds for national service [B 285].

By 1965 about seventy authorities had adopted or experimented with alternative school examination schemes. But as no further knowledge existed as to the design of the

schemes, Lunn undertook a survey to collect the requisite information [QRL 418]. Each
of the 174 principal school medical officers in England and Wales in 1967 completed a
questionnaire. Thus amassed were data on the stages in school life at which selective
schemes were used, the numbers of pupils involved in selective schemes and the methods
used to select children for examination. Evaluative assessments of selective as opposed
to routine examination systems were carried out in Birmingham by Asher [B 28], in
Colchester by Barrett [B 41] and by Lunn in Sheffield [B 292]. In all of these enquiries
the examination results of more than 1000 children were scrutinized. More recently, the
general question of the role of the school eye clinic was raised by Ingram with reference
to defects diagnosed in periodic examinations and referred to clinics held in North-
amptonshire [B 259].

Child-guidance services in England and Wales were independently surveyed in 1969
by the Child Guidance Special Interest Group, a group affiliated with the Association of
Psychiatric Social Workers [QRL 143]. The exercise was carried out in response to the
1968 Seebohm Report's [B 328] observation that an urgent assessment was needed of
the country's psychiatric services, their resources, function, relationship to the NHS,
and training of other workers, etc. Three types of child-guidance clinics have evolved as
a consequence of provisions in both the NHS and education services: hospital clinics,
local education authority clinics and integrated or 'joint clinics'. In all, staffing has been
by teams including a psychiatrist as medical director, educational psychologists, and
psychiatric social workers, but the emphasis in the hospital clinics has tended to be
medical, while the stress has been on educational factors in the community-based
clinics. Although the aims of the survey were orientated towards the place and function
of the psychiatric social worker in the Service, an overall picture of current clinic
organization and staffing was obtained. A piloted questionnaire was dispatched in
February 1969 to the head/senior or only psychiatric social worker in child-guidance
clinics and departments of child psychiatry listed in the membership book of the
Association of Psychiatric Social Workers. The response rates were considered satisfactory in the light of the uncertainties in the service at that time; 96 of a total of 134
local education authority clinics and 25 of the 43 hospital departments complied.
Tabulations covered characteristics of staffing and workloads for each type of team
member, sources of referral, waiting lists, provision for special groups of patients and
other facilities. Local education authority and hospital clinics were separated out and
the former grouped according to region.

In 1976 the report of the Committee on Child Health Services (chaired by Professor
S. D. M. Court) was published. The recommendations in Volume I [B 119] cover
aspects of the health care of all children, while Volume II [QRL 728] is a compendium
of statistics relating to the health of children and the provision and use of various
services, drawn from a range of published and unpublished sources.

5.4. Hospital accident and emergency and out-patient departments

5.4.1. *Assessments by individuals of their attendances at accident and emergency and
out-patient departments*

In the GHS of 1971 respondents were asked 'During the months of . . . . ,
. . . . and . . . ., did you (or any of your children under 15) attend as a

patient, the casualty or out-patient department of a hospital (apart from hospital ante- or post-natal clinics)?' [QRL 510]. The average attendance rate of 1·0 per person per year for Great Britain was slightly lower than might have been expected from official statistics provided by central government departments although comparisons were difficult for a number of reasons, notably the official policy of recording each departmental visit as a separate visit, plus the impossibility of calculating from the GHS data the number of multi-attendances. The incomparability of their findings with national workload statistics recorded via routine returns bothered OPCS. Reasons offered included the long reference period on memory for informants and more crit- ically the definitions of out-patient and casualty attendances which are much more precise in hospital terminology than the meanings given to them by the general public. So in a pilot exercise, informants were asked to separate out consultative out-patient attendances from casualty or emergency attendances and visits to ancillary departments such as physiotherapy. The study revealed 'quite extensive inability on the part of informants as a whole, to identify in official terminology the proceedings in which they had taken part when they went to a hospital, other than as an in-patient' (*ibid*.). The question applied in the main 1972 survey was slightly amended to clarify the reference period, but the 1973 question reverted to the original wording although with the age of children changed to 'under 16'. The latter survey included for the first time a series of questions on future out-patient appointments but relevant tabulations were not pub- lished. (The full review of the method adopted for the GHS appears in Subsection 2.2.1.2.)

Cartwright, too, admittedly from a very much smaller population sample, found that her 1964 data on out-patient attendances perceived by respondents suggested a lower average annual rate of attendances including casualty than indicated by the MoH estimates ([QRL 127] and Subsection 5.1.1). On the other hand, Palmer and his colleagues [QRL 521], reporting on the Lambeth population survey in which respon- dents were asked about in- and out-patient experience, commented that when sample results were checked against hospital records the general tendency was for more hospital experience to be reported than recorded. But this may have been a con- sequence of the Inner London population surveyed—validation showed that the hos- pital experience of men was better reported than that of women, especially elderly women, while that of Social Classes I and II was better reported than that of other classes.

5.4.2. *Accident and emergency services*

Accident and emergency departments have been the subject of a number of reviews in the past two decades. In the late 1950s the NPHT sponsored an enquiry by a committee chaired by Dr John Fry, to look at the delivery of services to casualty patients [QRL 252*]. A small team of investigators visited each hospital in fourteen areas of England (that is, twenty main hospitals plus smaller units). Information and impressions were gathered ranging over the topographical background of the areas, the organization and work of the A & E departments, and public opinion as represented by complaints and legal actions. The bulk of the report was descriptive with little of the material presented as statistical tables. A second enquiry was set up about the same time when the Standing Medical Advisory Committee of the Central Health Services Council established an A

& E sub-committee under chairmanship of Sir Harry Platt. The report was published in 1962 [B 325]. To provide this committee with statistics, a survey of NHS hospitals in England and Wales was carried out in the week of 24–31 October 1960. HMCs and Boards of Governors, whose annual returns to the MoH for 1959 showed any casualty work, were requested to arrange for the completion of survey forms in each hospital in the group which had an A & E department. Seven hundred and eighty-nine of the 896 hospitals circularized actually completed records of new patients during the reference period. Emergency admissions only were to be included. Items collected about each new patient at their first attendance were: age and sex; source of case; condition for which treatment was sought; disposal; and medical/nursing personnel seeing patient. In addition, the hospitals recorded the total number of patients attending the department during the survey period. The majority of the tables in the report were aggregated at national level but a breakdown of new patients by regional hospital boards/teaching hospitals and certain urban hospital groups was included.

The major recommendation of the Platt report was that services should be concentrated into units serving population of at least 150,000. These would be equipped and staffed to deal with major injuries and other emergencies day and night. This and other recommendations were adopted as policy by the MoH, and in 1966 the Ministry carried out another survey of A & E departments in England and Wales to assess the revised situation. The results, which were made available in a circular, HM(68)82, indicated that further rationalization in the geographic spread of units was warranted, and so a further directive to hospital authorities was issued in 1968. It stressed that departments treating fewer than 10,000 new cases a year should be the exception—a population of 150,000 was thought to give rise to at least 20,000 new cases annually.

A further national review of the level of provision of A & E departments took place in 1970, this time by the Accident and Emergency Services Sub-Committee of the British Orthopaedic Association [QRL 598]. (Meanwhile, a working party of the Accident Services Review Committee of the BMA was conducting a pilot study in which visits were made to five RHB/BG hospitals to collect evidence on which to base recommendations [B 3].) In this subsequent survey, the hospitals in the 1966 enquiry were recontacted, a questionnaire being addressed to the Consultant in Charge of the Accident Service. Three hundred and thirty-five hospitals were approached but twenty-nine were found to be inappropriate because the accident service had since been closed or amalgamated, or they were specialist hospitals. Questionnaires were returned by three-quarters of the remaining hospitals. Thus the analyses of populations served, workloads, staffing including GP involvement, and accident bed, X-ray, plaster room and operating theatre provisions, appeared to relate to 1969–70 and were usually for a base-line of 228 hospitals.

In September of the same year, yet another A & E survey was conducted in England and Wales, the secretaries of the RHBs and BGs being contacted by the DHSS in conjunction with the Welsh Office. Three forms were completed. Two dealt with regional rationalization and capital development programmes projecting forward until March 1973, while the third detailed the organization and medical staffing of individual major A & E departments and were completed by the relevant HMCs or BGs. (A major A & E department was defined as one normally staffed and equipped to deal immediately with major injuries and other emergency cases at any hour of the day or night.) There were 279 major departments identified as at 30 September 1970, and completed returns were received for virtually all of them. The tabulations related mainly to the existing and future provisions of departments, and various aspects of consultant staffing. The results of this survey were presented as evidence to a subcommittee of the House of Commons' Expenditure Committee, set up in June 1973 to enquire into the siting and staffing of A & E departments, the provision for minor casualty services, emergency road-accident-after-care schemes run by GPs, and the ambulance services [QRL 336]. The report and recommendations were published in the first volume while the second volume contained the minutes of evidence and submissions by many health professional and health administrative bodies including the BMA, RCGP, Casualty Surgeons Association, DHSS, various RHBs, etc. Incorporated in this second volume was an account of a research programme carried out by the Medical Care Research Unit at the University of Newcastle, to examine the social and medical characteristics of patients attending three A & E departments in the Newcastle upon Tyne area, and who were neither admitted to hospital nor had suffered a road accident [QRL 486]. In addition, a sample of patients attending their GPs for the treatment of trauma was interviewed [B 250, 251].

For 1 week in 1968, casualty departments of 126 hospitals in Greater London recorded the day and time of arrival of all new casualty attendances (33,250), plus age, sex, source of referral, type of case, disposal after treatment and whether brought by ambulance. The exercise was carried out on behalf of the Joint Working Group of London created by the Minister of Health to advise him on the co-ordination of the health services as a whole. In accord with the national policy at that time, the group felt that there was scope for some rationalization, particularly in central London, of the night and week-end accident services by concentrating accident services in a few hospitals. However, the paper by Fairley and Hewett [B 184] contained only one statistical table. In both the Southmead health centre treatment room and the nearby hospital A & E department, special records were kept during 26 weeks in 1970 of patients attending with new complaints who were registered with the health centre doctors. The findings were compared [B 160].

5.4.3. *Out-patient services*

5.4.3.1. Ad hoc *studies of the purpose and function of out-patient departments*. A series of studies intended to elaborate the purpose and function of out-patient departments was undertaken in English and Scottish hospitals during the early 1960s. The need for such was made clearly evident at a conference late in 1957 convened by the NPHT to discuss future trends in medicine and the organization of hospital and other health services. Since access to specialist opinion is dependent upon referral by general practitioners, almost all the studies incorporated a component on general practitioner referral patterns to both investigatory and out-patient departments. The study areas and the sponsoring agencies were: Edinburgh, and north-east Scotland by the NPHT; two non-teaching hospitals in south-east England, and Guy's Teaching Hospital financed by the King Edward's Hospital Fund for London; and the nationally-based study of eighty hospitals in nine hospital regions again by the NPHT. All but the last study were reported in 1966 in *Problems and Progress in Medical Care*, Second Series [B 299]. In addition, special analyses were made of out-patient attendances at the Reading hospitals over 3 months in 1958 ([QRL 53*] and Section 3.3) and St. Thomas's Hospital, London, during 6 months of 1964–5 [B 333].

The national study described in *Gateway or Dividing Line?* [QRL 244] by Forsyth and Logan was undertaken for the most part in 1962. The object was to ascertain how out-patient departments across the country functioned and whether they still performed the traditional roles attributed to them. For example, the out-patient department had been seen to serve as the venue for consultation between the personal doctor and the specialist about the patient. But as the GP was rarely present, an adequate system of communication was necessary if the consultation was to be effective. Again, the out-patient department had long served as a site for professional training, as well as enabling patients to be screened by the consultant for in-patient admission. The research team were anxious to see how closely reality matched these historical ideals. If they were now redundant, then the time had come to revise them.

The survey, administered by the Medical Care Research Unit of the University of Manchester, involved eighty hospitals in eleven HMC groups in nine hospital regions. The sampling method was not described in detail, but the aim was to select a minimum number of HMC areas that were representative of industrial and farming communities, communities expanding or declining in population, seaside and inland towns, and where in-patient provision was above and below average. All areas were some distance from teaching hospitals, self-contained, and served a total of two million people. The field work was multi-phased, but the major component was the monitoring of new out-patient workloads in eleven specialties over 1 year. Obstetrics, radiotherapy and dentistry were not covered. A definition of a *new* out-patient which differed slightly from the MoH definition was adopted, that is, a patient referred for the *first* time to a particular specialty, or one who had been referred *before* to the specialty but who had previously been discharged from hospital care or who had not attended for at least 12 months. Patients attending hospital for one episode of illness and referred again with a new complaint were classified as new referrals. Inter-specialty transfers of new patients were classified as repeat attendances rather than new as in the MoH conventions. However, transfers from the casualty department to a specialty qualified as new patients. On the whole these definitions gave little trouble.

Two samples of new out-patients were selected. Every new out-patient attending during every fourth week for a calendar year had data recorded on age, sex, area of residence and referral agent by the records room clerks. Simultaneous recording occurred in all survey areas and 50,000 patients were included. The second sample of new patients provided more detailed information. For fifty consecutive new out-patients referred to each specialist in each hospital group, data were recorded in two stages. On the first attendance, data on age, sex and occupation were collected. After 6 months, provisional and final diagnoses, the attendance pattern for the 6-month period, the rank of doctors consulted, and the disposal of the patient were extracted from the case notes. Further, a sample of those still attending at the end of 6 months was followed up for periods of up to 3 years. Thus these extensive data were available for 13,600 patients who were identical in age and sex distribution by specialty with the 50,000 patients sampled over 12 months.

General practitioners' use of direct access facilities was assessed by extracting from the daybooks of X-ray departments and pathology laboratories information about both the requests and the doctors concerned. This review took place over alternate months during 1962 but it was restricted to 369 family doctors practising within the boundaries of the major local government authorities in each hospital area. Another phase in the study was a survey of 190 consultants and Senior Hospital Medical Officers in ten of the survey areas. The questions covered the allocation and use of time for out-patients, the organization and facilities in out-patient departments, the clinicians' relationships with GPs in this area, and attitudes on domiciliary consultations. One hundred and sixty-four completions were received.

The analyses in the book covered the characteristics of the new patient attenders, appointment waiting times, descriptions of the case loads in the major specialties including use of investigations and outcome, communications between consultants and GPs, and consultant opinions. Referral rates for the 369 GPs were graphed. Analytical material was also presented on the conditions and organization of the out-patient departments in the study areas. Many inadequacies and deficiencies in the arrangements for out-patients in the early 1960s were demonstrated, but it was clear to the researchers that the problems were complex and could not be treated in isolation from the general question of hospital management.

Similar study designs to the national survey described above were adopted in the four regional studies published in the 1966 series of *Problems and Progress in Medical Care* [B 299]. Thus they are reviewed collectively with the emphasis being on the methodological stages. The Edinburgh study [QRL 599] undertaken by Scott and Gilmore covered hospitals administered by seven Boards of Management within the South-eastern RHB. In north-east Scotland [QRL 44], Backett and his colleagues investigated hospital out-patient clinics in the counties of Aberdeen, Kincardine, Banff and Moray together with those in the city of Aberdeen, an area considered to be relatively self-contained as the GPs referred very few patients to departments outside it. The survey of the two non-teaching hospitals in south-east England was carried out from Guy's Hospital Medical School and reported by Chamberlain [QRL 140]. The aim of this study was to assess out-patient care in two hospital groups serving very different areas, an Inner London working-class district and a prosperous provincial south coast area. As much of the data collected was comparable in definition with the fourth study, a concurrent survey of Guy's Hospital, some of the findings from the two exercises were compared in Chamberlain's paper. The Guy's Hospital study (Butterfield and Wadsworth, [QRL 112]) endeavoured to describe the work done in the out-patient departments of a teaching hospital and their relation with the local community and referring GPs. There had been a marked percentage decrease in out-patient attendances at this and other teaching hospitals which was contrary to the overall national trend. However, inter-specialty variations were evident, the more highly specialized clinics such as cardiology attracting higher proportions of new patients compared with the country as a whole.

Data on the personal and medical characteristics and the specialty of *new* out-patients were collected in all four studies. (The MoH definition of a new out-patient was adopted—briefly, a new out-patient was one whose first attendance of a continuous series for the same ailment or single attendance fell within the year under review. Inter-departmental transfers were new at the first attendance in each department, and likewise reattendances after discharge.) The material was either recorded specifically for the study as in Edinburgh where for 1 year *pro formas* were jointly completed by clinic secretaries and clinicians examining the patients, or was abstracted from the hospital records including the correspondence. The fieldwork of the various studies occurred during 1961–3 but over varying periods of time and with a wide range in totals of new patients surveyed—17,860 in north-east Scotland, 15,357 Edinburgh, 1700 approximately in the two southern hospital groups and 1556 for Guy's Hospital. There were variations too in the range of specialties covered in each study, the most restrictive being in north-east Scotland where six only were monitored. This difference must be taken into account if inter-study comparisons are attempted.

General practitioners' usage patterns of open access diagnostic departments were assessed in Edinburgh, the north-east of Scotland and the two south-eastern hospital groups. The last study also examined domiciliary consultation records. A further step in north-east Scotland was the recording of the outcome of investigations ordered at the first consultation for a subsample of 1096 patients at a specific hospital. Interviews were conducted with all but twelve of the 263 general practitioners in Edinburgh in 1963. Furthermore, thirty of these doctors known to be interested in research recorded over an 8-week period their reasons for each referral made together with the dates of the hospital communications. The 'referred' patients were then followed-up for a year and the doctors interviewed about each of them. Chamberlain, too, interviewed family doctors but only a small number in each area. Patient interviews were conducted in Edinburgh usually within 2 weeks of the patients' first visit to hospital. They were chosen at random from all referred patients each week for 2 months in 1962; 139 were interviewed. All the patients in the Guy's Hospital study were interviewed on arrival by lay and medical workers and then again at the point of departure to learn how their time in the department had been spent. Their names were selected from the appointment lists before the clinic sessions were due to begin. At one hospital in north-east Scotland, clinic records were scrutinized to see if DNA (did not attend) patients later appeared at the clinics. The findings suggested that non-attending newly referred patients should be taken into account when calculating GP referral rates from out-patient records. There are, though, inter-specialty variations in non-attendance rates, psychiatry having probably the highest—see the paper on non-attending new psychiatric patients by Hoenig and Ragg [QRL 326*].

There were some methodological problems discussed in the papers. In the Edinburgh study, the sample was based on one recording day weekly for a year, so representing one-sixth of all new patient attenders. But the only way of checking this was by comparing the survey figures with the monthly returns of new out-patients submitted by the hospital records departments to the RHB. Here there were discrepancies, the sample varied from the official recordings in different months from 9 to 15 per cent of the monthly returns. A greater proportion of the discrepancies was thought to be the result of anomalies in the methods used by the hospitals in compiling their returns. The working definition of a new out-patient was found to vary in different departments, as did the methods of providing the monthly data, so confirming the Tees-side experiences of Airth and Newell [QRL 11]. Again, it was the intention in the south-east England non-teaching hospitals study that 1000 patients attending each group should be sampled, but the target was far from reached primarily because of the inaccuracies in the SH 3 returns.

The contributions of the 'local' studies described above, when added to Forsyth and Logan's national description of out-patient activities, have provided a comprehensive overview of this sector as it was in the early 1960s. The north-east Scotland study added an extra dimension in considering the effect of distance from patients' homes and the use made by them of differing hospital clinics. Despite the variability in definitions applied and study designs, the evidence demonstrates the necessity to take into account inter-specialty variations when discussing out-patient services. However, there is now a need for a more interpretative evaluation of the workloads carried in the out-patient sector, especially as the organization of care provided by primary medical practitioners has been so transformed in the past decade. (Note that some sources relating to psychiatric out-patient departments appear in Subsection 5.1.2.9.) The application of Hospital Activity Analysis (HAA) to the monitoring of the workloads of out-patient departments has not yet progressed beyond experimental trials. One such attempt in the Chesterfield Hospitals, under the auspices of the Trent RHA and the DHSS, has been described in a series of reports, most notably [B 440, 441].

5.4.3.2. *Organization of out-patient departments*. The excessive lengths of time spent by patients waiting first, for an out-patient consultation date, and secondly, in the out-patient department to see the consultant or his deputy, have been recognized as problem areas since the inception of the NHS. (The concept of 'waiting time' being an indicator of unmet demand is developed in Section 3.3.) During 1952 thirty-four clinics in nine hospitals were observed—approximately 6800 out-patients. The study was sponsored by the NHPT and the University of Bristol [B 355]. It confirmed a number of impressions. Some patients were waiting for periods of over 1 hour in many clinics, the reception areas of which were often physically uncomfortable. What seemed to be needed was improved punctuality by doctors coupled with a more rational appointments system which was less intent in ensuring that the doctor was not kept waiting for patients. Eleven years later, a more exhaustive study was commenced to review the situation, for it was evident that waiting times still remained a controversial issue in public discussions of the hospital service. A research team from the Operational Research Unit of the NPHT visited sixty hospitals in England, Wales and Scotland [QRL 508]. In total, 12,485 patients were observed of whom 26 per cent were new patients. Also 913 doctors were observed. The number of clinics covered was 474 representing twelve specialties. The results reconfirmed the necessity for doctors to arrive punctually at the start of each clinic, and the need to re-examine appointment block-booking systems.

Soon afterwards, in 1964, the MoH issued a Circular on Management Problems, HM(64)102. One of its purposes was to stimulate HMCs to examine and, where necessary, improve the service offered in their out-patient departments. Two standards were suggested; first, that the waiting time for an appointment should not exceed 2 weeks and, secondly, that the waiting time before seeing the clinician in the out-patient department should be minimized. The NPHT survey (see above) found that in only eleven of sixty hospitals were average waiting periods in out-patient departments acceptable within the context of the Management Circular (that is 70 per cent of the patients were being seen within half an hour of their appointment times and not more than 3 per cent were waiting an hour). HMCs were asked to review their own situation and furnish reports to the RHBs who would then collate them and provide a summary to the Ministry. During 1965–6, Stewart and Sleeman interviewed administrators and nursing and medical staff (173 persons) in a random sample of thirty HMCs in England and Wales. Personnel in fourteen RHBs were also questioned. The researchers wished to know if the Circular was necessary, if it was treated conscientiously by the HMCs and RHBs, and if it made any difference. The findings revealed a considerable apathy amongst hospital authorities towards the workings of their appointment systems. The standard suggested in the Management Circular of a maximum wait of 2 weeks for a non-urgent appointment in all clinics was not met by any of the thirty HMCs. However, Stewart and Sleeman did not question this assumption by the MoH that 2 weeks was the limit of a reasonable time-span [B 425].

Note. Statistics on waiting times for out-patient appointments and time spent in out-patient departments are indexed in the QRL accompanying Chapter 3 on Unmet Demand.

5.4.3.3. *Peripheral consultant out-patient services*. The idea of siting some consultant out-patient sessions away from the confines of general hospitals has been mooted for many years. Lord Dawson of Penn with the members of the Consultative Council on Medical and Allied Services recommended in 1920 that primary health centres should accommodate out-patient clinics conducted by visiting consultants and specialists. A precedent for consultant involvement in decentralized clinics had already been established when the 1912 National Insurance Act encouraged local authorities to construct tuberculosis dispensaries by offering to meet four-fifths of the costs. The National Health Service Act, 1946 embodied the principle of health centres which were to be established by LHAs, and the possible services to be provided in these premises included specialist out-patient activities. Since then, various documents produced by professional bodies, government committees and health-care commentators have argued for the siting of out-patient clinics not only in health centres, but in general practitioner hospitals and in group practice premises. The advantages of such sessions are seen to encompass: convenience to the patients coupled with the reassurance of being seen in a setting already familiar to them; the promotion of personal contact between hospital and community personnel at the time of referral; and the opportunities for mutual education between doctors. The disadvantages cited are usually speculative: the possible dispersal of consultants' time and effort; the necessity to increase medical staff of all grades to provide sufficient cover while peripheral clinics are in session; and the general reluctance of the hospital clinician to leave the confines of the hospital. There are as yet no published statistics on the frequency that out-patient activities are performed at peripheral sites. The *British Health Centres Directory 1973* [QRL 98] indicated the health centres in which RHB consultant clinics were accommodated or planned. (See Subsection 4.1.5 for a description of the method of compilation.)

The out-patient facilities serving a dispersed population resident in the Scottish Border counties of Berwickshire, Peebles, Roxburgh and Selkirk were analysed by Gruer [QRL 285]. In the report Gruer attempted to relate the existing provision of out-patient facilities to the apparent 'demand' of a community. It was carried out in the Department of Social Medicine at the University of Edinburgh, and was financed by the SHHD. There were two parts to the investigation. In the initial stage, a survey of new out-patient referrals was conducted with the intention of first, documenting the existing distribution of out-patient facilities *within* the Border area, and secondly, to investigate the *total* use of out-patient facilities by the Border population. A follow-up survey constituted the second stage. Here the aim was to learn about the events in the year following the first out-patient attendance for a sample of patients referred during the first survey.

In 1969 out-patient clinics within the Border area were held at one general hospital (Peel), five GP hospitals, two other clinic sites administered by the Border Hospital Board of Management, and LHA clinics at fourteen sites. Out-patients from the Border counties were also seen in the departments of hospitals in Edinburgh the regional centre, and a few were referred to towns fringing the counties. A record form was completed jointly by the clinic secretaries and clinicians for each new out-patient attender (using the HS 10 definition) at the Border hospital clinics over a 3-month period, April to June 1969. Excluded were psychiatry, orthodontics, physiotherapy, X-ray, casualty and antenatal attenders. The medical records of the LHA clinics and the Edinburgh and East Lothian hospitals were searched retrospectively—in the hospitals, appointment clerks had assisted by noting patients with Border addresses. General practitioners with patients residing in the Border counties were asked to detail their referrals over a 2-month period to hospitals outside the study area. A validation check showed that it was reasonable to assume that all patients seen as new referrals in Border hospitals were recorded in the survey. However, in the only check that could be made in Edinburgh, in one clinic a discrepancy of 18 per cent was observed over the first 3 weeks of the survey. Thus it had to be assumed that the total number of referrals to Edinburgh may have been underestimated. In the second stage of the study, a retrospective survey was carried out on the hospital clinical records of a stratified random sample of patients from the Border counties 1 year after the date of their first out-patient consultation. The categories applied in the stratification were: patient discharged at first visit, patients with selected diagnoses, remaining patients referred to Edinburgh, and remaining patients referred to Border clinics subgrouped according to distance of clinic. There were 2106 patients in the first survey from whom 831 were sampled for the follow-up survey. The adequacy of the local clinic sessions to cope with the Border community's demands was estimated for each specialty. Only for orthopaedic surgery did the Border clinic scheduling appear to be sufficient to cope with all new referrals. Coupled with the movement of patients to Edinburgh clinics was a commitment by Edinburgh consultants to travel into the counties to hold clinics in six specialties. From the data, Gruer constructed models of alternative arrangements of out-patient facilities for the Border counties to estimate costs; first, to the NHS (that is, the time spent by consultants on travelling to clinics outside their base hospitals) and secondly, to the community by patients attending hospital.

5.5. Hospital diagnostic and pharmaceutical departments

5.5.1. *Pathology and radiology services*

Gross workload figures for pathology requests and radiology examinations are published annually and were reviewed in [B 14]. *Ad hoc* studies of hospital departments have been few if reviews of the workload component created by general practitioners in response to direct access policies are excluded (Subsection 5.1.2.7). In 1959 the Operational Research Unit of the NPHT considered the organization of diagnostic

X-ray departments [B 357]. The fieldwork consisted of examining in depth the operation of six departments serving hospitals of varying bed complements and included
were two teaching hospitals, one of which was in Scotland. Patients' progress through
the departments was timed, radiographers were studied in depth and a range of
supporting staff (for example, porters, dark-room technicians, filing clerks) were also
observed. From the material amassed, the research team was able to define nine
principles, the last being that 'there should be regard for the patients' point of view'. A
broad range of recommendations to local authorities was also devised.

The organization of hospital pathology departments was of concern to the Association of Clinical Pathologists' Committee on Hospital Organization. It was realized that
before answers could be given to questions about how new equipment could be used to
cope with increasing demands, it was necessary to have a greater understanding of the
current activities in pathology departments. With this purpose in mind, Rose and
Abel-Smith undertook an intensive enquiry into the use of pathology services in one
hospital group [QRL 577]. With finance from the DHSS, a random sample of the
records of over 3000 patients referred to pathology laboratories in 3 months of 1966
were analysed. The study area (unnamed) was a hospital group (without a teaching
hospital near by) serving 0·3 million people. The analysis of the hospital clinicians'
demands on the group's laboratory resources showed that they made two-thirds of all
requests but their patients constituted fewer than half of all investigated patients. There
were, however, marked variations in inter-specialty use and between in-patient and
out-patient demands. Even within specialties, clinicians' usage rates were noticeably
different.

Ashley, Pasker and Beresford took up this last point and endeavoured to see if
intra-specialty variations were due to the case mix of individual consultants [QRL 41].
They set up an enquiry into investigation usage which was disease oriented. Fifteen
common diagnoses were selected—six medical and nine surgical including orthopaedic
and genito-urinary diseases. In eight acute district general hospitals in the south-east of
England, cases were drawn from diagnostic indices and operating-theatre registers. The
sample size was unstated and there was no comment as to the source of the referral
(in-patient, out-patient or casualty). In all 1824 cases were examined and details of
pathology and radiology and their constituent tests were recorded. Significant
differences between hospitals were observed in their use of pathology in eleven diagnoses, and in the use of radiology in ten diagnoses. Although this was a small study, it
demonstrated how much still needs to be understood about the clinical activities of
hospital specialists before any system is designed to ration diagnostic facilities.

The sputum cytology service in England and Wales was surveyed by Oswald and his
colleagues [QRL 519]. Almost all of the 231 laboratories completed questionnaires
during 1972–3; they had been identified by the RHBs and then the director of each was
asked by telephone to collaborate in the study. The tabulations spanned workload
statistics for 1971 including source of specimens, staffing levels and laboratory procedures and results for 1971.

The functions of the chest services in Scotland were reported on by a subcommittee of
the Scottish Standing Medical Advisory Committee in 1973 [QRL 602]. Data on the
medical staffing in respiratory diseases and tuberculosis were obtained by members
visiting the five hospital regions. In addition, a survey was undertaken of chest clinics and
out-patient departments. The clinics were separated into four groups according to the

total number of attendances for 1969, and twenty-two were selected. In each the attendances were monitored over periods of 4 to 8 weeks early in 1971. Completed forms totalled 1591. Each patient record form incorporated the source of the referral, the principal diagnoses, type of attendance, investigations requested and disposal. Information was also collected on about 301 attendances during which the patient did not see a member of the medical staff (these being tuberculosis contact cases, patients receiving routine medication or attending for X-ray only). References have already been made in Subsection 2.5.33 to the review of the mass miniature radiography service in Scotland (1949–69) by Carstairs and Howie [QRL 124] and to Heasman's analysis of the first 3 full years of data (in the mid-1950s) relating to the mass radiography service in England and Wales [QRL 305].

5.5.2. *Pharmaceutical services*

Although the total annual expenditure on drugs by English hospital authorities was about £43 million in 1973–4, *ad hoc* statistics on the workloads borne by the hospital pharmaceutical service seem to be unpublished. There have, of course, been a number of investigations into the prescribing and administration of drugs in individual hospitals and psychiatric units for example [QRL 313*; B 127, 128, 331]. The report of a working party set up by the DHSS, SHHD and the Welsh Office to advise on the efficient and economical organization of the hospital pharmaceutical service contained a statistical appendix in which were detailed hospital pharmacists and pharmaceutical students, and pharmacy technicians and student technicians in post on 31 August 1968 ([QRL 197] and Section 4.4).

5.6. Hospital in-patient services

5.6.1. *Assessments by individuals of their contacts with hospital in-patient services*

Once more, the GHS for the years 1971, 1972 and 1973 have provided the largest enumerations of persons' experience with in-patient provisions ([QRL 510, 512, 513] and Subsection 2.2.1.2). In all the surveys respondents were asked if in 3 specified months, they or any children under 15 (under 16 in 1973) were in hospital as a patient, overnight or longer. Follow-up questions probed the numbers of days or nights in hospital altogether, the category of patient (medical, surgical, maternity) or cause, and, except in 1973, the name and town of the hospital. (Recording spaces for two to three visits were allocated on the schedule.) In the first survey, the dates of admittance were asked, for it was the intention to compare the GHS in-patient data on discharge during the reference period with official statistics. However, too few persons could remember the exact date they went into hospital so it was decided in the subsequent surveys merely to ask in which month the person left hospital. The 1973 survey enquired if patients were NHS or private. Only one table was published in each of the reports—the number of medical and surgical in-patient spells per 1000 persons in a 3-month reference period, and the average number of in-patient days per spell, by sex and age.

The most exhaustive attitudinal survey to date on patients and hospital care is

Cartwright's book, *Human Relations and Hospital Care*, first published in 1964 [QRL 126]. The main fieldwork funded by the NPHT was multi-phased and extended over 1960–2. In twelve randomly selected parliamentary constituencies in England and Wales, every twenty-second person on the electoral register was sent a letter. There was some stratification based on urban/rural characteristics and region in the selection of the constituencies. The letters requested knowledge about whether or not the individual to whom it was addressed had been to hospital as an in-patient at all during the 6 months October 1960–March 1961. A tear-off strip at the bottom of the letter form was to be completed indicating yes/no and where relevant, a new address. Altogether 29,400 persons were approached. Eighty-seven per cent replied of whom 3·8 per cent had been in hospital. Attempts were then made to trace each of these 1119 self-identified persons. On enquiry, 15 per cent were found to be ineligible usually because either their hospitalization occurred outside the reference period or, they had completed the form on behalf of another family member—a problem which bedevils many postal surveys. Despite the seemingly high overall non-response rate of 29 per cent, Cartwright was reasonably confident from other evidence that the estimated hospitalization rate derived from the people who did reply was reasonably accurate. Of the 739 patients who were interviewed, just under two-thirds were women. Sixteen per cent of these patients had been maternity cases, 47 per cent were surgical patients and the remainder, 37 per cent, medical patients.

Complementing the patient survey was an interview survey of general practitioners chosen from the same twelve constituencies as the patients. A random sample of twelve doctors per area was selected from lists supplied by ECs responsible for primary medical services in the local areas. Successful interviews were carried out with 124 doctors. The book is organized in sections integrating material from the two surveys. Assessments of in-patients usage were also made by respondents in the local surveys of Bermondsey [QRL 669], and Lambeth [QRL 521]. It was found in this latter study that respondents' recall of in-patient experiences was much more reliable than their assessments of contacts with out-patient departments.

5.6.2. Ad hoc *studies of the use made of non-psychiatric in-patient services*

The routine statistics from the Hospital In-patient Enquiry (HIPE) reviewed in [B 14], and now from the HAA have offered comprehensive analyses of how in-patient services are utilized. Consequently, the need for expansive (national or regional) *ad hoc* enquiries has been minimal. There have, of course, been *ad hoc* studies into the provision of in-patient resources to meet the demands of communities and these are reviewed in Subsection 4.1.2. They contained some material on the use made by local populations of existing services and drew attention to the variables most likely to affect demand—notably the current bed provision. Recently though, attention has been focused upon the question of *why* these services have been utilized in this way, and more pertinent, whether it represents the optimum use. In 1971 Heasman and Carstairs published a paper reviewing variations in some aspects of consultants' in-patient management in Scotland. Considerable variations were observable in the length of stay, the time spent in hospital before or after operations and the proportion of patients operated on in surgical units. The authors concluded that 'the differences could be due to great variation in the constraints encountered by the consultants in their work, or to wide differences of opinion about the optimum treatment for specific diagnoses' [B 242, page 495]. Their data were displayed graphically.

Certain studies have enumerated long-stay patients occupying beds designated as 'acute' and have sought to provide explanations using evaluation techniques—see both Section 3.5 and Subsection 6.2.4.3. One such exercise was in the extensive Liverpool investigation (reviewed in Subsection 4.1.2). The results were reported by Butler and Pearson in a separate publication, *Who Goes Home?* [QRL 109]. Patients staying in an acute ward for longer than 30 days were classified as long-stay. A point prevalence survey of each hospital in the Liverpool Region containing beds officially classified as acute was carried out and all long-stay patients in those beds at the time of the survey were enumerated. Information about each patient was collected from the case records and from interviews with the nursing staff, medical staff and, where appropriate, the social work staff. In addition, the nursing staff were asked to complete a Nursing Dependency Form for each patient relating to the day of the interview. Apart from personal details and clinical histories relating to eligible patients, the two-person interviewing team sought opinions about the most appropriate type of care to meet the patient's current needs and where this was not acute care, the reason that prevented the patient's transfer. Thirty-seven hospitals yielded 1106 eligible subjects.

The Scottish Hospital Centre conducted a study in forty-two hospitals in Scotland to assess the need for 'supporting' beds as demonstrated by the number of patients who might be more suitably accommodated in such beds rather than in 'acute' ward units [QRL 459]. The hospitals (which included eight teaching hospitals, eight district general hospitals (DGH) and 'convalescent' and small general hospitals) were surveyed in 1966–7. In all, 4350 beds were enumerated in representative wards undertaking general medical, surgical, orthopaedic and gynaecological work. As well as a census, assessments were made of the medical and nursing dependencies of patients from clinical and nursing records and discussions with staff, but it is not clear if all of the patients in the census were also viewed at the bedside. This exercise demonstrated the necessity to gather material supplementary to questionnaires completed by staff who may not be aware of their own influence in making a patient dependent.

Excess bed use (here defined as 50 days or more) of persons aged 65 years and over in acute, geriatric and mental illness hospital units was assessed by Downie in an analysis of hospital in-patient statistics for Scotland predominantly for 1966 [B 167]. Some comparative data with England and Wales were presented. Using the same definition of a long-stay patient as Butler and Pearson (see above), Sutherland surveyed long-stay admissions to eight acute medical wards of three Aberdeen hospitals between 1967 and 1968 [QRL 633]. A number of small studies have examined the possible substitution between general hospitals (consultant care) and GP-managed hospital beds. References to these are made in Subsection 5.6.4.

A special census of children and adolescents in non-psychiatric wards of NHS hospitals in England and Wales was taken on 24 June 1964, and repeated on 24 March 1965, to learn of 'welfare' practices implemented for this category of patient [QRL 474]. Two censuses close together were considered necessary as a check on reliability. Forms circulated to all non-psychiatric hospitals were completed for every ward where a patient under 17 years of age was occupying a bed on the morning of the census date. More than 22,000 patients were covered in each census of whom four-fifths were children under 12 and the remaining fifth adolescents aged 12 to 16 years. 'Welfare' questions included arrangements for parents to stay at hospitals with their children, and whether tuition was available to children and adolescents able to profit by it.

In Wales during 1971–2 a multi-disciplinary enquiry into the welfare of hospitalized children was undertaken. Included in the material amassed were two surveys, one of children who had been recently discharged and the other on families of long-stay in-patients (mental subnormality and chronic sick). The study was reported by the Welsh Hospital Board in 1972 [QRL 707], but in the research team were members of the sociology department of University College, Swansea, and they have prepared a further publication [B 173].

5.6.3. *Emergency bed services*

The Emergency Bed Service (EBS) covering the Greater London boroughs enables family doctors to admit promptly to hospital a patient suffering from an acute medical or surgical condition (other than an accident) if the doctor himself has not been successful in securing a bed. The organization of the service is such that if the EBS operation-room staff are unable to locate a bed in health districts nearest to the patient's home, the regional medical admissions officer on duty intervenes. The officer can suggest to the referring doctor that the case be held back overnight ('referral back') and the doctor then reapplies for a bed, or seeks a domiciliary consultation or an urgent out-patient appointment. Alternatively, for more urgent cases, the details of the case are passed to a medical referee who is a doctor nominated by the health district closest to the patient's address. This usually results in admission. In the mid-1960s Warren, Cooper and Warren [QRL 691] were concerned to learn of the frequency that cases were referred back (that is, the demand for in-patient care was unmet, see Section 3.3). They followed up all of these cases (395) over a 12-month period from April 1965 and compared their details with those of a one-in-ten sample of patients who were admitted after scrutiny by a medical referee (702), and a one-in-fifty sample of controls—persons who were directly admitted (935). (There were 46,600 admissions via the EBS during the year.) Basic information was collected from the EBS records within 4 days of the occurrence of the event and the GPs reponsible for the 'referred back' patients were contacted.

Trends, both monthly and annually, in the numbers, and sex and age composition of the applications to the EBS between 1966 and early 1975 were plotted by Bates and Sharratt [B 495]; they showed a gradual reduction in the total workload. (The EBS covers about 200 hospitals and is administered by the King Edward's Hospital Fund for London but receives financial reimbursements from the four Thames RHAs. There are comparable emergency services operating in Birmingham and Liverpool.)

5.6.4. *General practitioner hospital services*

The future of these units was first thrown into doubt by the recommendations in *The Hospital Plan for England and Wales*, 1962 [B 324] and this uncertainty (which was reinforced by a DHSS Memorandum on the role of community hospitals in 1974 [B 156]), coupled with closures of some hospitals, stimulated a series of workload studies.

Family doctors and independent researchers attempted to measure the appropriateness of hospital care managed by GPs for different categories of patients. Differing methodological approaches were adopted by Smith and colleagues, and Trevelyan and Cooke when making comparative studies of patients in general and community hospitals. In the former study [B 416] a sample of the patients (908) admitted in the course of a year to two DGHs was analysed and compared with a similar sample of patients admitted to a GP hospital. The aim was to assess if the type of care provided in the GP hospital was appropriate for the cases treated and an independent assessor was engaged. In the Basingstoke study, Trevelyan and Cooke followed the in-patient experiences of 171 persons who had been admitted to two acute wards in a local cottage hospital and a consultant medical ward in the newly completed Basingstoke District General Hospital [B 439]. Recordings were made about the patients' condition at the time of admission and discharge, and the services used, while the referring family doctor was invited to give reasons for the type of hospital care selected for each patient. In 1971 Robinson [B 391] conducted two censuses of patients in twenty-four of the twenty-five eligible GP hospitals in the South East Metropolitan RHB. Supplementary material from case notes, and from interviews with staff, was collected about 326 patients. In Oxfordshire a study evaluating the role of the community hospital was mounted by the Oxford RHB, later the RHA and the DHSS, with much of the research being conducted by members of the Department of the Regius Professor of Medicine, University of Oxford. The project was outlined in a paper by Oddie and his colleagues [B 359] while the cost effectiveness of the trial was reported by Rickard [B 387]. In another paper, Bennett reviewed the role of community hospitals from the evidence of various studies [B 46].

5.6.5. *Mental handicap and mental illness services*

Statistical data about the comprehensive hospitals and units (in non-psychiatric hospitals) serving the mentally ill and the mentally handicapped in England and Wales are collected as part of the MHE and are published regularly [B 157]. Maynard and Tingle [B 313] critically assessed the usefulness of these and other routine statistics relevant to the mental health services while Bone, Spain and Martin [B 56] paid particular attention to the uses and limitation of official mental-handicap statistics available up to 1968. Maynard also calculated the 1969 regional staffing ratios for both medical and nursing staff in psychiatric hospitals [B 312]. An exhaustive history of the mental health services from 1744 to 1971 by Jones was published in 1972 [B 267]. The tenet of current psychiatric policy in the NHS is the transference of the treatment and management of mental illness and mental subnormality from the specialist hospital to psychiatric units in DGHs and to 'community' facilities. Several documents have set out the objectives regarding future targets for bed provision in hospitals and community residential units, occupational opportunities and training programmes, and educational facilities for mentally handicapped children of school age—see *Better Services for the Mentally Handicapped*, 1971 [B 155]; *Hospital Services for the Mentally Ill*, 1971 [B 142]; *Services for Mental Illness Related to Old Age*, 1972 [B 146]; and *Better Services for the Mentally Ill*, 1975 [B 151].

Data collection for the MHE commenced in 1964 with the recording of patient statistics on forms SBH 112. Statistics relating to facilities and services were added to the forms in 1965. Immediately prior to the commencement of the MHE a census of patients in psychiatric beds was carried out on 31 December 1963 by the General Register Office, and reported by Brooke [QRL 97]. Enumerated were all patients in psychiatric beds—a psychiatric bed being defined as a bed under the care of a psychiatrist. Included were hospitals for both the mentally ill and the subnormal, and those in psychiatric units in general hospitals, including special teaching hospitals. Items requested for each patient were: sex, age, date of admission, type of resident, legal status, first or other admission, mental category, diagnosis and marital status. Censuses similar in design to this but specific to mental illness patients or the mentally handicapped were subsequently carried out and so they are separately detailed in the following subsections. Ten years previously, Brooke had undertaken a cohort study over a 2-year period of patients first admitted to mental hospitals in 1954 and 1955 [QRL 96*]. Age, sex and diagnosis were tabulated against area of residence of patients. The analysis was then repeated for the 1957 admissions [B 212].

5.6.5.1. *Censuses of mentally handicapped patients.* At the end of 1970 a census of mentally handicapped patients in hospitals in England and Wales was taken by the DHSS and the Welsh Office [QRL 188]. It was necessary for two reasons. First, the census of psychiatric hospital patients carried out in 1963 to serve as a base-line against which estimates could be derived from the MHE was somewhat dated. Secondly, with the increased awareness of the needs of these patients (see the Command Paper, *Better Services for the Mentally Handicapped* [B 155]) more meaningful statistics were required by planners—statistics on the range of physical, sensory, behavioural and other incapacities of the patients, and on their education, training and occupation. Amongst patients in mental handicap hospitals, a systematic one-in-three sample was selected, while there was a full enumeration of all mentally handicapped patients in other NHS hospitals and in contractual beds as identified by the RHBs. The actual number of returns made was 26,064 representing 65,520 patients.

The design of the questionnaire was governed by two factors. It was important to be able to relate the results to those from the MHE so certain questions had to conform. New questions on education, training and employment were asked as well as incapacity questions adopted practically unchanged from those developed and used in the Wessex Mental Subnormality Survey (Kushlick and Cox [QRL 381*] and Subsection 2.5.24); they were completed by the hospital staff from the knowledge of the patients. The grading of incapacities into degrees of severity was done from the recorded answers by the DHSS. However, the Department itself did not undertake any fieldwork to test the reliability of the answers. The report did not state how the census was managed within individual hospitals. Definitions were, though, provided. Also conducted in England and Wales during 1970 was an enumeration of mentally handicapped (and mentally ill) persons in residential accommodation provided by local authorities under Section 12 of the Health Services and Public Health Act, 1968, or run by non-profit-making organizations and registered under Section 19 of the Mental Health Act, 1959 [B 334].

There had been an earlier mental handicap census intended to fill the gaps in the knowledge about these patients. The sponsoring bodies—the National Association for

Mental Health, the National Society for Mentally Handicapped Children and the Spastics Society—felt that the 1963 base-line census for the MHE was very disappointing in its treatment of the mentally handicapped. So to fill the gaps, Bone, Spain and Martin enumerated retrospectively patients in all hospitals for the mentally handicapped administered by RHBs in England and Wales at the end of 1964. The questionnaires were dispatched to the hospitals in July 1965 and there was a 97 per cent coverage of the special interest group—the patients resident in hospitals for the mentally ill administered by RHBs [B 56].

The provision of services in an unidentified RHB for the mentally handicapped was examined by a multi-disciplinary research team [B 268]. The fieldwork, which commenced in 1971, was in stages, and one involved team members visiting each hospital and small unit to collect descriptive material via the completion of schedules and discussions with staff. Later detailed investigations were made of specific topics such as 'back wards' and community care.

5.6.5.2. *Census of mental illness patients.* This was carried out in mental illness hospitals and units in England and Wales at the end of 1971 [QRL 201]. It was a companion to the census of mentally handicapped patients in hospital undertaken 12 months previously (see above) and together they provided updated base-lines for the MHE. The need for a new census to supplant the data from the 1963 census described in Subsection 5.6.5 was accentuated by the falling rate in annual in-patient residents per 1000 population ($3 \cdot 4$ to $2 \cdot 3$ between 1954 and 1971), coupled with the practice of the DHSS of estimating the numbers of in-patients resident at the end of each year by using admission and discharge statistics from the MHE to extrapolate the 1963 results. Furthermore, only a few estimates of patient numbers according to characteristics were feasible; sex, age, length of stay in hospital and region. Thus new data collected in the 1971 census included diagnosis and the extent to which in-patients were engaged in some form of occupation.

An individual questionnaire was completed for all patients in the MHE in the special units or wards for children, adolescents, alcoholic addiction and drug addiction and all other patients under 20 years of age. But for adults aged 20 years and over who were resident or on short leave in mental illness hospitals and units other than those described above, a one-in-three sample was taken. The procedure was that the names of all in-patients at midnight 31 December 1971 were listed on one of three types of nominal rolls. The first two types related to patient groups requiring full enumeration and the third roll was used for selecting the sample of adults. On these sheets, an asterisk appeared against every third line. A questionnaire was completed for the person whose name was entered on the line. The brief description of the method in the report does not state whether the names were entered alphabetically, the definitions that applied to various questions (apart from the coding of the diagnoses and broad diagnostic groups) or which hospital staff were responsible for completing the questionnaires. In the report there is an important rider regarding the interpretation of the data from this and other censuses or point prevalence studies. The figures represent the situation at one point in time. They do not indicate the pattern of events over a period. An example was given where misinterpretation could occur: 65 per cent of in-patients in the census were shown to have been in hospital for 2 years or more, but this did not mean that about two-thirds of all in-patients stayed for at least 2 years. Indeed, during 1971, 85 per cent of patients discharged stayed less than 3 months. Appended to the report is a description of a census of mental illness *day* patients in England and Wales as at April 1972—see Subsection 5.7.2.

As a precursor to a detailed investigation of industrial therapy, all mental illness hospitals with over 100 beds in England and Wales were surveyed to establish the volume and variety of industrial therapeutic practice [QRL 685]. The exercise was conducted by Wansbrough and Miles under the auspices of the King Edward's Hospital Fund for London. Of the 122 hospitals to which a questionnaire was sent in 1967, seventy-four complied; twenty-two did not have an industrial unit. Collected were data on the type of work done, payment and usage figures.

5.6.5.3. *Long-stay patients and case registers.* The reservations about the NHS policy proposals to decentralize psychiatric care into general hospital units and community facilities have prompted some appraisals about the social and medical characteristics of mental hospital patients, particularly those identified as long stay (see, for instance, the review by Brown of the role of mental hospitals [B 72]). Bewley and his colleagues enquired about the outcome of patients 20 months after a census at the Tooting Bec Hospital, London [QRL 66* and B 199]. From the Camberwell psychiatric case register material Hailey investigated 6 years later those patients identified in the original 1964 census as being long stay (having already been an in-patient continuously for 12 months or more). Over half were still in hospital [B 227].

Longitudinal psychiatric case register projects, notably in Newcastle, Wessex, South-ampton, Nottingham, Aberdeen and Camberwell, have amassed a wealth of data about local communities' use of mental services. Both the Camberwell register (1964 to 1971) and the Aberdeen project (1963 to 1970–1) have been reviewed in collections of papers; [B 477] relating to the former register, and [B 37, 38] to the latter. Statistics from these projects on lengths of in-patient stay are indexed in the QRL accompanying Subsection 6.2.4.3.

5.6.6. *Non-central government routine in-patient statistics*

The Northern Ireland Hospitals Authority produced annual reports until September 1973 [QRL 503]. (The twenty-fifth report was for the year ended 31 December 1972, and the final report was published the following year.) The primary duty of the Authority was to administer the hospital and specialist services and ancillary services in Northern Ireland on behalf of the Minister of Health and Social Services. Thus it was responsible for: hospital accommodation; medical, dental, nursing, social and other services required at or for the purpose of hospitals; drugs, medicines and equipment needed by hospitals; invalid carriages or other similar vehicles; and appliances. The deployment of specialists' services, and the provision of accommodation and services under the Mental Health Act (Northern Ireland) 1961, were also the Authority's charge; likewise the facilities for clinical medicine/dentistry research and teaching at the Queen's University of Belfast. Other services which it administered were ambulance, pathology, diagnostic radiology, blood transfusions and tuberculosis care in hospital and clinics. The annual reports provided both a descriptive overview and statistical appendixes covering these areas of responsibility.

From October 1973 the Northern Ireland health and personal social services were restructured, so integrating the former hospital and specialist services with local health authority, port health, school health, local authority welfare, child-care and general health services. The management and delivery of these services rests with four health and social services boards, each of which is geographically co-terminous with a number of the new local government districts. The earliest of the annual reports prepared by the boards [B 174, 457] contained hospital workload statistics, for example, in-patient admissions and waiting lists, out-patient and A & E attendances, and units of work for physiotherapy and X-ray. Additionally, they included a wealth of community health and social services statistical tables—vital statistics, immunizations, school medical inspections, child health clinics and health centres, community nursing workloads, etc. Annual reports of the Department of Health and Social Services for Northern Ireland will be published in due course (see Chapter 4).

Prior to 1974, certain RHBs and BGs published annual reports detailing hospital in-patient, out-patient and other workload statistics for individual hospitals and clinics, as well as, in some regions, LHA/school health service clinics staffed by consultants in the employ of the RHB. The range of data corresponded closely to the SH 3 returns made annually to the DHSS. So for each specialty there might be statistics on: staffed beds allocated; average daily number of beds available and occupied; discharges and deaths; waiting list sizes; throughput per average available bed; annual number of out-patient clinics; new out-patients; and total attendances. Other inclusions could be data about radiology and pathology, day patient, and A & E statistics, plus a separate section on mental illness hospitals. Three of the RHBs producing such volumes were Sheffield, South Western and South East Metropolitan [B 413, 420, 418]. Some statistical material has been incorporated in the earliest available annual reports of certain RHAs and AHAs.

Health-service directories usually contain information about hospitals, clinics and health centres (including bed provisions where relevant), as well as detailing administrative arrangements and personnel. The *Hospitals and Health Services Year Book* issued annually by the Institute of Health Service Administrators is a 'directory' of the NHS [B 96] and it has often been used as the basis of a sampling frame. The edition for 1975 was considerably modified to take account of Reorganization in April 1974. Thus the contents include a directory of government departments with responsibilities for health throughout the United Kingdom, and a directory of statutory bodies concerned with the provision of health services. A series of sections detail the NHS organization in the health regions of England, the health authorities of Wales, the Scottish Health Boards, the Northern Ireland Health and Social Services Boards and the Isle of Man Health Services Board. In each section the administrative authorities are listed with senior officers in post identified. Classified according to health district (or health and social services district in Northern Ireland) are hospitals, day hospitals and health centres with their names and addresses. Further, for hospitals only, the type (for example, acute, geriatric, convalescent), the bed complement, the numbers of amenity and private beds at the hospital, and the existence of a major A & E department are coded. For each health district relevant information is provided on ambulance services, family practitioner services and community health services, nurse training schools, and community health councils. Three other sections cover first, Ministry of Defence Hospitals, Special and State Hospitals, and Department of Health Hospitals for War Pensioners; secondly, Boards of Governors of Specialist Post-graduate Teaching Hospitals; and thirdly, independent hospitals in the United Kingdom. The volume encompasses yet more directories, for example, a listing of hospital and health service organizations, and local authorities. Some RHAs have also produced comprehensive directories, for instance Trent [B 438] and South East Thames [B 419]. A directory of the Northern Ireland Health and Personal Social Services was published in 1976 [B 353]; previously there had been available hospital directories covering the Northern Ireland Hospitals Authority [B 354].

5.7. Day hospitals

5.7.1. *Geriatric day hospitals*

The function or role of geriatric day hospitals within the hospital service has been seen by the DHSS to encompass the rehabilitation of elderly people who have been ill and the maintenance of independence when it is threatened. Further, in day hospitals, assessments can be undertaken of patients who do not need to be admitted but who cannot be adequately assessed at home or in an out-patient situation. The majority of published studies have therefore attempted to evaluate the function of a single or small group of day hospitals in terms of these ideals. Brocklehurst's survey in 1969 of consultant geriatricians in the United Kingdom formed only one part of his review of geriatric day hospitals (see Subsection 4.1.3 and [QRL 95]). Besides this, he described five day hospitals in south-east England providing details of their history, physical amenities and staffing. Patient profiles were created from their social and physical characteristics, diseases, the reasons for their attendance and treatment received. To complement these cross-sectional data with material on the effectiveness of care, a retrospective search of case records was mounted in one hospital to learn, in particular, of the duration of attendance episodes and the frequency of weekly visits within each episode and the variations in clinical states. All patients (965) attending the Lennard Day Hospital in Bromley, Kent, between 1963 and 1968 were reviewed. (Note, that this technique and others which have been used in assessing outcome of medical care are discussed in Subsection 6.2.5.)

The relatively high readmission rates of former in-patients of the Sunderland Geriatric Unit who were known to be living alone prompted the setting up of a random controlled trial with approximately 250 experimental cases (after defaulters were excluded). The aim was to test if attendance for treatment in a day unit would reduce the demand for admission to hospital by the elderly living alone (Woodford-Williams *et al.* [QRL 724*]). The fieldwork was carried out in 1960–1. A paper published subsequently by Woodford-Williams and Albarez assessed the function of the Sunderland Geriatric Unit via the case histories of 100 patients [B 486]. However, assessment of a day-hospital function was considered by Martin and Millard to be extremely difficult to crystallize—the total attendance in a day is dependent upon the size of the unit and the availability that day of ambulance transport, while total attendances and new patient referrals over a year also do not give an adequate indication of the activity [B 309].

From a study of the rehabilitative and social-care activities in three day hospitals during 1973, they were able to suggest that the size of the unit affects all aspects of day care. Not only does it affect the provision of transport and staffing, but it affects the outcome of patients referred. They developed a planning index of day-hospital activity (New Patient Index) which related the number of new patients referred over a period to the total number of places available in the unit and the number of days worked during the period. The resulting figure was, therefore, a measure of 'throughput'.

5.7.2. *Psychiatric day hospitals*

Between 1946 and 1966, sixty-five day hospitals for psychiatric patients had been established and were identifiable by the MoH. By the latter date about 8000 new patients were attending such units and a similar number of new patients were recorded as day attenders at in-patient wards. A pilot study of day hospitals was mounted by the MoH to ascertain what kinds of patients were attending and the nature of the care they were receiving [B 140]. Fifteen day hospitals, each administratively associated with a mental illness hospital, participated in the study which extended for 1 year, 1 March 1966 to 28 February 1967. For each new patient attending in that period, a record card was completed. The definition of a new patient was that adopted in the compilation of routine mental hospital statistics. So patients who commenced more than one series of attendances during the survey period were enumerated as 'new' each time a series began. At the end of the enquiry fourteen of the fifteen consultants in charge of the day hospitals provided general information about their own hospital and made assessments of the outcome of treatment for patients who completed treatment during the year of study.

In April 1972 a complete enumeration was carried out of day patients attending mental illness hospitals and units under RHBs and teaching hospitals in England and Wales [QRL 201]. Thus covered were patients attending separate day hospitals and those using day facilities provided in conjunction with in-patient facilities. A day patient was defined as a person attending regularly at least one half day a week when the census was taken on 17 April 1972. Many of the categories in the questionnaire were similar to those administered in the 1971 census of mentally ill in-patients which was described in the same volume (see Subsection 5.6.5.2). But specific to this survey were the date of first attendance for the current spell of day-patient treatment, frequency of attendance, source of referral as day patient and psychiatric in-patient care in the preceding year. Again, in common with the companion census, the administration of the fieldwork was not described but the coverage of patients was thought to be complete.

It has been suggested that the diagnostic typification of patients attending psychiatric day hospitals is different from that characterizing day patients treated in in-patient wards. There was only one table in the report of the national census which related diagnosis to type of day unit attended (day hospital, main hospital or teaching hospital) and any measurement of treatment outcome was impossible because the statistics were representative of only one point in time. Cross, Hassall and Gath overcame this problem when they studied the seven psychiatric day care units in Birmingham, by combining the cross-sectional method with a retrospective survey over 12 months following a census week in November 1968 [B 129, 209, 235]. Material about 647 patients was assembled from hospital case notes, attendance registers and interviews with medical and nursing staff.

5.8. Other hospital services

Some statistics relating to patients attending artificial limb-fitting centres in Scotland (1965–9) and England (primarily for 1970) have been published in appendixes to two reports ([QRL 601] and [QRL 200] respectively). The former report was produced by a working party concerned specifically with the future of the artificial-limb service in Scotland. In the latter report were the recommendations of a subcommittee of the Central Health Services Council which was set up in 1968 to consider the future provision of rehabilitation services in the NHS, their organization and development. (Sir Ronald Tunbridge was the chairman.) To assist the subcommittee in its deliberations, the DHSS conducted a survey of rehabilitation arrangements in large hospitals. Some statistical results and a commentary were also appended to the report as well as information on industrial rehabilitation units and government training centres in England and Wales, and sickness benefit statistics.

The Tunbridge subcommittee was of the opinion that the concept of rehabilitation centres which were geographically separate was no longer appropriate; instead general rehabilitation departments should be located at DGHs. The report was published in 1972, and in this same year a team from the Health Services Research Unit at the University of Kent examined the role of one such regional centre, Princess Mary's Hospital, Margate, which was the largest rehabilitation hospital in England [B 286]. Apart from an enumeration of admission record cards, material was collected via interviews about patients' functional capacity and social background.

Finally, entered in the QRL are miscellaneous statistics about the emergency obstetric services in England and Wales for 1968, and routine statistics regarding appliances, blood transfusion, etc., for Northern Ireland prior to 1974.

CHAPTER 6

EVALUATION OF MEDICAL CARE

Malleson [B 302] has recently produced a book *Need Your Doctor be so Useless?*
Though written in a pejorative way and including many examples of defects in health
care in America as well as in the UK, it is indicative of the growing concern about the
functioning of the health services in developed countries. This chapter covers the issues
involved in quantitative and qualitative evaluation of health care; the emphasis is on
method in this field rather than description of particular studies that have generated
statistics.

6.1. Scope of the chapter

Though there is increasing lip service paid to the need for evaluation of health services
in general and of particular innovations in care, this is often promulgated without any
clear definition of the aims of the particular service. A specification of the aims of the
NHS is

1. medical care should be accessible to the population,
2. the various services provided should be acceptable to the potential recipients,
3. health care needs should be identified and alleviated, and
4. the use of resources (for manpower training, prevention of disease, treatment of
   illness, care of the chronic sick, administration, research) should be appropriately
   allocated to achieve the aims 1–3.

Thus evaluation of the service must identify how far progress has been made towards
meeting these aims or the objectives which are subsets of the general aims.

This chapter is primarily concerned with various techniques or methods used in
evaluating the service, for example, HESs, surveys of attitudes or disabilities, medical
audits and the application of record linkage. Studies incorporating these techniques
have been grouped into subsections dealing with: accessibility of services to the population; facilities available for use in delivering care; acceptability or uptake of services
by the public; the processes involved in delivering care; and the outcome of care.
However, such a framework leads to an oversimplification of the approaches that have
to be adopted in studying such a complex and dynamic system as that of medical care. A
further subsection briefly considers the use of overlapping approaches that involve two
or more of the basic techniques.

Evaluation can, of course, be aimed at a particular facet of medical care, such as the
broad one of 'Primary Medical Care' or a specific one of 'Communication between
General Practitioner and Hospital'. This is an approach to either locations or functions
of the service. Rather different are studies of patient groups (the pregnant women, the

elderly) or medical problems (blindness, hypertension); the important difference is that examination of such issues will require an approach that straddles administrative boundaries of location and function. The text deals briefly with some of the issues involved in such studies; however, irrespective of the topic, the studies involve the application of the techniques described in the subsections of 6.2.

The QRL for this chapter has been organized in a framework different from the ordering of the text (unlike the other chapters and accompanying QRLs which are in parallel). Thus the QRL topic headings relate to the location of services, their function, patient groups and, lastly, medical problems. It is felt that this is the appropriate axis for someone seeking statistics on evaluation of medical care, whilst the text can be used as a general background to the methods used. No attempt is made to provide a comprehensive description in the text of this chapter of the studies indexed in the QRL. Many of the major studies have already been covered in earlier chapters, depending on the relevance of other material present in their reports; the location of the description of these studies is indicated in the column 'Text reference'.

Alderson [B 20] has pointed out that monitoring the performance of the health service can be considered at three rather different levels: monitoring the public health at national level, reviewing the use of resources at district level and auditing the outcome of care at individual level (patients or doctors). Statistics relevant to the first two categories come within the remit of the present review, but the majority of studies at the individual level are beyond the scope—with the exception of some national studies that have looked at all maternal deaths, for example. The detailed and painstaking studies carried out by one of a small group of doctors have had to be excluded.

6.2. Techniques used in evaluating medical care

6.2.1. *Accessibility*

There is acknowledged variation in the accessibility of medical care in three rather different ways: first is variation in relation to quantified need within a particular health care group. Chapter 2 discussed the variation in attitudes of subgroups of the population to seeking care; in addition the family doctor may vary his referral patterns for reasons other than objective assessment of need (Social Class V psychiatrically disturbed patients may be less likely to seek help from their GP, and he may be less likely to refer such patients to hospital). Secondly, there is major variation in the allocation of resources to different health-care groups. For example, there is major variation in the 'hotel' costs for a week's in-patient stay for acute hospitals, long-stay hospitals, those for the mentally ill and subnormal.

The third category is area variation, which can involve variation between either urban and rural locations or between urban areas in different parts of the country. Routine statistics can be used at a fairly coarse level to identify the distribution of health services across the country. It is acknowledged that the distribution of hospital facilities is an historical accident rather than a rational outcome of location in relation to variation in identified need from one part of the country to another. This issue has been discussed in the subsections on Need (2.1.2) and Resources (4.1.2). The availability of routine data and their value for studying distribution of resources have been examined by Jones and his colleagues [B 265, 266].

Obviously the analysis of numbers of patients per GP in each district of the country provides a very imprecise indication of the variation in accessibility of primary medical care. Further sources of data are those relating to unmet demand (see Chapter 3); however, the routine data are scanty and only give a broad indication of the queue for in-patient care (though the length of a waiting list or the mean time spent waiting prior to admission gives a measure of accessibility of services, it must not be taken as an absolute yardstick). In discussing the use of measures of 'services rendered' as indicators of need in Chapter 2 it was stressed that queues for care can act as powerful determinants of the overt demand for care; the evidence for stifling of demand was reviewed in Subsection 2.1.2. It is suggested that any short cut to assessment of the availability of services has major disadvantages; this argues for the surveying of (1) the population to check on their views on the ease of access to primary medical care and hospital care, (2) the medical profession. Even where such studies have been carried out it must be remembered that there may be a difference between what (1) people think is a desirable level of provision, (2) the health professional's views, (3) the implication of providing the latest refinements from medical research in order to obtain ideal results from care, (4) the feasible deployment, bearing in mind availability of trained staff and finances for capital and revenue.

6.2.2. *Facilities available for care*

Examination of more specific details of provision and use of facilities (i.e. staff, capital plant and equipment) in relation to handling of particular medical problems provides a rather different examination of the health services to that of availability. It can be examined at a relatively superficial level, such as identifying the size and furnishings of waiting rooms in primary medical care or hospital out-patients, the availability of a wash-basin in the doctor's surgery or the latest available treatment plant in a radiotherapy department, to the availability of adequately experienced staff to provide anaesthetic cover for emergency obstetric work [QRL 516]. It must be emphasized that the mere quantification of facilities only provides one view of the health service and it does not automatically reflect function—let alone outcome (for example, though a surgery may have a wash-basin, this may not be used when the doctor is very busy, whilst use or non-use does not automatically reflect the risk of cross-infection, let alone other aspects of quality of care). In particular, the tendency to accumulate data on facilities—because they are so readily collected—must not be pursued at the risk of failing to consider or assess other issues. The QRL contains references to provision of diagnostic equipment in GPs' surgeries (5.1.2.1), whilst the use of facilities is discussed in Subsection 6.2.4.3.

6.2.3. *Acceptability*

There is no point in providing health-care facilities if these are not used; this extreme is unlikely to occur, but attention has already been drawn in Chapter 2 (2.1.2) to the inverse care law and the tendency of those at greatest need to make relatively low use of available facilities. This is an issue that cannot be readily studied through the analysis of routine data; the individuals who do not use the 'service' must be located and information gathered about the reasons for this.

In a study of parents of a random sample of births Cartwright [QRL 128] studied the obstacles to the use of effective contraception in England. In particular she obtained data about the reasons for not attending family planning clinics. Studies of other 'preventive' measures have identified major variation in uptake of the services and looked for the reasons for this. For example, considerable effort has been invested in studying factors influencing response to screening for cervical cancer. In general the response to population campaigns has been disappointing [QRL 590]. Osborn and Leyshon [QRL 518] showed that home visiting made a major impact upon the reluctant participant. Richards [QRL 568] has indicated the benefit to response amongst persons living in rural areas, when offered a 'Do-it-yourself' Davies kit. Other workers [B 433, 321] consider that personal approach is likely to make a considerable impact upon response rate; it is interesting to note that where family doctors, for example, take an enthusiastic approach to screening they obtain a much higher response rate. Some of the highest response rates in the UK have been obtained in Aberdeen, in a compact population of cohesive nature in north-east Scotland [QRL 425]; this area has a history of excellent co-operation between the population and its maternity and gynaecological services. Davison and Clements [QRL 182] suggest that fear of cancer can deter women from attending for screening.

Delay in attending the family doctor or the hospital when disease presents can jeopardize the chance of successful treatment. Both the confidential enquiry into maternal mortality [QRL 31] and post-neonatal deaths [QRL 187] identified patient or parent failure to take appropriate action as an important component of outcome of care. Aitken Swan and Patterson [QRL 12] interviewed a sample of patients attending hospital with malignant disease in order to quantify the various factors influencing delay in seeking care; in particular they examined the relative influence of ignorance about early symptoms and the inhibiting effect of fear of cancer.

Once a patient has been advised or provided with treatment, there is a proportion who will overtly or covertly fail to comply; this has been examined for a number of diverse issues. Gray and Parr [B 221] visited patients who had been provided with hearing aids and identified those who were not using their aid. Many workers have investigated the proportion of patients failing to take any or all of their prescribed medicines; this has been studied by Joyce [QRL 362], Bonnar et al. [QRL 77], Vere [QRL 666], Porter [QRL 546] and Dunnell and Cartwright [QRL 220]. Vere [B 444] has indicated how a patient's non-compliance can be a reflection of a bewildering regime of multiple-drug schedules. A rather different form of non-compliance is the patient who fails to attend when a first appointment is made or defaults from planned follow-up. Hoenig and Ragg [QRL 326] have studied this amongst referrals to psychiatric out-patients.

6.2.4. *Process studies*

Sanazaro [B 402] discussed the approaches to medical audit in America, defining medical audit as an objective and systematic way of evaluating the quality of care provided by physicians. He emphasized that the major effort had been on hospital care; there was a move to compare recorded care against agreed essential criteria for (1) establishing the diagnosis, (2) using the most efficacious treatment, and (3) avoiding procedures or treatments that are contraindicated. He acknowledged that undue emphasis on the processes of care was misplaced and that further effort was required to study outcome (see 6.2.5). This paper was accompanied by the reactions of two clinicians and a general practitioner from the UK [B 168, 434, 84]. Doll [B 161] has discussed various approaches to monitoring the NHS, emphasizing that this must involve the clinician and administrator in a partnership and advocating distinction between monitoring and comment about subsequent desirable action. Dunlop [B 170] has stressed how Beavan was adamant that doctors must control clinical practice; Greenwood [B 225] and Benjamin [B 44] have also identified the problems of making invidious comparisons between the performance of different doctors. McColl *et al.* [B 294] have discussed the value of 'death-and-complications' meeting in medical audit of an academic surgical department. This approach uses a subset of patients (i.e. those with an untoward outcome) as a source of clinical material to review for variation from accepted standards of care.

The consideration of process studies has been included in this chapter, as such work contributes to the overall methods used in evaluating medical care. However, the majority of such work is informal, at individual doctor level; this may be a profitable exercise, though making no contribution to the accumulation of published statistics on the (mal)functioning of the health service.

6.2.4.1. *Diagnostic procedures*. There are two aspects to the achievement of the correct diagnosis: (1) the use of the correct examinations, tests and special investigations in order to adequately substantiate the correct diagnosis, and (2) the avoidance of unnecessary investigations, which are expensive and may have occasional harmful side effects. This important aspect of medical care has required special examination of patients and the documentation of their care; this material then requires review against some agreed 'standards of practice', in order to define atypical or unacceptable levels of investigation. Descriptive studies indicate the presence of a 'problem'; Ashley *et al.* [QRL 41] abstracted data on investigations performed on patients with fifteen selected diagnoses in eight acute hospitals. Holland and Whitehead [B 249] advocated further studies to identify factors influencing the initiation of requests and the influence of such tests on further medical action and the outcome of care.

There are no routine published statistics on the use of laboratory and other diagnostic facilities by general practitioners. Some special studies have been carried out, particularly an examination of whether the introduction of these facilities has had any impact upon the laboratory or X-ray department workload [QRL 22]. Darmady [QRL 178] and Fry [B 202] have looked at the relationship between use of direct access facilities and referral to out-patients.

6.2.4.2. *Treatment*. This Section discusses two DHSS schemes for regularly monitoring treatment; one involves prescribing by GPs, the other treatment from general dental practitioners. Other studies include the consideration of treatment, but are dealt with in the text elsewhere because of their use of different method (i.e. the Hospital Advisory Service—HAS—see Subsection 6.2.6, covers many aspects of care of long-stay patients; the confidential enquiry into maternal mortality uses 'outcome' as its start-point—see Subsection 6.2.5.1; the system for monitoring adverse drug reaction also starts with 'outcome'—see Subsection 6.2.5.1).

For about one month in twelve, data are collected centrally about the prescriptions issued for each FPC; this material is costed and coded to each practitioner in the country. It is then possible to identify those practitioners whose prescribing costs are considerably above those of their colleagues. This system not only looks at the cost of the prescription issued, but is also an attempt to study any variation in trends in prescribing. Practitioners who prescribe certain drugs at much higher levels than their colleagues can be identified; a letter may then be sent to them identifying the extent of such prescribing. Mandrax is one such drug that is monitored; Brown [B 71] illustrated the rather violent reaction that can take place upon receipt of such a letter from the DHSS. The statistics that are produced from this system are predominantly confidential, though some material on costing of prescriptions is produced by the DHSS [B 14]. A number of special studies complement this national evaluation and are indexed in the QRL. An *ad hoc* study can examine in greater detail the use of various drugs for specific diseases; for example, Lee *et al*. [QRL 398] studied the records of 125 patients referred to out-patients with rheumatoid arthritis and checked the proportion who had been given the cheap safe drug of first choice.

The only regular check carried out by the DHSS of quality of care involving examination of patients relates to individuals who have had routine dental treatment under the NHS; a sample is recalled and a check examination carried out of the recent treatment. Whatever the historical reasons for this procedure, it presents a remarkable example of evaluation; the statistics are again confidential to the DHSS. The reports in the QRL are the result of private initiative.

6.2.4.3. *Appropriate use of treatment facilities*. It is important to distinguish three quite separate ways of considering facilities—first is the actual distribution of such resources (see Section 6.2.2), second is the use made of these facilities (Chapters 4 and 5 deal with this), whilst third is the evaluation of use being made of health service staff and equipment. This latter activity overlaps with the two previous subsections of 'Process Studies'; consideration of the use of acute hospital beds can illustrate this: there are two aspects to assessing whether a patient actually in hospital is correctly located: (i) was admission initially required, and (ii) could the patient by now be discharged to some other form of care? Detailed special studies have been done to see whether domiciliary investigation and treatment was initially appropriate or whether earlier discharge to second-line care (including home care) might have been implemented. Such studies may identify that inappropriate staff and equipment have been employed to care for the patient whether or not the appropriate investigations were carried out and the accepted specific treatment given. In many of these studies there is no clear right and wrong; conclusions will depend on opinions and this will often involve balancing a number of disparate factors. The example of concern over the use of acute beds is one that has been studied for many years; shortly after the start of the NHS there were a number of papers on the need for second-line and community facilities to avoid the undue stay in an acute unit of elderly patients [QRL 20, 338, 279]. These and subsequent work are indexed in the QRL.

6.2.5. *Outcome studies*

There are four rather different measures of outcome that can be considered: mortality, morbidity, 'satisfaction' (of patient/family/staff) and economic measures. A wide variety of different studies have been mounted, but the development of the regular assessment of outcome of all aspects of medical care is still relatively limited—particularly in comparison with the wealth of studies on use of the health service. There has been increasing disillusion with the possibility of identifying positive indices of health; this has been associated with re-emphasis upon the use of negative measures of outcome (such as untimely death), in order to assess the functioning of health care. Rutstein *et al*. [B 400] have identified and classified certain 'sentinel' events (i.e. events which, following appropriate preventive or curative measures, should not have occurred). Field trials are in progress and the *Lancet* [B 280] points out that assessment of the ease of implementation will be crucial to extended use of the system. The following notes discuss the ways in which available data have been used to monitor outcome and indicate some of the special studies performed.

It is important to emphasize that many clinicians have followed up patients under their own care and published 'clinical reports' of the response to various treatments; in addition to such individual studies there have been an increasing number of clinical trials reported since the late 1940s. Though such scientific work quantifies the response to treatment no further reference is made to such work, which is beyond the scope of this review.

6.2.5.1. *Mortality*. National mortality statistics have been used as a general monitor of the health of the country; for example, the age-specific mortality of males and females in early middle age has been examined through the century to indicate the relative improvement in the health of the female compared with the male. Such use of national mortality data has been discussed in the previous review [B 14]. The national publications make available mortality statistics for local authorities, whilst some MO'sH have collected material for their own authority and prepared tabulations of this in their annual reports (these reports are discussed in Chapter 5, Section 5.3). This national or local material can, of course, be examined by specific causes of death or by age group. In Chapter 2 (2.1.2) reference was made to the use of such material as an indication of 'need'—it may seem a twist in logic to argue at the same time that mortality data may provide an indication of outcome of care. The material in itself cannot distinguish whether variation in mortality is due to variation in: health need; delivery of preventive or curative care; or outcome of care.

Rang and her colleagues [QRL 552] have indicated how hospital discharge data on individual patients when routinely linked to subsequent mortality can provide information of value to the clinician, hospital administrator and clinical research worker. Special studies have been discussed in Chapter 2 of mortality in: pregnant women (Subsection 2.5.22), neonates (Subsection 2.5.10.1), the post-neonatal period

(2.5.10.1), sudden death and all deaths in infancy (2.5.10.3), and patients with malignant disease (2.5.8). Though individual clinical studies are beyond the scope of this review there have been one or two collections of extensive survival data for regions or for regional centres, treating malignant diseases. These have tabulated the survival curves on long term follow-up of large numbers of patients with malignancy of different sites [QRL 222, 692]. Because of the particular interest in monitoring the outcome of treatment with radium added to the general nature of malignant disease, there was a strong lead to record basic data about patients at first treatment and organize thorough follow-up. This resulted in the collection and analysis of survival data, which have not been so readily available for a number of other important 'chronic degenerative diseases' of the middle-aged.

Morris and his colleagues [QRL 397] used published HIPE tables (see [B 14]) to examine the mortality in in-patients treated in teaching and non-teaching hospitals. A persistent difference in case-fatality rates led to a detailed study of variation in patient and treatment characteristics in an attempt to identify the reasons for this difference. A comparable exercise has been carried out by Ashford and his colleagues, who have analysed routinely available data on obstetric services and associated perinatal mortality rates. This has been followed by a detailed examination of hospital records for three selected units in the country; a system for classifying patterns of antenatal care was devised and related to perinatal mortality. This enabled comments to be made about appropriateness of care in the different locations [QRL 240]. This is a somewhat simpler approach than the comprehensive national studies that have been described in Chapter 2 (2.5.10.1; [QRL 111, 110]).

6.2.5.2. *Morbidity*. Data on the level of morbidity in the population can be used as an indication of the influence of preventive and curative community care. For example, the population surveys on dental health (see Chapter 2, Section 2.5.12) provide detailed data on the amount of caries and gum disorders in the population; they can be used to monitor the influence of preventive campaigns, or to indicate the degree to which active disease is treated and cured by the dental service. Comparable surveys were carried out in the areas introducing fluoride and the control areas in the centrally sponsored study of the benefits from adding fluoride to domestic water supply [QRL 481, 198]. Chapter 2 discussed the application of HESs; the dental surveys just mentioned are the only existing example of national routine HESs in this country (though many special studies have involved examination of samples of the population). On a local level, however, a number of family doctors have themselves carried out surveys of the morbidity in their practice, and this can be used indirectly to indicate the prevalence of disease and the success in preventing disorders or identifying disease at an early stage and curing it. There are no routine data on workload at hospital out-patients that could also be used as a measure of the success of treatment. As with mortality data, it could be argued that routine data of hospital discharges provide some indication of the outcome of medical care; if a community or out-patient campaign for prevention and treatment of a specific condition was mounted one would anticipate a decline in the hospital in-patient discharge rates or rates of bed day usage. It must be emphasized that such use of material is a fairly tenuous example of an outcome study. The validity of such data is also influenced because the national scheme handles data on 'episodes' rather than 'people';

it is difficult to tell whether reduction in the discharge rate is due to fewer people being hospitalized or patients having fewer readmissions.

Acheson [B 4] has described how the Oxford Record Linkage Scheme has a number of operational applications; by linking repeat admissions to hospital into a cumulative file more meaningful hospital statistics can be produced and the readmission rates calculated for persons with chronic diseases. Adelstein *et al*. [QRL 9] linked the records, which identified mothers who had a virus infection in pregnancy to subsequent records of live-born children; those children who had subsequently died were noted and it was possible to compare the observed and expected mortality from cancer. If routine or *ad hoc* record linkage cannot be carried out a planned collation of retrievable records may be required. For example, in order to study the outcome of children notified as born with spina bifida, Weatherall [QRL 701] contacted the notifying LHA who obtained details of the place of residence and type of education of surviving children.

It has already been emphasized in Chapter 2 (2.3.2) that studies in a stable general practice provide an excellent opportunity for obtaining long-term follow-up of patients. This can provide data on the 'natural history' of a range of common diseases, as influenced by present methods of care (see, for example, Fry [QRL 254]). Many other prospective studies will provide important data on the outcome of care of individuals; Chapter 2 discussed cohort studies of national samples of children, some of whom have been followed for over 20 years (Subsection 2.5.10.1). Two other categories of epidemiological study are also highly relevant to the present topic: (1) follow-up of large groups of initially healthy individuals, in whom the development and progression or resolution of disease is recorded; (2) the follow-up of groups of individuals with a particular chronic disease, where the determinants of outcome are being examined. Such studies will not have been mounted in order to study the outcome of medical care *per se*, but relevant data will often have been accumulated as part of the general study design.

Some special studies have been carried out to define techniques for assessing indicators of outcome. Munday [B 343] investigated a range of physiological measures of anxiety in hospital patients, whilst Franklin [QRL 246] used a range of 'Psychological' questionnaires to assess patient anxiety. Huskisson [B 258] examined various methods of measuring pain, as a preliminary to assessing the effectiveness of various pain-relief treatments. An interesting extension of this work was the study by Hayward [B 239] who suggested that the provision of adequate information to patients prior to operation had a beneficial effect upon post-operative pain and anxiety. A rather different approach has been the search for a global indicator of well-being—which might then be measured at various stages of each patient's treatment in order to quantify response to care. Grogono and Woodgate [B 226] used an index derived from the sum of scores (on a three-point scale) for ten aspects of 'well-being'. Breslow [B 62] has discussed the combined use of questioning an individual about his health and the objective measurement of functional reserves in order to derive a measure of health status. Rosser and Watts [B 396] have tested a simpler approach which requires a physician to score a patient on two parameters: (1) disability on an eight-point scale and (2) distress on a four-point scale which incorporates a judgement of pain and/or mental disturbance and/or reaction to disability. More theoretical approaches to the measurement of health have been provided by Fanshel [B 185] and Chiang and Cohen [B 102]. Williams

[B 468] suggested that the major stumbling-block to progress in this field was the absence of an accepted standardized method of categorizing social functioning.

An important aspect of follow-up studies has been the identification of duration of incapacity; for example, Semmence [QRL 603] and Kinlen [QRL 378] have followed up patients who have had a hernia repair or in-patient care for coronary artery disease. At the present moment it is not possible to automatically link hospital statistics for individual patients with sickness absence statistics handled by the Social Survey Division of the DHHS. The two examples mentioned above involved painstaking special follow-up of individual patients, together with use of retrievable data. Other studies on absence from work after illness were discussed in the rehabilitation section of Chapter 2 (2.5.27).

One consequence of the thalidomide disaster was an increasing interest in methods of detecting the unwanted side-effects of medication. Inman [B 260] has described the scheme introduced in England and Wales for the voluntary notification of adverse reactions to drug therapy. All practitioners are invited to participate in the scheme, by the submission of limited particulars about identified adverse reactions; where appropriate, there is a mechanism for instituting special enquiries. The drug-monitoring scheme is directed by a subcommittee of the Committee on Safety of Medicines (CSM) and managed by two full-time physicians with supporting administrative and clerical staff. Procedures have been developed for (1) identifying drug-safety problems, (2) obtaining more detailed information from patients who have suffered specific adverse effects, (3) carrying out epidemiological studies and (4) disseminating knowledge about adverse reactions to drugs. Forty doctors are employed part-time for field enquiries; this provides a unique task force for exploration of rare events requiring a national study. Inman [B 260] has discussed a range of difficulties in the appropriate identification and investigation of a drug-safety problem. Despite a number of important sources of error and bias in the material, this information system now generates routine morbidity data and provides scope for a range of special studies. A check of the validity of the reports was made on a sample of eighty-two reactions; this suggested that 78 per cent were probably drug related and a further 13 per cent possibly drug related [B 260]. Regular reports are produced which relate the quantity of specific drugs used to the frequency of reported side-effects [QRL 192]. In addition to the production of a digest of statistics from the CSM, there are occasional reports where a 'cluster' of notifications has led to a special study. For example, Inman and Mushin [QRL 344] describe data from 130 reports of jaundice following halothane anaesthesia.

Christopher *et al.* [B 103] have described the system initiated in Aberdeen, in which a section for recording adverse drug effects has been incorporated into the standard Scottish hospital discharge summary sheet. All adverse reactions are extracted and records kept in a local register; appropriate reports are forwarded to the CSM.

6.2.5.3. *Satisfaction of patient/family/staff.* Reference has already been made to the studies by Cartwright on *Human Relations and Hospital Care* [QRL 126] and her study of *Patients and Their Doctors* [QRL 127]. Both of these studies looked at the use made of facets of medical care and the views of the patients of this contact with the health service. Information was also gathered from the GPs about the organization and functioning of the NHS. In both publications the author is careful to point out the problems of carrying out such an interview survey; there is no direct evidence that the factual information obtained is accurate and it is even more difficult to know whether the opinions are valid. A particular difficulty of collecting such data on opinions is in judging the relative strength of these.

Rather different has been the work of Raphael who has specifically restricted her studies to developing techniques for assessing patient's views on their hospital care—*Patients and Their Hospitals* [QRL 553] and *Psychiatric Hospitals Viewed by their Patients* [QRL 554]. The initial work commenced in 1965 with development of a questionnaire collecting views on five aspects of life in hospitals (the ward and its equipment, sanitary accommodation, meals, activities and general care). Following extensive use of the questionnaire this was redesigned in 1967 and the King's Fund has sponsored use of this questionnaire through many hospitals in the country. Data are published on the original results from twenty-eight hospitals, so that any individual hospital carrying out its own survey can check the distribution of responses against these results. A comparable technique was used in psychiatric hospitals, though some of the problems of collecting material were fresh. Some of the patients in long-stay wards could not see or did not speak English; others were apathetic and not pressed to participate. Because of this it was rather difficult to assess the actual response. In addition to these method studies the King's Fund sponsored two surveys on noise in hospitals, *The Most Cruel Absence of Care* (Hinks [QRL 316]). This work indicated the various sources of noise that were likely to impinge upon the patient and the impact of various measures to control this.

The Secretary of State for Scotland set up a working party on suggestions and complaints in hospitals, and Carstairs carried out a study in Scottish hospitals in 1967 to collect information from in-patients and out-patients [QRL 123]. A comparable enquiry was set up in England and Wales, and again a special survey mounted to collect factual information about patient satisfaction with hospital care [QRL 181]. One facet of these studies has been the consideration of methods of communication between patients and hospital staff. Fletcher [B 193] has reviewed the general importance of this topic, whilst Joyce *et al.* [QRL 362] have studied the failures of communication in a small group being treated as out-patients. The *British Medical Journal* [B 65] has discussed the method difficulties in assessing 'quality of life' of the elderly. Hall [B 228] has recently described the use of various subjective measures of 'quality of life' in Britain; the SSRC Survey Unit explored various approaches in 1971–5 and an instrument of a Health Symptoms index was thought to provide useful information.

The Central Health Services Council [B 94] has produced a report on the organization of the in-patients' day, after 5 years' deliberation. Many of the problems of avoidable nuisances are of long standing and the lack of apparent progress disappointing; the Secretary for State has identified communication and flexible visiting hours as priorities for improvement [B 66].

The subsection on GP workload (5.1.2) and the section on manpower (4.2) both discuss a number of studies which have included the collection of material on attitudes of staff to their work and on 'satisfaction'.

6.2.5.4. *Economics*. Cochrane [B 108] in his book *Effectiveness and Efficiency* has very clearly distinguished the relatively specific study of effectiveness (which examines the ability of a procedure to alter the natural history of a disease or symptom for the better) from the much more complex issue of assessing efficiency (which quantifies the ratio of the minimum resources required to achieve the effect to the resources used at present).

The health service has a relatively limited financial income (since 1948, in real money terms, the annual expenditure has very slowly increased), but all the time there are pressures for the extension of the service to provide new treatments or more modern methods of care and support. There are also the pressures to correct the inequalities in provision of care discussed in Subsection 6.2.1—usually by enhancing the service in low provision areas, rather than the reverse! There is great interest, therefore, in assessing the cost of particular facets of the health-care system and the benefits that result. In certain conditions it is relatively simple to measure the cost of treatment and, using an actuarial approach, assess the direct financial benefit of saving life or physical incapacity. However, it must be stressed that such calculations cannot be directly used to define the allocation of resources (saving a young child's life, reducing incapacity in a middle-aged wage earner, or prolonging life of an elderly person can be translated into financial terms—but not used to determine the ethical and moral issues of where to concentrate scarce resources). The role of economic assessment of outcome of medical care is to provide the 'decision-makers' with guidance as to the likely financial repercussions of any change in method of delivering medical care; they then have to weigh up many other factual and intangible issues when reaching a particular decision.

Consideration of economic aspects of medical care can lead to a whole range of literature very different from that covered in the review up to this point. Extension into this important area of work is beyond the scope of the text; a few general reviews of method are mentioned, whilst the QRL contains a very restricted number of studies from the medical literature that have included statistics on financial aspects of outcome of care. Fein [B 190] has briefly discussed the measurement of economic benefits of health programmes, Roberts [B 389] surveyed the economic evaluation of health care, whilst Ferster [B 192] reviewed the role of economic analysis in health services management. A specific patient group—the elderly—has been exposed to a cost-benefit analysis of their care by Wager [QRL 671]. Hospital costing and efficiency has been briefly described by Babson [B 30] and at greater length by Montacute [B 332]. Multi-author books on the economics of medical care have been edited by Hauser [B 236] and Cooper and Culyer [B 118].

A rather different aspect of economic evaluation is the scrutiny that the expenditure of the NHS receives in the Public Accounts Committee; Mr du Cann, in presenting the report to parliament, recently commented that 'there is something very wrong with the administration of the National Health Service' [B 82].

6.2.6. *Complex studies*

Separation of studies of the evaluation of medical care into various categories of method has a major disadvantage. The description of each approach is simplified, but the actual health-care system is complex and has often to be studied by a number of different overlapping techniques in order to look at need/unmet demand/use of resources/outcome of care.

A relatively recent innovation has been the establishment of an HAS in both England

and Wales and Scotland. Their aim is to provide constructive criticism and propagate good practices and new ideas in order to improve the management of individual hospitals. Their work has initially concentrated upon long-stay hospitals (for the mentally ill, mentally subnormal, elderly and young chronic sick) and associated units; the HAS operates through a sequence of multidisciplinary team visits to each hospital. A confidential report describing the hospital with recommendations (where appropriate) is sent to the health authority concerned. Whenever possible follow-up visits are made to discuss the translation of recommendations into practice. The published reports for the HAS [B 253–6, 409] describe the method followed and general aspects of findings and suggestions, but have not included any statistical analysis of the findings.

Cochrane [B 108] elaborated on the role of planned intervention studies; in particular, he stressed the value of Randomized Controlled Trials in assessing effectiveness and efficiency of health services. He indicated the application to preventive and curative regimes, but also to 'medical care' in the wider sense (e.g. the role of in-patient versus home care for a treatment of acute myocardial infarction). Dollery [B 164] suggested that Audit of Health Care should be established in this country through an (initially voluntary) Committee of Health Care. This would explore the feasibility of audit of hospital and general practice. Techniques comparable to those of the confidential enquiries into maternal and post-neonatal mortality and of the HAS might be used, but spanning total health care. In addition he advocated a special research effort in this field through a Health Care Research Board. General reviews of the techniques and their application to evaluation of health care have been provided by Cartwright [B 89], Adler et al. [B 7], Ashford [B 29], Knox [B 276] and Taylor [B 430]. Considerable experience has been gained in America over various techniques for audit; it is therefore salutary to note McSherry's conclusions of the value of the approach [B 301]. He considered that utilization-review and medical-audit programmes had not worked in his hospital and that much more reliance should be placed upon the inbuilt concern of doctors for high-quality care. The validity of his conclusions has been questioned by McColl and Fernow [B 293].

The evaluation of psychiatric services was clearly delineated by Wing [B 476]; he was rather disparaging about descriptive studies, emphasized that a case register was a foundation for special studies, whilst suggesting that greatest value was obtained by a series of planned evaluative studies of increasing complexity [(i) comparison of service statistics, (ii) comparison of statistics where the service has developed along different lines in two or more locations, (iii) contrast progress in subgroups of patients identified by differences in innate or acquired characteristics, (iv) controlled trials, (v) population-based epidemiological studies, (vi) combination of population-based statistics with planned intervention]. Sainsbury [B 401] has described the approach used to evaluate a comprehensive community psychiatric service. Though both these authors were dealing with the problems of psychiatry, the methods they describe are likely to be relevant to a wider range of medical care issues.

There has been increasing interest in the evaluation of primary medical care. Obviously the application of specific methods of evaluation will have to be tailored to the particular problem being studied; however, the general framework of examining availability/facilities/accessibility/process/outcome is equally suitable for hospital or primary care. A number of general method papers have discussed the issues of evaluating primary medical care: Mansfield [B 303], Hodgkin [B 247], Marson [B 308], Buck *et al*. [B 76] and Curtis [B 131].

6.2.7. *Caveat*

A number of papers have stressed the need for information and (if regular evaluation is to take place) information systems to generate the appropriate data [B 30, 123, 64]. What should be obvious is that all statistics are not suitable for this and that even accurate statistics may only permit a limited probe of complex issues. The need for accurate data has been discussed in Chapter 1 (Subsections 1.7.1–1.7.9); the general points raised there are equally relevant to evaluation. In addition it is worth bearing in mind the warning of Finagle's Laws: (1) the information you have is not what you want, (2) the information you want is not what you need, (3) the information you need is not what you can obtain.

CHAPTER 7

INFORMATION SYSTEMS—THE FUTURE

In preparation for this review the authors had to consider (i) what the managers required in the way of information for their work, (ii) what was presently available and acceptable. This led on to consideration of the gaps in the present information; this issue has been touched on in earlier chapters which have referred to defects in method and lack of hard data. This final chapter attempts to crystallize consideration of these issues. A comparable section 'Towards a unified Health Information System' (H Inf S) was inserted in the previous review [B 14]. This chapter begins with a paradigm 'Four steps in establishing a H Inf S'; it must be pointed out that the authors have not followed these four steps, as their primary task was rather different; the comments that follow stem predominantly from the work undertaken during this review (involving an examination of published statistics) rather than research directed at the development of improved information systems. However, Alderson has discussed a number of the points made in this chapter in greater detail elsewhere [B 13, 16, 17].

The second section in this chapter reviews in general terms managements' requirements for information, indicating in the broadest terms the various categories of information that are required for day-to-day management and planning. The third section then discusses the specific gaps which have been highlighted during the preparation of the review. This is followed by a section on some practical considerations. One cannot blindly advocate an extension of routine data collection or the mounting of a range of specific studies. The dilemma entailed in considering extension of the present information system is indicated and some priorities for future action identified.

A H Inf S is defined as a mechanism for the collection, processing, analysis and transmission of information required for organizing and operating health services, and also for research and training [B 15]. At its lowest level, in terms of a national health system, a H Inf S may be associated with the collection and processing of information for a single and specific treatment unit or service facility for the investigation of patients. Other systems may be located at local, regional or national levels of health care. There is a relationship between the location of the system and the uses to which the information is put, with emphasis on management at local level and strategic planning at national level. There is also an important relationship between the use of the system and the timeliness required of the data; a faster speed of processing is required for information used in management.

The primary objectives for such a system are to provide the managers involved in operating the health services at local level with relevant information, to provide at periodic intervals data that will show the general performance of the health services, and to assist planners in studying their current functioning and trends in demand and workload. As one of the main sources of data coming into a H Inf S is material concerning patients, it is essential that the system assists and interests clinicians by feeding back to them data that facilitate the study of clinical problems. Managers, planners and clinicians will frequently require detailed data, and the H Inf S should serve as a framework for a range of research studies in these fields.

7.1. Four steps in establishing a H Inf S

There are four basic steps in setting up a model intelligence system in the health service:

(i)   Examination of the resources for the intelligence system, both resources of data, staff, expertise and equipment for handling the information.

(ii)   Review of the problems faced by all levels of management in the health service; this includes study of the problems facing those responsible for administering the hospitals, and community health services, at national, regional and local level.

(iii)   Having identified the problems that management face, one wants a detailed study of how information is currently used and whether decisions on current problems are reached without need for or use of information.

(iv)   Consideration of the extent to which more efficient handling of presently available data can be used for a more profitable examination of problems faced by management, and review of the need to alter the collection of routine or *ad hoc* information.

Providing there is acceptance in the basic solution derived under step (iv) one then requires to introduce an innovation in provision of information; if possible the introduction of this should be monitored so that the outcome of the provision of information is observed. Unless this is carefully done it will be impossible to determine whether the provision of information has aided management and justified the cost of the system.

It has already been pointed out that this chapter is not based upon a careful study that has involved activity within each of the above four steps. The main task has been to review published statistics, i.e. only a small component of the total resources indicated in (i) above. However, consideration of the relevance of the statistics for inclusion in the QRL has involved (at least at second hand, with some direct experience stemming from the rather different work in which each author has been involved) contact with problems faced by management and observation on their present use of information.

7.2. Management requirements from information systems

It is suggested that the information system should assist in general management of the health service and in planning at all levels from health care planning teams within districts to strategic planning at regional level. To play an effective part in this range of work requires the production and presentation of rather different sets of output. In general terms [B 16] management requires data for the examination of current resources and current demands for the short-term reallocation of these resources in order to meet more effectively these demands 'tomorrow'. This imposes constraints as it necessitates data that are up to date and relevant to local issues. Quite different are the information needs for planning; this requires data which will facilitate the process culminating in decisions regarding the future provision of the correct balance of domiciliary, out-patient and in-patient facilities for the investigation treatment, and care of all 'perceived health needs' of the community. The planning process involves a lengthy time-scale and is particularly concerned with planning for the health needs of the next generation.

The rather separate requirements of management and planning are discussed in the next two subsections.

7.2.1. *Classes of data required for management*

7.2.1.1. *Trends in demand for services*. Information should be available to gauge the change in demand for health services. Simple indices of this change are in themselves useful, even if the complex issues responsible for such change cannot be clarified. Ideally the system should present data on new attendances at family practice, fresh requests for use of ancillary staff in the community (such as requests for health-visitor support or district nursing), direct-access investigations requested by family practitioners, new referrals to out-patients, numbers of emergency/booked/planned/waiting-list admissions to hospital, and workload of service departments such as pathology, X-ray, etc., in the hospital. Comparable data are also required for dentistry.

7.2.1.2. *Trends in bottlenecks*. At periodic intervals there should be presentation of material on the queues and waiting-lists for various services such as: numbers of patients awaiting deployment of resources in the community (such as patients requiring but not receiving routine visiting from the district nurse or other supporting services); the numbers of patients waiting and the mean waiting-time for urgent and non-urgent appointments at out-patients; the waiting-lists for in-patients (preferably tabulated by individual consultant and diagnostic category with the waiting-list converted from a count of patients to an estimate of bed days required by the patients on the waiting-list); delay time for complex investigations such as cardiac catheterization, respiratory function tests, etc.; the number of patients in acute beds in hospital awaiting transfer to long-stay care in chronic hospitals, admission to sheltered accommodation in the community, or discharge to their own or relatives' homes upon mobilization of community resources.

7.2.1.3. *Use of resources*. Ultimately it would be advisable to have a profile that indicates the complete deployment of staff and physical facilities, not just as an inventory of resources but in relation to services provided. For instance, there should be information about the work of the family practitioner and the ancillary staff in the community; this should not be just a count of items of service performed, but should relate the workload to specific patient-care groups. Similarly one requires information which quantifies the use of out-patient facilities, in-patient facilities and service units in hospital. The collection and presentation of this information on use of resources should be problem-orientated rather than collated by location of care.

7.2.1.4. *Outcome of care*. Judicious manipulation of the data from HAA may extend the currently available case fatality rate to indices of complication rates, recurrence rates and readmission rates. At its simplest this can be achieved by bringing together readmissions of individual patients to a hospital using the unit number. Much more difficult to obtain will be indices of recovery, reablement and patient satisfaction; some of this mateial will have to be collected by special studies which cannot be replicated in every region for even the major patient care groups, let alone specific diagnoses. Data must be collected not only on patient satisfaction, but also on staff 'morale' (especially on aspects of distaste for present duties and signs of overwork).

7.2.1.5. *Monitoring of innovations in health care*. It is essential that any new developments in medical care (whether these are gradual evolution in the way of delivery of health care, or more major change due to innovation and the introduction of fresh programmes of care) are monitored to demonstrate the impact of the change. For instance, with preventive schemes such as immunization and cervical cytology it is essential that statistics are presented on the uptake of these procedures, identifying the subgroups of the population who do not participate in the programmes, and contrasting the subsequent morbidity and mortality in the protected and non-protected. With the introduction of administrative or medical changes in the care of patients, such as the use of peripheral out-patients, or introduction of day-surgery, it is important to monitor the impact of these changes upon the functioning of the remainder of the hospital, as well as the outcome of those handled in the new system.

7.2.2. *Information requirements for planning*

The simplest way to plan is to identify the current workload, quantify the resources used to meet this workload, and relate this to the population in the catchment area; in this way 'norms for provision of care' can be derived. These norms can then be applied to the projected population figures in order to obtain anticipated requirements. Such an approach is likely to perpetuate the fault in the current system. In order to produce a more precise approach one requires detailed information about the diseases currently affecting the population, and on to this one needs to build estimates of: trends in the incidence of disease; possible changes in the attitudes of the population to health and health care; future variations in delivery of care; impending changes in therapy; and the effect that any new therapy is likely to have on the prognosis of disease. These data on trends are required in addition to the basic information (on need, unmet demand, use, outcome) that were discussed in the previous subsection. Two rather different types of change can occur in the delivery of medical care. First are minor alterations and the gradual shift due to the steady evolution of medical care; second are major changes resulting from innovation and advances in knowledge or technology. Examination of trends in patterns of working provides indication of the former, whilst discussion with the deliverers of medical care can provide estimates of change in practice.

7.3. Towards a health information system

In the past there has been a tendency to examine in isolation separate sets of data on (i) workload in the health service, (ii) deployment of staff and (iii) departmental unit costs. Estimates of workload plus unmet demand have been taken as indicators of need [B 32], whilst the volume of official complaints has been a yardstick of satisfactory service rather than any more specific measures. Attention has already been drawn to the necessity for bringing together data on need/unmet demand/use/outcome into a composite whole in order to build an improved picture of the functioning of the health service.

In order to assist management it is suggested that the information system has available the following sets of data: (i) demographic and environmental information (the census and other sources of data provide considerable information on these aspects); (ii) mortality and morbidity of the community; (iii) estimates of the health care needs of the population (such data are difficult to collect, and require special surveys of samples of the population); (iv) health resource data, including manpower; (v) health facilities data; (vi) medical care utilization information; (vii) indices of the outcome of medical care. The current challenge is to identify how available data contributing to the above seven classes can be brought together so that a total picture can be made available as soon as possible. This may seem 'pie in the sky', but Florence Nightingale [B 351] advocated the regular collection of a wide range of standard particulars to ascertain the results of particular treatments and special operations. She suggested that the whole question of hospital economics as influenced by diets, medicines and comforts could be brought under examination; she was also keen to study data on out-patients. Recently the Specialist Group on Management Services and Statistics of the Working Party on Collaboration between the NHS and Local Government advocated a move towards the accumulation and examination of data such as is indicated above [B 422]. The following subsections indicate the changes that might occur in information gathering and handling.

7.3.1. *Evolution of present activities*

The following subsection indicates some general development that can occur in the collection, presentation and use of information for management purposes. Six rather different items are identified; there is, however, overlap between some of these items and also from this subsection to the two following ones on the collection of fresh data and development of new methods for handling data.

7.3.1.1. *Precise specification of aims.* It is clearly recognized that for any study the aim must be identified in precise terms. When a report is subsequently prepared it is essential that the aim of the study is described; any variation from this aim, that occurs during the conduct of the study or in the analysis phase, must be identified. Though this seems a very trivial point to mention—as one would expect it to be well known—it is surprising the number of publications that do not clearly specify the aim; sometimes when brief and conflicting particulars are given about the method and interpretation of the study it is open to question whether a clear-cut aim had ever been identified even implicitly in the planning phase.

7.3.1.2. *Relationship of aim of study to possible course of action.* One would anticipate that all special studies conducted have been planned in such a way that the material that it is anticipated will become available from the study should be linked not only to the specified aim but the possibility that the particular results can be applied in some logical fashion in the management of the health service. This point is, of course, linked to the need to specify the aim, but is really concerned with one step beyond this; it is suggested that in considering the aim of the study the research workers should identify not only the contribution to fresh knowledge that should be derived from the study but have clearly in mind how health-service management should implement the findings from the study.

7.3.1.3. *Improved relationships between the research staff, NHS staff, and management.* Alderson [B 16] has discussed at some length the traditional gap that exists between research workers and both the clinical and health-service staff who might implement the findings or management who might use the results from studies in considering their decisions. There is often some hidden antipathy between research workers and these other groups, and Alderson was exploring the various ways of breaking down these acknowledged barriers. It is essential that relationships are developed to a satisfactory level and contribute both at the planning phase, during the conduct of the study, and when the analyses are being discussed prior to implementation. A comparable point was made by Cherns *et al.* [B 101], who point out that too few social scientists have served on both sides of the utilization fence; ability in research does not *ipso facto* equip a person with the knowledge needed to advise governments or other organizations. A rather different point was made by Glennerster [B 216] who pointed out the difference between the findings from commissioned research and subsequent recommendations of the committee requesting the research.

7.3.1.4. *Enhanced quality of definitions.* Chapter 1 (Subsection 1.7.8) touches on the problems that can arise where definitions vary or are imprecise in two or more studies which have attempted to collect data on the same general problem. It is essential in any *ad hoc* study that the definitions are clear and understandable to the field workers, so that capture and interpretation of the material is feasible. Where comparable data are collected for a similar problem either in different locations or at different points in time, it is essential that the definitions of items being collected in the study are comparable or at least permit translation of the findings from one study into the terms used in the other study. The problem of clarity of definition also, of course, applies to routine data-collection systems. An additional problem with such studies is the difficulty in having definitions that are simple and understandable by the staff responsible for capturing the basic data, without introducing the degree of complexity necessary to maintain standardization across the country. Once satisfactory systems have been developed there is then some built-in inflexibility which can create difficulty when the health service activity evolves and the original definitions no longer remain applicable.

7.3.1.5. *Dual record systems*. Greenfield [B 224] discussed the application of dual-record systems, which have been used in a number of countries where complete registration of vital events is either absent or incomplete. Their purpose is to provide a correction for the under-recording of events, through obtaining dual observations on the same sample members of the population during a given time. This concept could be applied in the data-collection systems that exist within the health service where two or more systems are handling items that overlap from one system to another. Greenfield concluded that an efficient subsampling procedure was preferable in order to obtain optimum efficiency rather than an attempt to duplicate records entirely.

7.3.1.6. *Collection of data as a by-product of operational systems*. The two rather different approaches to this are manipulation of clerical systems or the obtaining of data from computer systems as a spin-off of other activities. Either approach is predominantly of value in the collection of workload data, where the manual or computer systems are required as part of the health-care system; the data required for this activity are also filtered off into the information system. There are, however, comparable opportunities in the manpower planning field; the possibility has been examined of using payroll systems to generate a core of data for manpower planning.

7.3.2. *Gaps in presently available data*

The following comments are listed in the same order as Chapters 2–6; within these the material is again dealt with in a logical order comparable to that used in the text of these chapters. This means therefore that the material is not ordered by priority for collecting data to 'plug' the identified gaps; this issue of priority for action is discussed further in the final section, 7.4.

7.3.2.1. *Need*. Consideration should be given to expanding the GHS which already provides a basic H Inf S. The main deficiency of the GHS at present is the fact that the lowest geographical level that it comes down to, even on an annual basis, is national planning regions. These regions are not comparable to boundaries used within the health service; for application for management purposes one would need data at area level presumably (apart from the potential use of the GHS data as part of the Resource Allocation System, from country to region level). In addition, further thought should be given to the possibility of collecting additional particulars about determinants of need. It would be helpful if additional particulars could be collected that are linked to measures of need; one could then possibly use other sources of data by locality—such as the census—to identify the make-up of the constituent population in terms of the distribution of these determinants or indicators of need. For example, if a close relationship was found between overcrowding or some other demographic characteristic and need for health care for a particular set of diseases the decennial census could be used to identify the variation in need in relation to this determinant at local level, even down to level of enumeration district. The strength of the GHS should be its ability to collect data that are otherwise quite unobtainable through the present activity data-collection systems that exist within the Health Service. In particular it is suggested that the GHS should concentrate on linking with NHS activity systems; it might complement these by the collection of information on (1) reasons for taking certain actions, and (2) opinions about the subsequent contacts with the Health and Welfare Services.

This country has never had an HES and consideration should periodically be given to this issue. There are some national systems which include examination of subsamples of the population (for example: virtually all pregnant women are examined; data are available through the National Birthday Trust's periodic studies on the care of the pregnant women and newborn throughout the country; the majority of newborn children are now examined in hospital by medical staff prior to discharge and a proportion of children are seen at routine examination and clinic, and also on school entry). Consideration needs to be given to the mounting of a sample HES aimed at other risk groups of the population, such as the elderly or very elderly, one-parent families, or the families where one member is in contact with the psychiatric services.

Chapter 2 discussed the use of the National Morbidity Survey as a source of data on need. This application is one of the grounds on which the NMS could be extended and continued. Its extension is advocated because the present coverage is somewhat limited and the smaller the number of doctors that are involved the greater the suspicion that their method of behaviour is likely to be different and to a lesser extent that the patients that they draw into their practices are atypical; such biases suggest that the extrapolation of the data from this survey at present to the community as a whole becomes doubtful.

7.3.2.2. *Unmet demand*. In addition to collecting data on queues for care that are presently not documented consideration needs to be given to the method issues of studying the bottleneck effect of a queue in stifling overt demand. In addition attention should continually be paid to the accuracy of the statistics on queues for care (for example, for waiting-list patients, what proportion of entries are duplicates, or relate to patients who have died, or for other reasons would not enter hospital even when called up).

7.3.2.3. *Use*. Chapter 4 indicated a series of topics for which there were only presently available limited data. There seems to be inadequate information about the organization of primary medical care, with particular reference to the use of health centres. With the growing number of health centres comparable data are required for practice within and without such centres. This should relate to the functioning of these centres, including detailed data about the use of ancillary staff. The material collected on workload by different members of the Primary Medical Care Team should be organized by patient and the patients should be identified by their particular health-care group. These data must be formulated in such a way that material on health care of given individuals by different facets of the health service can be linked and also collated data can be made available on the total workload in caring for particular categories of health problem in different locations. Other facets of the community care that require additional data are community dentistry and also the school health service and care of the children (it is unlikely that radical alteration in data-collection systems will occur for these latter areas of work until the recommendations from the Court Report [B 119] have been implemented).

The present changes in health care include growing emphasis on the use of services that bridge the community/hospital junction. This includes the increasing use of day hospitals, community hospitals, day centres, peripheral out-patient clinics and surgery carried out on a day basis. Again statistics (as indicated in earlier sections) are required on these activities.

Routine data for the health service contain a relative abundance of information on work carried out caring for hospital in-patients. Complementary data are required on the direct access use of diagnostic facilities, care of patients at out-patients (including diagnosis, referral for other care, treatment, or referral back to family doctor) and the facilities available for rehabilitation following treatment.

Resource data presently provide fairly specific data on the capital and equipment available within the health service (though this cannot be necessarily linked to detailed data on health care by client-group within these facilities). There seems to be still lack of data on manpower, which must indicate the activities of the different categories of worker in hospital and in the community.

7.3.2.4. *Outcome measures.* Chapter 6 indicated the need to collect additional particulars on mortality, morbidity, rehabilitation (including return to work where applicable or return to activities of daily living), the side-effects following treatment, and patient and staff satisfaction. A considerable body of data is available on these measures, but not routinely collated with data on health care—so that it is impossible to monitor the side-effects in relation to specific treatments, or patient satisfaction in relation to variation in patterns of care. It is difficult to be precise about how much of this material should be available as a routine for all patients, how much effort should be invested in developing improved systems for assessing outcome, and where special studies of outcome will always be required in order to evaluate the impact of innovation in treatment. The general point being that where innovation in treatment occurs without a planned randomized control trial it becomes extremely difficult to evaluate the impact of the innovation. For conventional treatment some form of routine monitoring of outcome is required at least on a sample basis across the country in order to determine whether levels of care are maintained to an appropriate degree.

7.3.3. *The development of new methods*

In order to supplement the present information systems with the collection of additional routine 'facts' it is suggested that the only solution will be a move towards the use of master patient registers and associated subfiles.

A recent report from Scotland confirms their rather different approach to medical computing [B 220]. This article describes the progress in the establishment of a master patient index for Tayside, the reasons for this and the approach selected. The basic demographic data for each member of the population served are to be supplemented with minimal information on his or her previous medical history and the linkage of repeated contacts with the health service. The index should then provide a basic identifying and linking mechanism for the build-up of a range of other specific files of information. It is argued that this information is required for the day-to-day management of existing services and for longer-term planning; specific examples are given of the contribution that the files should make to the family doctor service and the hospital service. This work has application at district or area level; Heasman [B 241] has described the use of the national (Scottish) record linkage file as a tool of the central health organization.

The complexity of the general proposals described by Graham [B 220] poses a number of problems of logistics, but these cannot be resolved merely by clear thinking and discussion; evaluation of such activity can be achieved only by piloting such work on a fairly extensive basis. This should identify: the problems involved in setting up, maintaining and running the system; the costs; the benefits that stem from such systems. Alderson [B 19] has stressed that the attraction of fully developed master patient indices with associated subfiles is their potential for producing as a by-product information that is more complete, accurate, up-to-date, appropriate, acceptable and possibly cheaper than data from other approaches. As mentioned earlier, this requires major experiments to test and evaluate (including investment of effort in exploring full use of resulting information); the limited ventures in this field in England seem inadequate—watching Scotland progress has its advantages—but those interested in such activities can only sharpen their approach on the grindstone of practical experience.

The problems of using routine data were briefly indicated in Chapter 1 (Subsection 1.7.8). One particular issue that is raised by the consideration of a master patient index is confidentiality. This is likely to be a continual source of misunderstanding and friction in the present climate of opinion even if safeguards on storage and release of data are spelt out.

In addition to collecting additional particulars on 'facts' on need, unmet demand, and use there is a requirement for additional special studies. These special studies will have to cover rather different topics. First are the opinions of the population and medical staff—assessing their knowledge, attitudes and practice in certain circumstances. For contact (or failure to make contact with the health service where there are indications) one requires special studies to collect reasons why various decisions are made at each contact or referral point. Reference has already been made in the preceding subsection to the need for 'experiment' or randomized controlled trials in order to evaluate new treatment. In addition to surveys and such controlled trials there is an increasing place for Operational Research studies to identify variation in the functioning of the health service and in particular imbalance between different facets of the system. Matthew [B 311] has pointed out that it is impossible to contemplate the mounting of special studies to illuminate all the problems that exist in the organization and delivery of medical care throughout the country. There is a place therefore for the collection of basic data as a routine, the identification of major issues that warrant special study, and the supplementation of both these approaches by the use of simulation and modelling techniques to identify either imbalance in the functioning of the service, or the possible impact of various changes in the delivery of care.

Consideration of these new methods obviously brings one far beyond the feasible changes that could occur as a routine within the health service. The following section therefore attempts to define to what extent the information systems within the health service can be adapted in the coming few years, and which are the major issues to which research staff should devote their attention.

7.4. Some practical considerations

The preceding section indicates the potential range of items that may be called for; the wealth of data is not required in order to bury statisticians in statistics, but stems from consideration of management information requirements. Before responding to suggestions that additional data be collected every item presently collected must be reviewed to see if there is redundant material, or whether changes are required in the way current items are collected, coded and processed. The next step is to consider which of the following courses of action is appropriate:

(i) Addition of items to the list for routine collection on a 100 per cent basis.

(ii) Collection of relevant data on a sampling basis, where the sampling frame may be fixed (e.g. 10 per cent of all 'pathology' reports) or variable (collection of 100 per cent haematology one year, 100 per cent clinical chemistry next year, etc.).

(iii) Collection of relevant data in a purpose-designed once-off study.

(iv) Handling of available data (and perhaps opinions of experienced staff, particularly on unmet health needs and anticipated changes in health care) in a simulation or other dynamic model.

(v) Combination of two or more of the above approaches.

Implicit in the above is the need to plan any change in relation to clear-cut requirements of potential users. It is essential that repeat collection of identical items does not occur for different purposes and that the total H Inf S is viewed as an interlocking set of subsidiary systems. Many *ad hoc* surveys will benefit from being mounted as a temporary extension of the routine data-collection system, perhaps using the latter as a sampling frame.

The Office of Health Economics [B 360] has pointed out that those planning the new organizational pattern of the health service have misidentified the major health-care problems. It was suggested that administrative changes can do little to affect the quality of health care in any group in the population, and emphasis on the role of professional managerial expertise in the NHS is misplaced. Cartwright *et al.* [B 92] consider that the application of epidemiological techniques to determine medical policy will be more important than the adoption of new management methods. Systems such as described above are an approach towards the assessment of need, demand, workload, use of facilities and outcome of health care; when data covering these different aspects of health care are available it should be possible to monitor the functioning of the health service and plan the future. The present knowledge of the optimum approach to health information systems is deficient, despite the lip-service paid to identifying need, monitoring functioning of the health service, and optimizing allocation of resources. It is also important to acknowledge that hard information only provides a background against which decisions are made, often after considering a wide range of subtle but important attitudes and pressures. Yates [B 491] has clearly shown how the application of information can aid management and planning, but has indicated the investment of effort required in analysing and presenting data. There is thus a chicken and egg situation: lack of retrievable routine information (and staff to handle this information) prevents the development of refined methods for using an extended range of information of management and planning. 'Managers' are thus unlikely to put high on their priority information systems, when the present state of development of such systems costs money and yet provides limited value because of inadequacies of the systems.

The previous section (7.3.3) listed a range of gaps in the presently available information. It is felt that the major imbalance in availability of data is lack of workload data on out-patient care, the junction between the community and the hospital (day surgery, day hospitals, peripheral out-patient clinics, direct access investigation) and routine information about care delivered in the community. It is suggested that these gaps are the priority for attention, followed by or accompanied by research work on improved measures for assessing need, improved techniques for assessing functioning of the health-care system and relating data on function to outcome.

An important consideration in deciding where to invest further effort in information for management and planning is assessment of the likelihood of valid data being collected and implemented. Some judgement is required about the benefit that should stem from improved information. Some complex (and perhaps rare) problems might require major research investment in order to provide improved information—the impact of which would be slight. Also if alteration in the health-care system would be resisted by key personnel one must question the priority of collecting data relevant to such problems. As a generalization it is suggested that information that will improve the judgements made in planning are of higher priority than information for day-to-day management—which can be carried out with skill and judgement in the absence of factual data.

QUICK REFERENCE LIST

Description

The Quick Reference List is ordered in approximately the same way as the text. It covers statistics on: population needs for health care; unmet demand for health care; resources; use of services; evaluation of health care. The following table of contents indicates the order of entries in the QRL. However, if a user cannot immediately locate an entry in the QRL (either using the contents list as a guide or directly scanning the QRL) it must be remembered that some publications cover several topics. As discussed in Chapter 1 (Section 1.5) it has not been feasible to include multiple entries to certain publications in several locations of the QRL.

The QRL segment on 'Need' first discusses national population studies and then local population studies. These are followed by entries on general practice from national, regional and local work. Statistics derived from industry are then inserted. These are followed by entries on specific medical problems which are arranged in alphabetical order. Within this general framework national studies take precedence over local studies, whilst studies that were carried out a number of years ago are ordered before more recent work. (This convention also applies to the remainder of the QRL.)

The entries on 'Unmet Demand' cover general practice, casualty department, out-patients, in-patients and private care. Within these segments the general order follows the sequence of events that patients might pursue during their contact with the health services.

The QRL segment on 'Resources' spans facilities, manpower (medical and dental, nursing and midwifery, professional and technical) and other resources. Within each of these main topics the types of data are arranged alphabetically. The following entries on 'Use of Services' are divided into the various services patients might encounter—general practitioner and dental practitioner, community health, A & E, out-patient, diagnostic, in-patient and day patient, and other. Again within each, the types of data are ordered alphabetically. In both of these segments, tables of previously unpublished routinely collected statistics have been indexed. Usually these special tabulations have been prepared by central government departments for committees of enquiry.

Coverage on evaluation of medical care deals first with evaluation of general practice, then out-patients, in-patients, day and residential care. These entries are again ordered in general in a sequence that a patient may follow throughout their contact with the health service. There are then a number of entries each dealing with specific medical problems. Finally there is a short section on evaluation of preventive medicine.

The geographical cover of the studies is indicated in the column headed 'Area'. In the segments on 'Resources' and 'Use of Services', parts of the entries in the 'Area' column have occasionally been enclosed in brackets; these indicate that only a minority of the tables covered by the entry are broken down to this level. The indication of geographical coverage needs to be interpreted in conjunction with consideration of the sample size. The sample size is indicated in the 'Remarks' column using a five-point scale.

Sample size has been coded as follows:

$$
\begin{aligned}
VS &= \quad\quad 1-\quad 199 \\
S &= \quad 200-\quad 999 \\
M &= \quad 1000-\ 4999 \\
L &= \quad 5000-24999 \\
VL &= 25000 +
\end{aligned}
$$

This indication of the sample size needs to be treated with caution in certain complex studies as there may be different subsets of the data derived from different samples. The sample size is the recorded number of individuals (or units) from whom data have been obtained—and as indicated in Chapter 1 (see Subsection 1.7.6) the proportion responding may be as important as the actual number of respondents, due to the bias introduced by low response. The time period of data collection is indicated in the column 'Year'; the majority of studies clearly state the period from which data were collected, though again this can be less precisely identified in some work.

The 'Remarks' column indicates the relevant section in the text where the topic is dealt with. Not every study for which there is an entry in the QRL has been discussed in the text. For the latter entries the cross-reference in the 'Text' column is in brackets.

As explained in Chapter 1, it has not been possible to provide copies of the data-collection forms for the 700 studies included in the QRL. However, where the published report contains a copy of the data-collection documents, this has been indicated by a Q in the 'Remarks' column.

QUICK REFERENCE LIST—TABLE OF CONTENTS

Need 220

 Morbidity 220

  National population studies 220

  Local population studies 220

  General practice—national 221

  General practice—regional 222

  General practice—local 222

  Estimated requirements for hospitals 222

  Statistics from industry 223

  Specific studies 224

   Abortion 224

   Accidents 225

   Addiction 226

   Addison's disease 226

   Adverse drug reactions 226

   Alimentary disease 226

   Arthritis 227

   Blood diseases 228

   Cancer 228

   Cardiovascular disease 228

   Children 230

   Deafness 232

   Dental health 232

   Diabetes 233

   Elderly 233

   Environment 235

   Epilepsy 235

   Eye diseases 235

   Family planning 236

   Feet 236

   Genito-urinary disease 236

   Handicap 236

   Maternity 237

   Mental illness 237

   Mental subnormality 238

   Migraine 239

   Nutrition 239

   Physique 239

Rehabilitation   239
Respiratory disease   240
Screening   242
Self-medication   242
Sexually transmitted disease   242
Skin disease   242
Smoking   243
Terminal care   243
Thyroid disease   244
Tuberculosis   244

Unmet demand   244
General practice   244
Casualty   245
Out-patients   245
Special problems   246
Private care   247

Resources   247
Facilities   247
Ambulances   247
Bed provisions   247
Day hospitals   248
General practitioner hospitals   249
Health centres and clinics   249
Medical and dental manpower   249
All grades of hospital doctors   249
Community doctors   250
Community physicians   250
Consultants   250
Dental practitioners   251
General practitioners   251
Junior hospital dentists   252
Junior hospital doctors   252
Medical migration   253
Student doctors   254
Women doctors   254
Nursing and midwifery manpower   254
All nurses and midwives   254
Community nurses of all types   255
Health visitors   256
Home nurses   256
Hospital nurses   257
Midwives   257
Nurses—general practice   258
Professional and technical manpower   258
Chiropodists   258

Dental technicians　258
Dietitians　258
Helpers　258
Occupational therapists　258
Ophthalmic personnel　259
Orthoptists　259
Pharmaceutical staff　259
Pharmacists　259
Physiotherapists　259
Radiographers　260
Remedial gymnasts　260
Speech therapists　260
Other resources　261
Prescribing costs　261
Radiography costs　261

Use of services　261
General practitioner services　261
All inclusive GP attitudinal studies　261
All inclusive GP workload studies　262
Allocation of consultation time　263
Allocation of working time　263
Appointment systems　263
Assessments of use by individuals　264
Assessments of use of GP family planning services　265
Deputizing services　266
Family planning and abortion　266
Home visiting　266
Investigations　267
Maternity medical claims　267
Medical records　267
Prescribing　268
Referrals　269
Sickness certification　270
Dental practitioner services　270
Assessments of use by individuals　271
Dental practitioner surveys　271
Dental practitioner workload statistics　272
Community health services　272
Annual and *ad hoc* statistics　272
Assessments of use by individuals　273
Referrals by doctors　274
School dental service　274
School health service　275
Hospital A & E and out-patient services　275
Assessments of use by individuals　275
A & E services　276

  Out-patient services   276
Hospital diagnostic services   278
  Pathology services   278
  Radiology services   279
Hospital in-patient services   279
  Assessments of use by individuals   279
  Ad hoc studies   280
  Emergency bed services   282
  General practitioner hospital services   282
  Gynaecology services   282
  Maternity services   282
  Mental-handicap and mental-illness services   283
  Northern Ireland routine in-patient statistics   284
Day hospital services   284
  Geriatric day hospitals   284
  Psychiatric day hospitals   284
Other hospital services   285
  Appliances and hearing aids   285
  Blood-transfusion service   285
  Domiciliary consultations   285
  Emergency obstetric services   285
  Limb-fitting centres   285
  Operations   285
  Physiotherapy   285
  Rehabilitation   285

Evaluation   286
Evaluation of general practice   286
  Ancillary staff   286
  Appointment systems   287
  Compliance with drug therapy   287
  Direct-access investigation   287
  Home visiting   287
  Introduction of a transport service   288
  Night calls   288
  Overall functioning   288
  Prescribing   288
  Views of patients   289
  Views of staff   289
Evaluation of general practice/hospital links   289
  Communication   289
  Direct-access investigation   290
  Referral to out-patients   290
Evaluation of out-patients   290
  Ambulance transport   290
  Communication doctor/patient   290
  Compliance with drug therapy   291

Consultants' views   291
Non-attenders   291
Out-patient referrals   291
Out-patient surgery   291
Evaluation of in-patient care   291
Admission systems   291
Alternative location of care   292
Investigations   293
Lengths of stay   293
Miscellaneous   295
Mortality   295
Morbidity   295
Nursing dependency   295
Patients' views   295
Prescribing   297
Staff views   297
Evaluation of day care   297
Evaluation of residential care   297
Evaluation of specific medical problems   297
Abortion   297
Addiction   298
Adverse drug reactions   298
Alimentary disease   299
Blood diseases   299
Cancer   299
Cardiovascular disease   300
Childhood   301
Dental disease   301
Diabetes   301
Eye disease   302
Family planning   302
Genito-urinary disease   303
Haemorrhoids   303
Maternity   303
Mental illness   305
Rehabilitation   305
Respiratory disease   305
Terminal care   305
Evaluation of preventive medicine   306
Anti-smoking campaigns   306
Cervical cytology   306
Fluoridation   307
Immunization and vaccination   307
Mass radiography   307

ABBREVIATION LIST FOR QRL

AC	Administrative county
A & E	Accident and Emergency
AEA	Atomic Energy Authority
AHA	Area Health Authority
Ann.	Annual report
BG	Board of Governors
BP	Blood pressure
Br.	Britain
Br. Isles	British Isles
BsM	Boards of Management
C	County
CB	County borough
CNS	Central nervous system
CO	Carbon monoxide
DCH	Diploma of Child Health
DCP	District Community Physician
DGH	District General Hospital
DN	District Nurse
DR	Doctor
DVT	Deep vein thrombosis
E	England
E. Anglia	East Anglia
EC	Executive Council
ECG	Electrocardiograph
ENT	Ear, Nose and Throat
E & W	England and Wales
FEV	Forced expiratory volume
FU	Follow up
GB	Great Britain
GHS	General Household Survey
GLC	Greater London Council
GP	General practitioner
HA	Health Authority (Northern Ireland)
Hb	Haemoglobin
HMC	Hospital Management Committee
hosp.	Hospital
Hosp. Reg.	Hospital Region
H&SS Board	Health and Social Services Board (Northern Ireland)
HV	Health Visitor
IHD	Ischaemic heart disease
IP	In-patient
IQ	Intelligence quotient
L	Large (sample size)
LA	Local Authority

lab	Laboratory
LHA	Local Health Authority
LOS	Length of stay
M	Medium (sample size)
MCHC	Mean corpuscular haemoglobin concentration
Met.	Metropolitan
MOH	Medical Officer of Health
MS	Marital status
MSW	Medical Social Worker
N	North
NE	North East
NHS	National Health Service
NI	Northern Ireland
NI Certificate	National Insurance Certificate
NMS	National Morbidity Survey
NW	North West
O/E	Observed over expected
OP	Out-patients
Parl. Const.	Parliamentary constituency
PCV	Packed cell volume
PTC	Phenyl-thio-carbamide
Q	Questionnaire
R	Region
Regist. District	Registration District
RHA	Regional Health Authority
RHB	Regional Hospital Board
RSCN	Registered Sick Children's Nurse
S	Small (sample size)
SC	Social class
Scot.	Scotland
SE Engl.	South East England
SEG	Socio-economic group
SEN	State Enrolled Nurse
SHMO	Senior Hospital Medical Officer
SMR	Standardized mortality ratio
SO_2	Sulphur dioxide
SR	Standard Region
SRN	State Registered Nurse
SW	South West
S Wales	South Wales
UK	United Kingdom
VL	Very large (sample size)
VS	Very small (sample size)
W	Wales
WP	War pensioner
wt	weight
WTE	Whole time equivalent

Topic and type of data	Detail of analysis	Area	Year	Publication (see QRL key)	Text reference	Remarks
Need						
Morbidity: National population studies						
Absence from work or education	Sex; age; SEG; job satisfaction; employment status; sick pay	GB; Planning Reg.	1971–3	[QRL 510, 512, 513]	2.2.1.2	VL; Q
Bedfast days	Sex; age	GB; Planning Reg.	1971–3	[QRL 510, 512, 513]	2.2.1.2	VL; Q
Chronic and non-chronic sick	Household size, type, heads' income; tenure, age, and amenities of accommodation	GB; Planning Reg.	1971–3	[QRL 510, 512, 513]	2.2.1.2	VL; Q
Limiting long-standing illness	Sex; age; marital status, employment status, SEG; condition, quarter	GB; Planning Reg.	1971–3	[QRL 510, 512, 513]	2.2.1.2	VL; Q
Limiting long-standing illness or acute restricted activity	Sex; age	GB; Planning Reg.	1971–3	[QRL 510, 512, 513]	2.2.1.2	VL; Q
Long-standing illness (with or without limitation)	Observed and age adjusted rates; sex; marital status; employment status; SEG	GB; Planning Reg.	1972–3	[QRL 512, 513]	2.2.1.2	VL; Q
Restricted activity in 2-week period	Sex; age; marital status; condition, quarter	GB; Planning Reg.	1971–3	[QRL 510, 512, 513]	2.2.1.2	VL; Q
Restricted activity in 2-week period	Sex; age; SEG	GB; Planning Reg.	1972–3	[QRL 512, 513]	2.2.1.2	Q
Self-medication	Category of medicine; sex; age; number of times; number of tablets	GB; Planning Reg.	1972–3	[QRL 512, 513]	2.5.29	VL; Q
Smoking	Sex; age; type of products; type of cigarette; number of cigarettes; marital status; highest qualification reached; SEG	GB; Planning Reg.	1972–3	[QRL 512, 513]	2.5.29	VL; Q
Morbidity: Local population studies						
Disease in male workers	Age; abnormalities; per cent requiring treatment	Midlands	1938–9	[QRL 490]	2.2.2.1	M
Housing	Type of tenancy, number of rooms; persons per room; overcrowding	Luton	1945	[QRL 287]	(2.2.2)	L

Prevalence of abnormalities	Blood group; PTC tasting ability; finger ridge patterns; skull variation; mental defects; mental illness; causes of hospitalization; cause of death; multiple sclerosis	Shetland Islands	1955–74	[QRL 63]	(2.2.2)	L
Ailments and action taken	Active complaints by type; chronic complaints; respondents/doctor diagnosed; action taken; details of digestive, nervous, rheumatic, respiratory, and skin complaints, and tiredness	Bermondsey & Southwark	1962–3	[QRL 670]	2.2.2.3	M
Chronic disease and disability	Per cent reporting disability, sex, age; final estimates of disability; impairment category; diagnoses	Lambeth	1966–8	[QRL 62]	2.2.2.4	L
Chronic cardio-respiratory disease	Sex; age, MS, SC, work status, smoking; severity of symptoms; proportion having medical care	Lambeth	1966–8	[QRL 10]	2.2.2.4	M; Q

Morbidity: General practice—national

Consultations and patients consulting	Sex, age, urban/rural location; diagnosis; frequency of illness; months of year; reasons other than sickness	E & W; Reg.	1955–6	[QRL 408]	2.3.2.1	VL; Q
Care for specific diseases	Sex, age, SC, occupation, urban/rural location; diagnosis—psychiatric; nervous system, digestive tract, skin, bones and organs of movement, genito-urinary, obstetric, cardiovascular, children, elderly	E & W; Reg.	1955–6	[QRL 564]	2.3.2.1	VL; Q
Consultations	Sex, age, occupation, SEG, SC, diagnosis	E & W; Reg.	1955–6	[QRL 408]	2.3.2.1	VL; Q
Consultations by children	Sex, father's occupation, SEG, SC, diagnosis	E & W; Reg.	1955–6	[QRL 408]	2.3.2.1	VL; Q
Episodes of illness	Sex, age, diagnosis, type of episode	E & W	1971–2	[QRL 511]	2.3.2.2	VL; Q
Home visits	Sex, age, diagnosis	E & W	1971–2	[QRL 511]	2.3.2.2	VL; Q
Surgery consultations	Sex, age, diagnosis, consultation rates for those registered throughout or for part of study	E & W; Reg.	1971–2	[QRL 511]	2.3.2.2	VL; Q
Referrals	Sex, age, diagnosis, type of referral	E & W; Reg.	1971–2	[QRL 511]	2.3.2.2	VL; Q
Consultations—married women, 15–44	Age, parity, years on 'pill', diagnosis	UK	1968–72	[QRL 365]	2.3.2.3	VL

Topic and type of data	Detail of analysis	Area	Year	Publication (see QRL key)	Text reference	Remarks
Need—*contd.*						
Morbidity: General practice—regional						
Consultations	Sex, age, characteristics of practice	SW Engl.	1964–5	[QRL 726]	2.3.2.3	VL
Home visits	Sex, age, severity, follow-up	SW Engl.	1964–5	[QRL 726]	2.3.2.3	VL
Indirect consultations	Sex, age, characteristics of practice	SW Engl.	1964–5	[QRL 726]	2.3.2.3	VL
Consultations	Diagnosis, location of practice	S Wales	1965–6	[QRL 713]	2.3.2.3	VL
Morbidity: General practice—local						
Consultations and visits	Sex, age, MS, SC, household and family size, smoking, full-time education	Exeter	1966–7	[QRL 37]	2.3.2.3	VL
Episodes	Diagnosis; sex, age	Inner London	1951–2	[QRL 333]	2.3.2.3	M
Consultations	Diagnosis; sex, age	Beckenham	1947–73	[QRL 253]	2.3.2.3	L
Morbidity: Estimated requirement for hospitals						
National study	In-patient requirements by specialty	E & W	1942–3	[QRL 469]	2.1.2	VL
Local study	Out-patient and in-patient requirement by specialty	Stirlingshire	1946	[QRL 504]	2.1.2	VL
Local study	Out-patient and in-patient requirement by specialty	Ayrshire	1948	[QRL 505]	2.1.2	VL
Local study	Out-patient, in-patient, and diagnostic facilities required by specialty	Northampton and Norwich	1950–1	[QRL 506]	2.1.2	VL
Local study	In-patient requirements	Reading	1956	[QRL 52]	2.1.2	
Local study	Out-patient and in-patient requirement by specialty	Barrow	1958	[QRL 243]	2.1.2	VL
Local study	Out-patient and in-patient requirement by specialty	Tees-side	1957–8	[QRL 11]	2.1.2	L
Local study	'Second-line' beds required	Scot.	1966–7	[QRL 459]	2.1.2	M
Local study	In-patient requirements by specialty	Liverpool R	1966–8	[QRL 245]	2.1.2	L
Local study	In-patient requirements for elderly; influence of sex, age, SC, urban/rural residence	NE Engl.	1970	[QRL 260]	2.1.2	L
Factors influencing hospital usage	Diagnosis, age, sex; MS, SC, household size, smoking, full-time education, family size	Exeter	1966–7	[QRL 37]	2.3.2.3	VL

Factors influencing hospital usage	Hernia and varicose veins: length of stay, SC	Liverpool R	1966–8	[QRL 403]	2.1.2	M
Factors influencing hospital usage	Prevalence of bunions, haemorrhoids, hernia or varicose veins on interview; severity, desire for operation	Warrington	1967–8	[QRL 403]	(2.1.2)	S

Morbidity: Statistics from industry

National Dock Labour Board	Number treatments; category of employer	UK	1947–75	[QRL 599]	(2.4)	L
Post Office employees	Sex, age, MS, category of work; sickness rates, working time lost, duration of spells, uncertificated absence; medical retirements, deaths; diagnosis	GB	1955–75	[QRL 548]	(2.4)	VL
British Rubber Manufacturers	Spells and days lost, cause, sex, age, MS; occupational group	UK	1958–9	[QRL 523]	(2.4)	VL
National Coal Board	Prevalence of pneumoconiosis, area of work; other prescribed diseases, diagnosis	UK	1959–75	[QRL 498]	(2.4)	L
UK Atomic Energy Authority	Accidents, location, site, cause; sickness absence, days lost, location, cause; deaths in employees and pensioners, cause	UK	1962–75	[QRL 665]	(2.4)	VL
UK Atomic Energy Authority	Certified absence, cause, sex; age, grade, deaths by cause; whole body γ-dose	UK	1964–8	[QRL 219]	(2.4)	VL
Civil service	Certified and uncertified sick leave, age, staff group	UK	1967–8	[QRL 646]	(2.4)	VL
Manual workers	Absence in pairs matched for sex, age, workplace, occupation; certified, uncertified and other absences, diagnosis, influence of shift system	UK	1968–9	[QRL 640]	(2.4)	M
Post Office employees	Sex, age, grade of work; sickness, retirement and death rate	UK	1972–5	[QRL 548]	(2.4)	VL
British Steel	Sickness absence spells and days lost; treatment room attendances, special department attendances; location within corporation	UK	1972–5	[QRL 93]	(2.4)	VL
Local industry employees	Industrial and non-industrial attendances by cause and condition	Slough	1974–5	[QRL 164]	(2.4)	VL
Manual workers	Sickness absence: age, occupational group, shift; O/E cause of death	E & W	1956–68	[QRL 638]	(2.4)	L
Engineering works plus government departments	Short-term absences: sex, age, MS, length of service; distribution of medical and non-medical absence and lateness, day of week, period of year	NI	1955–8	[QRL 249]	(2.4)	M

Topic and type of data	Detail of analysis	Area	Year	Publication (see QRL key)	Text reference	Remarks
Need—*contd.*						
Morbidity: Statistics from industry—*contd.*						
Refinery workers	Number and length of certified absences, lateness and other absences; length of service, shift/day work	Shell Haven	1946–65	[QRL 636]	(2.4)	M
Office workers	Sickness absence: sex, MS, job grade, duration of journey to work, type of transport	London	1969–70	[QRL 639]	(2.4)	M
London Transport	Sex, age, job; days of sickness, inception of spells: broad diagnosis	London	1949–71	[QRL 551]	(2.4)	VL
Morbidity: Specific studies						
Abortion	Age, MS, SC, method termination, use of contraceptives	Kingston	1964–9	[QRL 204]	(2.5.1)	M
Abortion	Trends by quarter of year, place operation	GB	1968–71	[QRL 385]	(2.5.1)	VL
Abortion	Grounds for termination, MS, SC	E & W	1970	[QRL 73]	(2.5.1)	M
Abortion	Gestation, consultation GP, first OP visit, at termination, place operation	E & W	1972	[QRL 385]	(2.5.1)	M; Q
Abortion	Gestation, age, MS, parity, SC, use of contraceptives	E & W	1972	[QRL 131]	(2.5.1)	S; Q
Abortion	Year of age under 16, pregnancies, per cent aborted, region residence/treatment, comparison observed/expected numbers	E & W; Hosp. Reg.	1970	[QRL 385]	(2.5.1)	M
Abortion—repeat	Number repeat abortions, age, MS, SC, parity, within 1 year previous abortion	E & W; Hosp. Reg.	1970–2	[QRL 385]	(2.5.1)	M
Abortion— complications	Type of complication	London	1970	[QRL 461]	(2.5.1)	S
Abortion— complications	Type of complication, type of operation	Oxford	1968–70	[QRL 625]	(2.5.1)	VS
Abortion— complications	Haemorrhage	London	1969–70	[QRL 413]	(2.5.1)	M
Abortion— complications	Type of complication	Kingston	1964–9	[QRL 204]	(2.5.1)	M
Abortion— complications	Readmission required, type of complication	E & W; Hosp. Reg.	1972	[QRL 385]	(2.5.1)	M; Q

Abortion—sterilization	Proportion having sterilization, parity, SC, place operation	E & W; Hosp. Reg.	1968–71	[QRL 385]	(2.5.1)	VL
Accidents—home	Age, sex, MS, SC, household size; type, month, day of week, time of day, length incapacity	Aberdeen	1955–7	[QRL 442]	(2.5.2)	L; Q
Accidents—home	Sex, age, pre-existing disability, social circumstances; cause, place and type of accident, time of day	GB	1960–1	[QRL 92]	(2.5.2)	M
Accidents—home, to children	Age, sex, SC, time of day, type of accident	Norfolk	1971–2	[QRL 496]	(2.5.2)	S
Accidents—home, to children	Age, family circumstances, evidence for stress in home	Surrey	1972–3	[QRL 342]	(2.5.2)	VS
Accidents—home, to elderly	Type of accident, type of fall; general health, injury severity and duration	Wolverhampton	1959	[QRL 609]	(2.5.2)	S
Accidents—home, to middle aged/elderly	Fractures: site of fracture, sex, age, type of accident, duration hospital stay	Oxford, Dundee	1954–8	[QRL 379]	(2.5.2)	L
Accidents—home	Child poisoning: sex, age, SC (numbers and rates); type of substance, last time used in household, symptoms, severity, confirmation of diagnosis	Bristol	1970–3	[QRL 117]	2.5.2	VS
Accidents—road	Killed, injured (numbers and rates): class of road user, age, built-up areas, weather, darkness, street lighting, road surface, type of road, month, use seat belts, skidding; breath test failures after accident with injury	GB	1934–74	[QRL 186]	2.5.2	VL
Accidents—road	Type of injury, class of road; category of road user; age, interval to death; object causing injury	W Midlands	1959–63	[QRL 269]	(2.5.2)	S
Accidents—road	Type of injury; severity, source of injury; car component causing injury; direction of impact; impact speed; class of road	W Midlands	1965–9	[QRL 431]	(2.5.2)	S
Accidents—road	Type of injury; class of road, direction of impact, category of road user, interval to death	W Midlands	1959–68	[QRL 270]	(2.5.2)	S
Accidents—road	Raised blood alcohol in Road Traffic Accident casualties; category of road user, time of day; age of drivers	Manchester	1960	[QRL 137]	(2.5.2)	S
Accidents—road	Seat belt wearing (number and per cent): injury, category of road user; object hit; type of impact; vehicle speed	E & W	1962	[QRL 401]	(2.5.2)	S

Need—*contd.*

Morbidity: Specific studies—*contd.*

Topic and type of data	Detail of analysis	Area	Year	Publication (see QRL key)	Text reference	Remarks
Accidents—road	Crash-helmet wearing: age, SC, driving experience; club membership; reasons for wearing/not wearing helmet	E	1957	[QRL 594]	(2.5.2)	M; Q
Accidents—road: motor cyclists	Age, driving experience, accident details	E & W	1958	[QRL 595]	(2.5.2)	M; Q
Addiction: alcohol	Prevalence, sex, offences for drunkenness	GB; Planning Reg.	1956	[QRL 525]	(2.5.2)	S
Addiction: alcohol	Age, sex, SC, MS, occupation, urban/rural residence; contact with GP, psychiatrist, AA; serious injury, attempted suicide, adverse effects on work, family, community	Cambridgeshire	1961–4	[QRL 495]	(2.5.2)	VL; Q
Addiction: alcohol and teenagers	Age, religion, pocket money; prevalence of drinking, circumstances and location of consumption	Glasgow	1970	[QRL 180]	(2.5.3)	M; Q
Addiction—heroin	Persons known to Home Office, age, first registered, present state, for deaths age	E & W	1947–66	[QRL 65]	(2.5.3)	M
Addiction—heroin	Prevalence of users; category of use, source of information	Crawley	1967	[QRL 15]	(2.5.3)	VS
Addiction—heroin	Prevalence of users; parents' SC	'Town' in E	1967–8	[QRL 380]	(2.5.3)	VS
Addiction—drug-taking amongst students	Prevalence in medical students; sex, smoking, characteristics of home	Glasgow	1971–2	[QRL 429]	(2.5.3)	M
Addison's disease	Prevalence: age, sex, tuberculous/non-tuberculous	NE Met. RHB	1960	[QRL 452]	(2.2.2.5)	VS
Adverse drug reactions	Specific reactions, specific drug within class of drug; deaths; estimated total numbers of prescriptions	E & W	1964–73	[QRL 192]	2.5.4	VL
Alimentary disease—perforated peptic ulcer	Age, sex, site perforation; monthly, weekly, daily, hourly distribution	W Scot.	1924–63	[QRL 430]	(2.5.5)	L
Alimentary disease—peptic ulcer	Perforation, site ulcer, mortality; sex, age; monthly, daily, hourly distribution	W Scot.	1938–43	[QRL 343]	(2.5.5)	L
Alimentary disease—peptic ulcer	Perforation, site ulcer; sex, age, SC, occupation, urban/rural	NE Scot.	1946–56	[QRL 705]	(2.5.5)	M

Condition	Details	Place	Years	Ref	Section	Size
Alimentary disease—peptic ulcer	Prevalence at autopsy, sex, age, site of perforation	NW London	1952–3	[QRL 361]	(2.5.5)	M
Alimentary disease—peptic ulcer	Prevalence at autopsy, diagnosis, sex, age	UK	1956	[QRL 698]	(2.5.5)	L
Alimentary disease—peptic ulcer	Hospital discharges, complications, mortality, sex, age; teaching/non-teaching hospital	E & W	1956–7	[QRL 355]	(2.5.5)	L
Alimentary disease—peptic ulcer	Incidence, complications, sex, age, SC, urban/rural residence	York & environs	1952–7	[QRL 550]	(2.5.5)	S
Alimentary disease—peptic ulcer	Diagnosis; complications; sex, age, SC, occupation, urban/rural	SW Scot.	1957–9	[QRL 402]	(2.5.5)	M
Alimentary disease—duodenal ulcer	Incidence in men, confidence of diagnosis, age	UK	1947–65	[QRL 456]	(2.5.5)	S
Alimentary disease—peptic ulcer	Prevalence in men; age, SC; dyspepsia, blood group 'O', secretor status, serum pepsinogen	Lambeth	1967–9	[QRL 147]	(2.5.5)	S
Alimentary disease—gastrointestinal haemorrhage	Sex, age, SC; diagnosis, confidence of diagnosis, severity of bleeding, blood group	NE Scot.	1967–8	[QRL 358]	(2.5.5)	S
Alimentary disease—Crohn's disease	Hospital admission, site; sex, age, SC, blood group, urban/rural	NE Scot.	1955–68	[QRL 382]	(2.5.5)	VS
Alimentary disease—Crohn's disease	Estimated incidence, sex	Nottingham	1958–72	[QRL 465]	(2.5.5)	VS
Alimentary disease—gall bladder	Prevalence at autopsy, sex, age	Dundee	1902–73	[QRL 56]	(2.5.5)	M
Alimentary disease—gall bladder	Operations, sex, age, per cent of all operations	Bristol	1933–70	[QRL 327]	(2.5.5)	M
Alimentary disease—gall bladder	Operations, age	Luton	1961, 71	[QRL 541]	(2.5.5)	S
Alimentary disease—acute pancreatitis	Sex, age, incidence, deaths, cause, recurrences	Bristol	1950–67	[QRL 659]	(2.5.5)	S
Alimentary disease—abnormal radiology	Sex, age; diagnosis	NE Scot.	1967–70	[QRL 537]	(2.5.5)	VL
Arthritis—rheumatoid	Prevalence by diagnoses, joints involved, clinical grade, X-ray, differential agglutination test, sex	Leigh	1949–54	[QRL 368]	(2.5.6)	S
Arthritis—rheumatoid	Prevalence, X-ray, differential agglutination test; sex, age	Rhondda	1953–5	[QRL 462]	(2.5.6) 2.2.2.2	L
Arthritis—rheumatoid	Prevalence, certainty of diagnosis, X-ray, sex, age	Leigh and Wensleydale	1954–6	[QRL 390]	(2.5.6)	M
Arthritis—rheumatoid	Prevalence, certainty of diagnosis, X-ray	Annandale	1955	[QRL 392]	(2.5.6)	VS
Arthritis—disc degeneration	Prevalence, symptoms, X-ray, sex, age, occupation	Leigh, Rhondda, Watford, Wensleydale	1953–6	[QRL 391]	(2.5.6)	M

Need—*contd.*

Morbidity: Specific studies—contd.

Topic and type of data	Detail of analysis	Area	Year	Publication (see QRL key)	Text reference	Remarks
Arthritis—Paget's	Hospital discharge rates; mortality	E, W, S: Hosp. Reg.	1961–72	[QRL 51]	(2.5.6)	M
Blood diseases— anaemia	Prevalence of anaemia, diagnosis, Hb, PCV, MCHC, sex, age, miners/non-miners	Rhondda Fach	1958	[QRL 375]	(2.5.7) 2.2.2.2	S
Blood diseases— anaemia	Prevalence of anaemia, diagnosis, Hb, PCV, serum iron, sex, age	Wensleydale	1958	[QRL 374]	(2.5.7) 2.2.2.2	S
Blood diseases— anaemia	Symptoms, Hb, PCV, sex, age	Cardiff	1963	[QRL 723]	(2.5.7) 2.2.2.2	S
Blood diseases— pernicious anaemia	Prevalence of pernicious anaemia	GB; Reg.	1957	[QRL 596]	(2.5.7)	VL
Cancer: mortality	Sex, age, site, calendar period	E & W	1911–70	[QRL 136]	(2.5.8)	VL
Cancer: incidence	Sex, age, site	Manchester	1932–64	[QRL 222]	2.5.8	L
Cancer: incidence	Sex, age, site	Birmingham	1960–72	[QRL 692]	2.5.8	VL
Cancer—breast: relative risk	Age, MS, duration schooling, age at marriage, age at first pregnancy, parity, lactation history	S Wales	1965–7	[QRL 416]	(2.5.8)	S
Cancer—cervix	Age; interval first coitus to positive smear; category of preclinical cancer	NE Scot.	1958–67	[QRL 425]	(2.5.8)	VL
Cancer—cervix	Age; SC, clinic/home smear	Derby	1964–5	[QRL 518]	(2.5.8)	M
Cancer—cervix	Prevalence of positives: age, SC, place of screening	Nottingham	1966–70	[QRL 526]	(2.5.8)	L
Cervix cancer— aetiology	Prevalence *in situ* carcinoma and SMR by occupational order of husband	Manchester R	1965–72	[QRL 675]	(2.5.8)	VL
Cardiovascular disease— IHD	Incidence and mortality, activity at work	London	1948–52	[QRL 493]	(2.5.9)	VL
Cardiovascular disease— IHD	Incidence and mortality, BP, serum cholesterol, physique, family history, age	London	1956–65	[QRL 494]	(2.5.9)	S
Cardiovascular disease— IHD	Prevalence symptoms, ECG changes, mortality, age, miners/not miners	Rhondda	1958	[QRL 308]	(2.5.9) 2.2.2.2	S
Cardiovascular disease— IHD	Prevalence of symptoms, ECG changes, BP, physique, age, smoking, respiratory function	E.	1963	[QRL 562]	(2.5.9)	S
Cardiovascular disease— IHD	Prevalence symptoms, ECG changes, confidence of diagnosis, physique, age, occupation, smoking, respiratory functions	Staveley	1966	[QRL 310]	(2.5.9) 2.2.2.2	S

Topic	Description	Place	Years	Reference	Section	Size
Cardiovascular disease—IHD	Prevalence symptoms, ECG changes, BP, wt, diabetes, per cent having medical care	London	1968–72	[QRL 560]	(2.5.9)	L
Cardiovascular disease—IHD	Incidence infarction, previous history smoking, age, leisure activity	E & W	1968–72	[QRL 491]	(2.5.9)	S
Cardiovascular disease—IHD	Incidence and mortality, previous history, sex, age	Edinburgh	1967–8	[QRL 257]	(2.5.9)	M
Cardiovascular disease—IHD	First/subsequent attacks, mortality, sex, age, place of birth	Tower Hamlets	1970–2	[QRL 533]	(2.5.9)	S
Cardiovascular disease—IHD	Incidence, mortality, promonitory symptoms, sex, SC	Tees-side	1972–3	[QRL 159]	(2.5.9)	M
Cardiovascular disease—IHD	Male civil servants: age, smoking, physique, BP, cholesterol and blood glucose, other risk factors: relationship to incidence of angina and ECG changes	London	1968–75	[QRL 563]	(2.5.9)	L
Cardiovascular disease—hypertension	Distribution of blood pressure: sex, age, correction for arm circumference	W London	1951	[QRL 289]	(2.5.9)	M
Cardiovascular disease—hypertension	Distribution of blood pressure: sex, age, index groups and relatives	W London	1951	[QRL 290]	(2.5.9)	S
Heart disease—hypertension	Systolic and diastolic pressure in population sample and first-degree relatives; sex, age	Rhondda Fach	1954	[QRL 464]	(2.5.9) 2.2.2.2	M
Heart disease—hypertension	Initial and subsequent BP, cardiovascular and renal morbidity, mortality, sex, age	Rhondda Fach and Vale	1954–71	[QRL 463]	(2.5.9)	M
Cardiovascular disease—hypertension	Sex, age, parental mortality; distribution of BP	Birmingham	1960	[QRL 415]	(2.5.9)	L
Heart disease—hypertension	BP, cardiac width; age, sex	Tyree, Glasgow & Clackmannan	1969	[QRL 300]	(2.5.9)	M
Heart disease—hypertension	BP, sex, age	Renfrew	1972–3	[QRL 301]	(2.5.9)	M
Cardiovascular disease—stroke	Incidence; sex	S London, N Surrey	1962–3	[QRL 170]	(2.5.9)	VS
Cardiovascular disease—varicose veins	Population sample and first-degree relatives: sex, age, family history, parity, heavy lifting, prevalence of varicose veins	Cardiff	1966	[QRL 704]	(2.5.9)	S
Cardiovascular disease and blood group	Atherosclerosis patients: diagnosis, blood-group distribution	London	1958–70	[QRL 376]	(2.5.9)	M
Cardiovascular disease and blood group	Venous thromboembolism patients: diagnosis, blood group	Nottingham	1961–70	[QRL 634]	(2.5.9)	S
Cardiovascular disease and diet	Sucrose intake, heart diagnosis, smoking, sex	S Wales	1968	[QRL 230]	(2.5.9) 2.2.2.2	M
Cardiovascular disease and diet	Myocardial infarction and control patient, sugar intake, smoking, weight, activity at work, SC, MS	E & Scot.	1968–9	[QRL 542]	(2.5.9)	S

Topic and type of data	Detail of analysis	Area	Year	Publication (see QRL key)	Text reference	Remarks
Need—*contd.*						
Morbidity: Specific studies—*contd.*						
Cardiovascular disease and diet	Myocardial infarction, control patients, relatives: lipid profiles, sex, age	London	1970–1	[QRL 530]	(2.5.9)	S
Cardiovascular disease and diet	Myocardial infarction and control patients, lipid profiles, sex, age	London	1972–3	[QRL 399]	(2.5.9)	S
Cardiovascular disease and family history	Patients with IHD and controls: sex, age, observed and expected deaths from arteriosclerotic heart disease, myocardial degeneration, stroke	London	1964–5	[QRL 615]	(2.5.9)	M
Cardiovascular disease and hardness of drinking water	Average annual mortality rates for heart disease and all causes; change in death rates, change in water hardness; sex	E & W	1948–64	[QRL 169]	(2.5.9)	L
Cardiovascular disease and hardness of drinking water	Persons dying from accidents: macroscopic state of coronary vessels, calcium and magnesium content	London & Glasgow	1964–5	[QRL 171]	(2.5.9)	S
Cardiovascular disease and hardness of drinking water	Males living in six hard-water and six soft-water towns: age, physique, smoking, heart rate, BP, cholesterol, respiratory function	E & W	1971–2	[QRL 631]	(2.5.9)	S
Children: perinatal loss	Maternal age, parity, SC; obstetric history, care in pregnancy, details of delivery	GB; Planning Reg.	1958	[QRL 111]	2.5.10.1	VL; Q
Children: perinatal loss	Maternal age, height, smoking, parity, SC; care in pregnancy, details of delivery	GB; Planning Reg.	1958	[QRL 110]	2.5.10.1	VL; Q
Children: neonatal death	Sex, SC, birth wt, delivery characteristics	Newcastle	1960–7	[QRL 500]	2.5.10.1	L
Children: post-neonatal deaths	Age of infant; maternal age, parity, pregnancy history, country of birth, avoidable factors, cause of death	E.	1964–6	[QRL 187]	2.5.10.3	S; Q
Children: infant deaths	Sex; maternal age, parity, SC; cause of death, multiple births, legitimacy	E & W; Reg. conurbations urban/rural aggregates	1949–50	[QRL 304]	2.5.10.3	VL
Children: infant deaths	Maternal age, parity, SC, legitimacy, cause of death	E & W; Reg.	1964–5	[QRL 624]	2.5.10.3	L

Children: infant deaths	Sudden deaths in infancy: sex, age, month of death; illness in preceding fortnight, type of bedding	E.	1954–63	[QRL 472]	2.5.10.3	S; Q
Children: infancy	Illnesses, accidents, congenital malformations, use of health services; SC, housing, child care	Newcastle	1947–8	[QRL 623]	2.5.10.1	M
Children: 1–5	Illnesses, accidents, physical and emotional development, use of health services; age, SC, housing	Newcastle	1948–53	[QRL 468]	2.5.10.1	S
Children: 1–5	Illnesses, accidents, development, use of health services; sex, age, SC, separation from parents, prematurity	GB; Reg.	1948–50	[QRL 212]	2.5.10.1	M; Q
Children: school children	Physical and emotional abnormalities at 6; sex, SC	GB; Reg.	1952	[QRL 212]	2.5.10.1	M; Q
Children: school children	Disturbed behaviour, mental ability; SC	E & W	1954–7	[QRL 211]	2.5.10.1	M
Children: school children	Illnesses, physical and emotional development, IQ, use of health services; SC, child care	Newcastle	1952–62	[QRL 467]	2.5.10.1	S
Children: school children	Sex, SC, family characteristics; obstetric history; intellectual and educational retardation; psychiatric disorders; physical disability	Isle of Wight	1965	[QRL 588]	2.5.10.5	S
Children: under 8	Sex, SC; hospital admissions, cause; other ailments requiring hospital care; psychological and social adjustment	GB; Stand. Reg.	1958–65	[QRL 179]	2.5.10.1	L; Q
Children: aged 11	Prevalence of enuresis, asthma, bronchitis, visual defects; hospitalization, reason; stage of puberty, number requiring special education, handicap	GB	1958–69	[QRL 532]	2.5.10.1	L
Children: aged 15	Minor illnesses reported by cause; asthma and bronchitis; skin conditions; eneuresis: migraine; hearing, speech and vision; pubertal development; obesity; medical reasons for school absences	GB	1973–5	[QRL 241]	2.5.10.1	L
Children—home care of acute illness	No. of patients, month of year, source of cases, procedures involved, expenditure	W London	1954–5	[QRL 400]	2.5.10.3	S
Children—congenital abnormalities	Incidence, age at ascertainment, combined malformations	Birmingham	1950–9	[QRL 394]	2.5.10.2	L
Children—congenital abnormalities	Incidence, diagnosis, age and method of diagnosis; maternal age, parity, occupation, illness in pregnancy	Watford & St. Albans	1952–5	[QRL 422]	2.5.10.2	M

Topic and type of data	Detail of analysis	Area	Year	Publication (see QRL key)	Text reference	Remarks
Need—*contd.*						
Morbidity: Specific studies—*contd.*						
Children—congenital abnormalities	Incidence, diagnosis, mortality in infancy and stillbirth	Exeter	1954–60	[QRL 687]	2.5.10.2	S
Children—congenital abnormalities	Incidence, diagnosis; rate/thousand births	Liverpool & Bootle	1960–4	[QRL 618]	2.5.10.2	M
Children—congenital abnormalities	Incidence, type; multiple defects; source of notification	S Wales	1964–6	[QRL 567]	2.5.10.2	M
Children—congenital abnormalities	Incidence of CNS defects, type, live or still-birth, sex, month of birth	NI	1964–8	[QRL 225]	2.5.10.2	M
Children—non-accidental injury	Incidence, type of injury, age, sex; father's occupation, home circumstances, attitude of parents	NE Wiltshire	1965–73	[QRL 514]	2.5.10.4	VS
Children—non-accidental injury	Parents' age, personality, neurosis, IQ, criminal record	Birmingham	1971–2	[QRL 617]	(2.5.10.4)	S
Children—asthma	Sex, age, family size, SC; allergic manifestations, respiratory functions	Aberdeen	1964	[QRL 184]	(2.5.10.5)	VS
Children—louse infestation	Prevalence, age, sex, social character of school	E	1975	[QRL 208]	(2.5.10.5)	S
Children—deafness	Incidence in children under 6; sex, year of birth; family history	NI	1953	[QRL 629]	(2.5.11)	S
Deafness	Hearing loss, sex, age, audio-frequency	Annandale	1957	[QRL 314]	(2.5.11)	S
Deafness	Age, sex, acoustic trauma from rifle fire and occupation; prevalence of presbycusis, conductive deafness, diagnosis	S Wales, Annandale	1957–8	[QRL 315]	(2.5.11)	S
Dental health	Sex, age, MS, SC, SEG; number of teeth per person, proportion decayed, proportion restored, proportion denture wearers; subjects' opinions of dental health and dental care, frequency of dental care	Salisbury, Darlington	1963	[QRL 105]	2.5.12	S; Q
Dental health	Sex, age, SC; state of dental health; treatment, attitudes and practice of dental hygiene	E & W	1968	[QRL 282]	2.5.12	M; Q
Dental health	Sex, age, SC; state of dental health; treatment knowledge, attitudes and practice of dental hygiene	S	1972	[QRL 652]	2.5.12	M; Q

Dental health of children	Age; parents' SC and education; state of dental health: mother's attitude, knowledge and practice of dental hygiene	E & W	1973	[QRL 650]	2.5.12	L; Q
Diabetes	Glycosuria; diabetic	Salford	1955	[QRL 107]	2.5.13	M
Diabetes	Glycosuria; diabetic, lag-storage, renal, transient, and childhood glycosuria	Newcastle	1957	[QRL 558]	2.5.13	M
Diabetes	Glycosuria, age, sex; blood sugar, sex; diagnoses	Halstead	1960	[QRL 292]	2.5.13	L
Diabetes	Glycosuria; glucose tolerance tests; family history; obesity; age	Birmingham	1960	[QRL 70]	2.5.13	L
Diabetes	Glycosuria; blood sugar; glucose tolerance tests; 'borderline' diabetics	Bedford	1961	[QRL 606]	2.5.13	VL
Diabetes in children	Incidence, age, sex	GB	1972	[QRL 670]	(2.5.13) 2.5.10.1	L
Elderly—national studies	Sex, age, MS, SC, income; morbidity; incapacity; sensory impairment; illnesses; self-evaluation of health; loneliness; contact with health and welfare services	GB	1962	[QRL 658]	2.5.14	M
Elderly—national studies	Requirement for home helps, rehousing, district nursing and health visitor	GB	1965	[QRL 296]	2.5.14	M; Q
Elderly—local studies	Sex, age, MS; assessment of health; specific disabilities; social circumstances; recent medical care	Wolverhampton	1945–7	[QRL 608]	2.5.14	S; Q
Elderly—local studies	Sex, age, MS, occupation, social circumstances; physical disabilities, recent medical care	NI	1949	[QRL 7]	2.5.14	M; Q
Elderly—local studies	Sex, age, MS, SC; physical abnormalities on examination; mental state; nutrition; mobility; recent medical care	Sheffield	1949–51	[QRL 321]	2.5.14	S; Q
Elderly—local studies	Sex, age, MS, SC; prevalence of health and welfare needs; mobility, isolation, mental state, severity of illness	Edinburgh	1954	[QRL 278]	(2.5.14)	M; Q
Elderly—local studies	Sex, age, MS; social isolation, mobility; recent medical care; support required when ill	E London	1954–5	[QRL 656]	2.5.14	S; Q
Elderly—local studies	Sex, age, social characteristics; diet, recent illnesses, mobility	Dundee	1955	[QRL 443]	(2.5.14)	S; Q
Elderly—local studies	Sex, age, MS, SC, housing, social isolation, activities; physical illnesses, mobility, care required when ill; persons in institutions, reasons for admission; mortality cause	Stockport	1956–7	[QRL 94]	(2.5.14)	M
Elderly—local studies	Sex, age, MS; mobility; contact with GP; isolation and loneliness	Orkneys	1957	[QRL 571]	(2.5.14)	S

Topic and type of data	Detail of analysis	Area	Year	Publication (see QRL key)	Text reference	Remarks
Need—*contd.*						
Morbidity: Specific studies—contd.						
Elderly—local studies	Sex, age, social isolation, housing; use of community services; proportion requiring admission to institutions; mobility	Barrow	1961	[QRL 223]	(2.5.14)	S
Elderly—local studies	Sex, age, MS, social isolation, loneliness, mobility	Harrow, Northampton, Oldham, S Norfolk	1963–4	[QRL 663]	2.5.14	S; Q
Elderly—examination of GP's patients	Sex, age; mean haemoglobin; prevalence of iron deficiency anaemia by cause; folate and B12 levels	Kilsyth and Glasgow	1969–70	[QRL 438]	(2.5.14)	S
Elderly—local studies	Sex, age, MS, SC; housing and amenities; mobility, physical and mental illness, use of health and welfare services	Scottish Border Counties	1971–2	[QRL 286]	(2.5.15)	S; Q
Elderly—examination of GP's patients	Men aged 60–69; SC; prevalence of various diseases or disabilities; smoking; per cent in employment; reasons for retirement	Birmingham	1956	[QRL 102]	(2.5.14)	M
Elderly—examination of GP's patients	Sex, age, SC; mobility, symptoms; physical and emotional illness; contact with health services; need for further care	Aberdeen	1962	[QRL 561]	(2.5.14)	S; Q
Elderly—examination of GP's patients	Sex, age; known and unknown disabilities; physical and mental illness	Edinburgh	1962–3	[QRL 714]	(2.5.14)	S
Elderly—examination of GP's patients	Sex, age; disabilities detected; need for four community services	Kilsyth	1969	[QRL 25]	(2.5.14)	S
Elderly—in institutions	Sex, age, family; mobility, ability for self-care, specific handicaps, mental impairment	E & W	1958–60	[QRL 657]	(2.5.14)	L; Q
Elderly—in hospital	Sex, age; diagnoses; multiple pathology	Aberdeen	1957	[QRL 715]	(2.5.14)	S
Elderly—in hospital	Sex, age, MS, social characteristics; available care at home; duration of dependency, diagnosis	Glasgow	1966–7	[QRL 350]	2.5.14	S; Q
Elderly—receiving community services	Age, housing, finance, isolation; mobility and handicaps; frequency of care from community services; need for specific services	S London	1951	[QRL 139]	(2.5.14)	M

Topic	Variables/details	Location	Year	Reference	Section	Code
Elderly—receiving community services	Sex, age, finance, isolation; mobility	W Hartlepool	1962	[QRL 47]	(2.5.14)	S; Q
Elderly—receiving community services	Sex, age; nutrition, socio-medical assessment, diagnoses of physical and psychiatric disorders	S London	1965–6	[QRL 274]	2.5.14	S; Q
Elderly—mental disorders	Sex, age; diagnosis of psychiatric disorders; previous treatment and institutional care	Newcastle	1960	[QRL 366]	2.5.14	S
Elderly—mental disorders	Sex, age, MS; psychiatric assessment; learning test scores, peripheral arteriosclerosis, generations in household; neuroses; GPs' awareness of illness	Swansea	1961	[QRL 528]	2.5.14	S
Elderly—osteoporosis	Sex; height and weight, cortical thickness, biochemistry	S Wales	1956–67	[QRL 8]	(2.5.14) 2.2.2.2	VS
Elderly—anaemia	Sex, age; haematological values	S Wales	1968–9	[QRL 227]	(2.5.14) 2.2.2.2	S
Elderly—hospital bed requirement	Sex, age, SC, urban/rural; beds required, specialty	NE Engl.	1967	[QRL 260]	(2.5.14)	L
Environment—air pollution	SO_2 and smoke levels; secular trend; variation in residential, commercial, industrial, and smoke control areas	UK, SR, C, CB	1961–71	[QRL 202]	2.5.15	L
Environment—air pollution	Rural and urban locations: smoke, hydrocarbon levels	NW Engl. N Wales	1956–7	[QRL 160]	2.5.15	L
Environment—air pollution	Smoke, SO_2, specific hydrocarbons, secular variation; CO, hourly variation	City of London	1961–3	[QRL 683]	2.5.15	L
Environment—air pollution	Smoke, specific hydrocarbons; monthly variation	Belfast	1961–2	[QRL 682]	2.5.15	M
Epilepsy	Sex, age, MS, SC; prevalence, incidence, age at onset, frequency attacks, aetiology	E	1958	[QRL 545]	(2.5.16)	S
Eye diseases—blindness	Sex, age; diagnosis, aetiology, degree of blindness	E & W	1948–62	[QRL 619–622]	2.5.17	VL
Eye diseases—blindness	Sex, age: mobility, residual sight, use of aids, need for aids; Braille reading ability; use of talking books	E & W	1965	[QRL 281]	2.5.17	M; Q
Eye diseases—blindness	Registered handicapped: sex; age, MS, SC; cause of blindness; ability to work; contact with statutory services; need for home help; other handicaps	GLC	1968–70	[QRL 2]	2.5.17	S
Eye diseases—glaucoma	Sex, age; ocular pressure; prevalence glaucoma by type	S Wales	1964	[QRL 332]	(2.5.17) 2.2.2.2	M
Eye diseases—glaucoma	Sex, age; ocular pressure; further assessment required; prevalence glaucoma	Bedford	1964–6	[QRL 48]	2.5.17	L

Need—*contd.*

Morbidity: Specific studies—*contd.*

Topic and type of data	Detail of analysis	Area	Year	Publication (see QRL key)	Text reference	Remarks
Eye diseases—lens opacities in steel workers	Age: prevalence of cataract; occupation type and length	Ebbw Vale	1969	[QRL 680]	2.5.17	S
Family planning	Age, SC, religion, family size; knowledge, attitudes and practice of family planning	E & W	1967–70	[QRL 128]	2.5.18	S
Family planning	MS, characteristics of women; knowledge, attitudes and practice	E & W	1970	[QRL 76]	2.5.18	M; Q
Family planning	General practitioner's age, sex, religion; attitudes to: role in birth control, changes needed in services; contraindications and side effects of pill; sterilization; methods used and changes 1967–71; high parity and illegitimacy in locality	E & W	1970–1	[QRL 133, 134]	2.5.18	S; Q
Family planning—students	Age, sexual experience, type of partner, use of contraception; views on: contraceptive advice+pregnancy; reasons for not using contraception	Aberdeen	1971	[QRL 421]	(2.5.18)	M
Feet	Sex, age, SC; prevalence of abnormalities, duration of symptoms, self-treatment	E & W	1966	[QRL 146]	2.5.19	M; Q
Genito-urinary disease—dysuria	Women, age; prevalence of dysuria, renal function, BP, contact with health services	S Wales	1967	[QRL 696]	(2.5.20) 2.2.2.2	M
Genito-urinary disease	Women, age; urinary symptoms, renal function, consumption of analgesics	S Wales	1967–8	[QRL 695]	(2.5.20) 2.2.2.2	M
Genito-urinary disease	Renal failure requiring dialysis or transplant; sex, age, diagnosis, presence of other disease	Scot.	1968–9	[QRL 534]	2.5.20	S
Genito-urinary disease	Renal failure requiring dialysis: sex, age, diagnosis	NI	1968–70	[QRL 424]	2.5.20	S
Handicap—national study	Sex, age, household composition, income; cause of disability; limitation of household, leisure, work activity	GB	1968–9	[QRL 297]	2.5.21	L; Q
Handicap—national study	Sex, age, MS, education; occupational status, limitation of work activity	GB	1968–9	[QRL 104]	2.5.21	L; Q

Handicap—local studies	Sex, age; prevalence of disability, diagnosis	Peterborough	1953	[QRL 49]	2.5.21	M
Handicap—local studies	Sex, age; prevalence of disability, diagnosis	Lambeth	1966–7	[QRL 62]	(2.5.21) 2.2.2.4	L
Handicap—local studies	Sex, age, MS; disability, cause, limitation of activity	E London	1967	[QRL 614]	2.5.21	M
Handicap—local studies	Sex, age, MS; young chronic sick known to GP, disability, IQ, diagnosis, support required	W Scot.	1970–1	[QRL 437]	2.5.21	VS
Handicap—young chronic sick in hospital	Sex, age; type hospital, length of stay, diagnosis	E & W	1967	[QRL 475]	2.5.21	M
Maternity	Age, parity, SC; work in pregnancy, expenditure on equipment, premature labour	GB	1946	[QRL 210]	(2.5.22) 2.5.10.1	L; Q
Maternity	Age, parity, SC; toxaemia, place of booking and delivery, gestation; bleeding; delivery method, supervision, duration, analgesia, episiotomy	GB	1958	[QRL 111]	(2.5.22) 2.5.10.1	L; Q
Maternity—mortality	Age, parity, MS; place of booking and delivery; cause of death, avoidable factors	E & W	1952–72	[QRL 29–31] [QRL 676–679]	2.5.22	L
Mental illness	Sex, age, occupation; prevalence contact with various health and welfare agencies	S Wales	1951–6	[QRL 121]	2.5.23	S
Mental illness	Sex, age; persons known to GP with psychiatric symptoms: contact with hospital and welfare services, including admission	Anglesey	1951–63	[QRL 359]	2.5.23	L
Mental illness	Sex; patients with and without psychiatric morbidity, illnesses, grade illness, frequency of consultation	S London	1956–67	[QRL 369]	2.5.23	S
Mental illness	Sex, age, SC, length of residence, social factors; self-assessment of medical diagnoses and nerves; GP, OP and IP contacts	'Newtown, E'	1957–60	[QRL 635]	(2.5.23)	M
Mental illness	Sex, age, MS, SC, social circumstances; general health, personality, physique, neuroses	Croydon	1960–1	[QRL 291]	2.5.23	M; Q
Mental illness	Sex, age, MS, SC, ecological and demographic factors; general health, GP consultation rates, diagnoses, personality, treatment	London	1961–2	[QRL 610]	2.5.23	L; Q
Mental illness	Sex, age, psychiatric symptoms, diagnosis, use of health services	London	1973	[QRL 299]	(2.5.23)	S
Mental illness	Women with and without psychiatric illness: previous life crisis, severity of crisis, SC, family composition, relationship with husband	London	1973	[QRL 100]	(2.5.23)	S

Need—*contd.*

Morbidity: Specific studies—contd.

Topic and type of data	Detail of analysis	Area	Year	Publication (see QRL key)	Text reference	Remarks
Mental illness	Patients consulting GP: proportion with psychiatric illness on screening	Bradford	1973–5	[QRL 356]	(2.5.23)	M
Mental illness— general out-patients	Patients attending various specialties: sex, age, per cent with psychiatric illness on screening	London	1958	[QRL 174]	(2.5.23)	S
Mental illness— admissions	Total admissions, first admission rates, diagnosis, LOS, type of hospital, disposal, sex, age	London	1947–51	[QRL 501]	2.5.23	M
Mental subnormality	Prevalence: sex, age, severity; place of care	Anglesey	1951–63	[QRL 359]	(2.5.24) 2.5.23	L
Mental subnormality	Prevalence: age; severity; diagnosis; known to educational authority	London: Middlesex	1960	[QRL 277]	2.5.24	M
Mental subnormality	Prevalence: severity; family background, details of pregnancy	Newcastle	1960–72	[QRL 500]	(2.5.24) 2.5.10.1	L
Mental subnormality	Prevalence: sex, severity, diagnosis, social grade; aetiology; parental intelligence	Edinburgh	1962–4	[QRL 216]	2.5.24	S
Mental subnormality	Clinical categories; associated diseases; particulars of pregnancy and delivery	Edinburgh	1962–4	[QRL 215]	2.5.24	S
Mental subnormality	Prevalence: sex, SC, family characteristics; IQ, neurological abnormality, psychiatric status; educational placement; details of pregnancy	Aberdeen	1962	[QRL 69]	2.5.24	VS
Mental subnormality	Prevalence: place of care; day school, occupation centres	NI	1962	[QRL 593]	2.5.24	M
Mental subnormality	Prevalence: age, severity of clinical diagnosis; aetiology; behavioural category; place of care	Wessex	1963	[QRL 381]	2.5.24	M
Mental subnormality	Prevalence: age, sex; grade; area of origin; agency of care	NE Scot.	1966	[QRL 346]	2.5.24	M
Mental subnormality	Prevalence: sex, age, social and physical incapacity; agency of care	Camberwell	1967	[QRL 720]	2.5.24	VS
Mental subnormality	Grade; age; type of care; aetiology; dependence on others	NE Scot.	1968–70	[QRL 727]	2.5.24	M

Topic	Variables	Place	Year	Reference	Section	Source
Migraine	Prevalence: age, sex, vision	S Wales	1968	[QRL 693]	2.2.2.2	M
Nutrition—infants	Age, vitamin D intake	E & W	1960	[QRL 81]	2.5.25	M
Nutrition—children	Sex, age, family size, income, maternal education, SEG; physique, nutrient intake	GB	1963	[QRL 475]	2.5.25	S; Q
Nutrition—children	Sex, age, family size, income, maternal education, SC; physique, nutrient intake	GB	1967–8	[QRL 196]	2.5.25	M; Q
Nutrition—elderly	Sex, age, income, expenditure on food; anthropometric, medical and biochemical values; energy and nutrient intake	GB	1967–8	[QRL 189]	2.5.25	S; Q
Nutrition—elderly	Sex, age, MS, SC, housing, income, expenditure on food; consumption of food items; energy and nutrient intake	Sheffield	1951	[QRL 82]	2.5.25	S
Nutrition—elderly	Age, household, mobility; nutrient intake; physique	N London & Herefordshire	1970	[QRL 233]	2.5.25	VS
Nutrition—elderly	Place of birth, anthropometry, haematological and biochemical values	Coventry	1970	[QRL 226]	2.5.25	S
Physique—adults	Sex, age, height, weight	S Wales	1954, 1958	[QRL 33]	(2.5.26)	M
Physique—males	Age, height, weight	Birmingham	1960	[QRL 371]	(2.5.26)	L
Physique—adults	Sex, age, height, weight, occupational category	London	1964–6	[QRL 485]	(2.5.26)	L
Physique—males	Sex, age, height, weight; occupational category	S Wales	1965	[QRL 371]	(2.5.26)	L
Physique—males	Age, smoking, height, weight	London	1970	[QRL 681]	(2.5.26)	M
Physique—pregnant women	Age, SC, calendar period, height, weight	Aberdeen	1950–64	[QRL 645]	(2.5.26)	L
Physique—cohort born 1947	Sex, age, birth rank, family size, subjects' occupation, parents' SC, age at menarche, height, weight	Newcastle	1947–69	[QRL 466]	(2.5.26) 2.5.10.1	S
Physique—school children	Sex, age, family size, height, weight, skinfold	London	1959	[QRL 597]	(2.5.26)	L
Physique—school children	Sex, age, skinfold	Aylesbury	1971	[QRL 156]	(2.5.26)	M
Rehabilitation— hospital in-patients	Sex, specialty, prognosis, outcome	London	1950	[QRL 662]	2.5.27	M
Rehabilitation— hospital in-patients	Males, age, SC, previous employment, diagnosis, prognosis, outcome	Glasgow	1950–3	[QRL 238]	2.5.27	S
Rehabilitation— hospital in-patients	Males, age, LOS, prognosis, outcome	Glasgow	1957–9	[QRL 177]	2.5.27	S
Rehabilitation— hospital in-patients	Sex, age, MS, SC, housing, diagnosis, length of stay, prognosis, outcome	Dundee	1957–60	[QRL 293]	2.5.27	S
Rehabilitation— hospital in-patients	Males: age, diagnosis, length of stay, prognosis, outcome	Aberdeen	1957–9	[QRL 706]	2.5.27	S

Topic and type of data	Detail of analysis	Area	Year	Publication (see QRL key)	Text reference	Remarks
Need—*contd.*						
Morbidity: Specific studies—contd.						
Rehabilitation— hospital in-patients	Sex, age, household, MS, SC, prognosis, outcome	Aberdeen	1972	[QRL 75]	2.5.27	VS
Respiratory disease— national sample	Sex, age, MS, SC, urban/rural residence, smoking; phlegm production, prevalence of chronic bronchitis, respiratory function	GB	1959	[QRL 256]	(2.5.28)	M
Respiratory disease— population study	Sex, age, SC, urbanization, air pollution, smoking; prevalence of respiratory disease	GB	1965	[QRL 383]	(2.5.28)	L
Respiratory disease— national sample	Postmen: incidence of respiratory disorders, secular trend temperature and fog, air pollution index	UK	1950–7	[QRL 561]	(2.5.28)	M
Respiratory disease— national sample	Civil servants: age, sex, indoor/outdoor work, population density, overcrowding, 'fog index', sickness absence bronchitis and other respiratory diseases	GB	1948–54	[QRL 234]	(2.5.28)	L
Respiratory disease— four area sample	Postmen: age, smoking, prevalence of respiratory symptoms, respiratory function, sputum production	London, Gloucester, Norwich, Peterborough	1960–1	[QRL 330]	(2.5.28)	S
Respiratory disease— local study	Men 55–64: occupation, SC, smoking, prevalence of respiratory symptoms, respiratory function, X-ray abnormality, physique	Leigh	1954	[QRL 311]	(2.5.28) 2.2.2.2	S
Respiratory disease— local study	Sex, age, smoking, occupation, dust exposure, respiratory symptoms and function, X-ray abnormality	Staveley	1957	[QRL 307]	(2.5.28) 2.2.2.2	S; Q
Respiratory disease— local study	Nine-year follow-up; original age, occupation, smoking, respiratory function, X-ray, subsequent respiratory function, mortality	Staveley	1966	[QRL 309]	(2.5.28) 2.2.2.2	S
Respiratory disease— local study	Sex, age, SC, smoking, prevalence of chronic bronchitis	Cheshire	1964–5	[QRL 574]	2.5.28	VL
Respiratory disease— local study	Males: age, prevalence of chronic bronchitis; non-bronchitics: smoking, medical history, physique, respiratory function	S Wales	1964–5	[QRL 417]	2.5.28	VL

Respiratory disease—local study	Male: age, smoking, dust concentrations SO_2; prevalence of respiratory symptoms and chronic bronchitis, FEV	S Wales	1964–5	[QRL 416]	2.5.28	L
Respiratory disease—local study	Civil servants (male): age, prevalence of respiratory symptoms, respiratory function, X-ray abnormality	London	1969–71	[QRL 560]	(2.5.28)	L
Respiratory disease—children	Attack rates acute coryza, chronic catarrh, sore throat, pneumococci and streptococci, tonsillectomy; sex, age, social factors	W London	1952–3	[QRL 84]	(2.5.28)	M
Respiratory disease—children	Cohort born 1946 studied when 15: previous disease in infancy, school absences, hospitalization, SC, air pollution; prevalence of respiratory and ENT disease	GB	1961	[QRL 214]	(2.5.28) 2.5.10.1	M; Q
Respiratory disease—children	Cohort born 1946 studied when 20: sex, SC, smoking, air pollution, respiratory disease as child, prevalence of respiratory symptoms	GB	1966	[QRL 157]	(2.5.28) 2.5.10.1	M
Respiratory disease—children	Sex, age, SC, urban/rural residence, prevalence of respiratory and ENT disease, respiratory function	EW	1966	[QRL 158]	(2.5.28)	L
Respiratory disease—children	Sex, age, SC, no. children in house, no. persons in bedroom, history and prevalence of respiratory disease, respiratory function	Sheffield	1963–5	[QRL 419]	(2.5.28)	S
Respiratory disease—children	Four-year follow-up of 5-year-olds in previous study: previous respiratory state, prevalence of respiratory disease	Sheffield	1967–9	[QRL 420]	(2.5.28)	S
Respiratory disease—children	SC, no. of siblings, parents' smoking and winter phlegm, prevalence of respiratory symptoms	Aylesbury	1971	[QRL 155]	(2.5.28)	M
Respiratory disease—emergency admission	Referrals for admission: sex, age, indices of air pollution and weather	London	1955–62	[QRL 331]	(2.5.28)	L
Respiratory disease—bronchitis patients	Index of degree of illness, indices of air pollution and weather	London, Manchester	1955–68	[QRL 393]	(2.5.28)	M
Respiratory disease—bronchitis patients	Sex, age, smoking, age onset and length history, bronchitis, mortality	London	1951–63	[QRL 520]	(2.5.28)	S
Respiratory disease—bronchitis patients	Age, parents' SC, patients' SC during working life	London	1960	[QRL 457]	(2.5.28)	VS
Respiratory disease—bronchitis patients	Smoking, respiratory function, subsequent deaths over 10 years	London	1963–74	[QRL 357]	(2.5.28)	VS

Topic and type of data	Detail of analysis	Area	Year	Publication (see QRL key)	Text reference	Remarks
Need—*contd.*						
Morbidity: Specific studies—*contd.*						
Screening—adults multiphasic	Sex, age, SC, smoking; health worries, recent use health services, prevalence defects of breast, anaemia, diabetes, ocular pressure, hearing, vision, BP, ECG, respiratory function, sputum production	Rotherham	1962–6	[QRL 268]	2.3.1	(L); Q
Screening—general practice—middle-aged men	Age: prevalence previously undiagnosed conditions	Birmingham	1971	[QRL 539]	(2.3.1)	(VS)
Screening—general practice—middle-aged women	Age; main pathological findings	Edinburgh	1966–7	[QRL 600]	2.3.1	(S)
Screening—school girls	Urinary tract infection—prevalence: radiological findings, year of birth	Cardiff, Oxford	1972	[QRL 42]	(2.3.1) 2.2.2.2	L
Screening—school entrants	Prevalence of neurodevelopmental defects: speech, epilepsy, squint, testicle descent, asthma; school progress	Isle of Wight	1967	[QRL 57]	(2.3.1)	S
Self-medication	Sex, age, SC, personal characteristics; general health, recent symptoms; prescribed and non-prescribed medicines taken, reasons for medication	GB; Reg.	1969	[QRL 220]	2.5.29	M; Q
Self-medication	Sex, age, prescribed and non-prescribed medicines taken, category and frequency of medicine taken	GB	1972–3	[QRL 512, 513]	(2.5.29) 2.2.1.2	VL; Q
Sexually transmitted disease—gonorrhoea	No. cases treated, sex, country of origin, size of town where treated, location in country	GB	1952–69	[QRL 85, 88, 89]	2.5.30	VL
Sexually transmitted disease—syphilis	No. cases treated, sex, country of origin, size of town where treated	GB	1963–9	[QRL 86, 87, 90]	2.5.30	M
Sexually transmitted disease	No. cases treated, diagnosis, country of origin	E & W	1945–68	[QRL 711]	2.5.30	VL
Skin disease	Prevalence of skin disease, diagnosis, severity; sex, age, SC, previous medical care	Lambeth	1967–9	[QRL 556]	2.2.2.4	M

Topic	Details	Area	Date	Reference	Section	Code
Smoking—adults and adolescents	Sex, age, SC, smoking habits: knowledge/attitude/practice of respondent, parents, friends and school of smoking; church attendance; attempts to stop smoking	E & W	1964	[QRL 432]	2.5.31	M; Q
Smoking—adults and adolescents	Sex, age, highest qualification attained, SEG, per cent current smokers; type and amount of product smoked	GB	1972–3	[QRL 512, 513]	2.5.31 2.2.12	VL; Q
Smoking—adults and adolescents	Sex, age, SC, occupational group, urban/rural residence; smokers, ex- and non-smokers; age starting; product smoked, consumption, inhaling	UK, E, S, W	1956–71	[QRL 649]	2.5.31	VL
Smoking—students	Smoking habits; medical, non-medical students' knowledge and attitudes of health hazards; attempts to stop smoking	E & W	1965–6	[QRL 114]	2.5.31	M; Q
Smoking—school children	Smoking habits; age, SC, academic ability, personal characteristics; type of school; knowledge/attitudes/practice of respondent, family, friends	E & W	1966	[QRL 115]	2.5.31	L; Q
Smoking—health hazards	Male doctors: age, smoking category, inhaling, years since stopped smoking; mortality rates by cause	GB	1951–71	[QRL 206]	(2.5.31)	VL
Smoking—health hazards	Males—age, occupation, smoking habits; prevalence of respiratory symptoms, and chronic bronchitis; respiratory function	S Wales, Leigh, SW Scot.	1952–5	[QRL 307]	(2.5.31) 2.2.2.2	S
Smoking—health hazards	Pregnant women: influence on perinatal mortality	GB	1958	[QRL 110]	(2.5.31) 2.5.10.1	VL
Smoking—health hazards	Pregnant women: influence on birth weight	UK	1970	[QRL 141]	(2.5.31) 2.5.10.1	VL
Smoking—health hazards	School children: amount smoked, respiratory symptoms	SE Engl.	1965	[QRL 329]	(2.5.31)	M
Smoking—use of health services	Sex, age, smoking habits; GP contacts, OP attendances, days in hospital	Exeter	1966–7	[QRL 34]	(2.5.31)	VL
Terminal care	Sex, age, MS, household composition, no. living children, housing; cause of death, course of fatal illness, place of death, support for community care	E & W	1969	[QRL 130]	2.5.32	S; Q
Terminal care—elderly	Sex, age, MS, SC; cause of death, place of death, duration symptoms, dependency	Glasgow	1969	[QRL 350]	(2.5.32) 2.5.14	L; Q
Terminal care	Sex, age, place of death, dependency	Manchester	1969	[QRL 16]	(2.5.32)	VS

Topic and type of data	Detail of analysis	Area	Year	Publication (see QRL key)	Text reference	Remarks
Need—*contd.*						
Morbidity: Specific studies—contd.						
Thyroid disease	Sex, age, parents, siblings, cousins, residence history, water supply, diet, prevalence thyroid disease, diagnosis	S Wales	1956	[QRL 660]	2.2.2.5	M
Tuberculosis	Notification rates: sex, age, occupation, abnormality detected	E & W; ACs, CBs	1938–55	[QRL 406]	2.5.33	VL
Tuberculosis	Abnormalities at mass X-ray: sex, age, SC, occupation, examinee group; activity of lesion detected	E & W; ACs	1955–7	[QRL 305]	2.5.33	VL
Tuberculosis	Abnormalities at mass X-ray: detection rate, active cases, type of unit, notifications	Scot., Aberdeen, Dundee, Edinburgh, Glasgow, Lanark	1949–69	[QRL 124]	2.5.33	VL
Tuberculosis	Prevalence of infective tuberculosis, progressive massive fibrosis, and positive tuberculin tests; sex, age, miners, ex-miners, non-miners; proportion newly discovered lesions	S Wales	1950–1	[QRL 151]	(2.5.33) 2.2.2.2	VL
Tuberculosis	Prevalence and incidence of infective tuberculosis, positive tuberculin tests; sex, age	S Wales	1953	[QRL 152]	2.5.33 2.2.2.2	VL; Q
Tuberculosis	Prevalence infective tuberculosis; sex, age	S Wales	1955	[QRL 153]	(2.5.33) 2.2.2.2	L
Tuberculosis	Prevalence tuberculosis, proportion new; sex, age	Annandale	1956	[QRL 148]	2.5.33 2.2.2.2	L
Unmet demand						
General practice						
Waiting time at GP's surgery	Time waited; appointment system	E & W	1964	[QRL 127]	(3.1)	M; Q

Waiting time at GP's surgery	Average waiting time, per cent waiting 30 minutes, appointment systems	'GB'	1963–5	[QRL 64]	(3.1)	S; Q
Waiting at GP's surgery	Average and maximum numbers in waiting room, appointment system	'GB'	1963–5	[QRL 64]	(3.1)	S; Q
Request for home visit	Time taken when doctor 'wanted in a hurry'	E & W	1964	[QRL 127]	(3.1)	M; Q
Request for night visit	Percentage terminally ill having night visit, possession of telephone	E & W	1969	[QRL 130]	(3.1)	S
Community nursing	Assessment of patients' unmet requirements	GB	1970–1	[QRL 265]	(3.1)	S
OP referral	Interval until referral to OP	E & W	1961	[QRL 126]	(3.1)	S; Q
OP referral	Interval consultation to OP attendance	Edinburgh	1962	[QRL 599]	(3.1)	S

Casualty

Delay before arrival	Time lapse between injury and attendance	E & W	1959	[QRL 252]	(3.2)	S
Failure to contact GP	Source of referral; skill required for care	E & W	1959	[QRL 252]	(3.2)	S
Failure to contact GP	Source of referral; need for hospital care	London	1961	[QRL 74]	(3.2)	S
Description of attenders	Reason for self-referral; medical care and procedures performed; patients' expectations of GPs' actions; SC	Newcastle	1972	[QRL 486]	(3.2)	S

Out-patients

Delay to appointment	Waiting time; specialty	Reading	1960	[QRL 53]	(3.3)	M
Delay to appointment	Average wait; specialty	Ayrshire	1962	[QRL 120]	(3.3)	S
Delay to appointment	Distribution by wait in weeks; specialty, diagnosis; per cent urgent	E & W	1962	[QRL 244]	(3.3)	L
Delay to appointment	Mean wait in days; specialty	SE Engl.		[QRL 140]	(3.3)	M
Delay to appointment	Waiting time; specialty	Aberdeen	1963	[QRL 44]	(3.3)	M
Delay to appointment	Waiting time; specialty	London	1962	[QRL 112]	(3.3)	M
Delay to appointment	Wait by specialty; GPs' views	S Wales	1965–6	[QRL 713]	(3.3)	VS

Topic and type of data	Detail of analysis	Area	Year	Publication (see QRL key)	Text reference	Remarks
Unmet demand—*contd.*						
Out-patients—*contd.*						
Delay to appointment	Waiting time; routine or priority referrals; NHS or private	Leicester	1970	[QRL 248]	(3.3)	M
Child guidance clinic: delay until seen	Per cent waiting by time for different clinics	6 clinics in E	1964	[QRL 648]	(3.3)	M
Ambulance transport	Waiting at home and out-patients for transport	Harrow	1972–3	[QRL 59]	(3.3)	S
Wait in out-patients	Time spent in out-patients	Edinburgh	1962	[QRL 599]	(3.3)	S
Wait in out-patients	Per cent non-attenders; unpunctuality of patients, mode of travel; unpunctuality of start of clinics; patients' waiting time; specialty	GB	1963–4	[QRL 508]	(3.3)	VL
Wait in out-patients	Time waiting in out-patients	Oxford RHB	1955, 1965	[QRL 54]	(3.3)	VL
Emergency admissions	Number of hospitals approached; number rejected, age, sex, diagnosis; time of day	London	1965–6	[QRL 691]	(3.4)	M
Emergency admissions	Percentage accepted immediately, reluctantly, or refused; time spent on telephone	Leicester	1970	[QRL 248]	(3.4)	VS
Admissions of terminally ill	Difficulty in obtaining admission; characteristics of patient, type of care required	E & W	1969	[QRL 130]	(3.4)	S
Waiting list	Delay prior to admission; hospitalization rate in area	E & W	1961	[QRL 126]	(3.4)	S; Q
Waiting list	Average waiting time, coefficient of variation	E & W	1964–71	[QRL 175]	(3.4)	CVL
Special problems						
Abortion—requests for termination	Action when request refused by NHS consultant	E & W	1970	[QRL 131]	(3.4)	S; Q
Abortion—request for termination	Action taken, MS	E & W	1972	[QRL 385]	(3.4)	M
Abortion—request for termination	Interval GP consultation/treatment	E & W	1972	[QRL 385]	(3.4)	M

Abortion—request for termination	Proportion refused by GP and consultant; subsequent action	Somerset	1972	[QRL 527]	(3.4)	VS

Note: See entries in EVALUATION (Chaper 6) for other references on care that has not met the patients' expectations

Private care

Consultations	Population sample: per cent consulting doctor privately; GPs: number of private patients/Dr	E & W	1964	[QRL 127]	(3.6)	S; Q
In-patient care	Hospital in-patients: per cent having private care; fees paid	E & W	1961	[QRL 126]	(3.6)	S; Q
Care of handicapped	Handicapped and impaired: per cent seeking medical advice privately; per cent seeking non-medical advice	GB	1968–9	[QRL 297]	(3.6)	L; Q
Consultations	Hospital referrals: per cent patients opting for private consultation; reasons for request	Leicester	1970	[QRL 248]	(3.6)	M

Resources

Facilities

Ambulances	Number of persons and cost per person carried, cost per vehicle mile	E & W; LAs	Ann. to 1974	[QRL 348]	4.1.1	VL
Ambulances	Type, other vehicles by location; mileage, numbers of journeys and patients carried, ambulance station	NI	Ann. to 1974	[QRL 503]	(4.1.1) 4	VL
Bed provisions—acute	Hospital groups, BGs—sizes according to total allocated beds; wholly psychiatric groups	GB; Hosp. Reg.	1968	[QRL 197]	(4.1.2)	VL
Bed provisions—acute	Critical bed numbers, various specialties, 6 RHBs, surveys	E & W	1956	[QRL 243]	4.1.2	VL
Bed provisions—acute	Demand and supply of beds, specialties, selected RHBs	E & W	1957	[QRL 11]	4.1.2	VL
Bed provisions—acute	Acute bed provisions 1960 to 1975; bed allocations 1969; medical and geriatric beds 1969	E & W; Hosp. Reg.	1960–75	[QRL 403]	4.1.2	VL
Bed provisions—acute	Present beds, critical bed numbers, specialties; beds needed to clear surgical waiting lists	Barrow	1957–8	[QRL 243]	4.1.2	VL
Bed provisions—acute	Survey hospitals, beds available, in-patient data; specialties; population at risk; critical bed numbers, selected diagnoses, comparisons with other surveys	Tees-side	1957–8	[QRL 11]	4.1.2	VL

Topic and type of data	Detail of analysis	Area	Year	Publication (see QRL key)	Text reference	Remarks
Resources—*contd.*						
Facilities—*contd.*						
Bed provisions—acute	Bed provision rates for surgical specialties 1967; rates for various types 1969; av. bed ratios surgical specialties; beds in different types of hospital 1968	Liverpool	1967–9	[QRL 403]	4.1.2	VL
Bed provisions—for children	Paediatrics, special care baby units, infectious diseases, psychiatry, ear, nose and throat; average number of available beds per department; hospital beds per 10,000 population 0–14 years; duration of stay of special-care babies	E & W; Hosp. Reg. (AHAs)	1974, 1975	[QRL 728]	(4.1.2)	L
Bed provisions—gynaecology and obstetric	Gynaecology beds, indices of provision and use	GB; Hosp. Reg.	1958–71	[QRL 385]	(4.1.2)	L
Bed provisions—gynaecology and obstetric	Gynaecology beds, types of wards; additional facilities needed for abortion work	GB; Hosp. Reg.	1972	[QRL 385]	(4.1.2)	L; Q
Bed provisions—gynaecology and obstetric	Obstetric and GP maternity beds, indices of provision and use	GB; Hosp. Reg.	1958–71	[QRL 385]	(4.1.2)	L
Bed provisions—gynaecology and obstetric	Staffed consultant maternity beds, GP staffed maternity beds	E & W; Hosp. Reg.	1968	[QRL 199]	(4.1.2) 4.3.6	L
Bed provisions—gynaecology and obstetric	Estimates of maternity bed requirements, 1981	E & W	1968	[QRL 199]	(4.1.2) 4.3.6	VL
Bed provisions—NI	General and psychiatric bed complement	NI; HMCs, named hosps.	Ann. to 1974	[QRL 503]	(4.1.2) 4	L
Day hospitals—geriatric	Units existing or planned, supporting social and medical services; staffing; old people's welfare committees	UK	1969	[QRL 95]	4.1.3	VS
Day hospitals—geriatric	Individual hospitals, date opened, days open per week 1972, and total attendances 1968	UK; Hosp. Reg., HMCs, BsM, Teaching Hosps.	1968, 1972	[QRL 95]	4.1.3	VS

General practitioner hospitals	Beds, maternity/other, type of unit	UK	1969	[QRL 351]	4.1.4	L
General practitioner hospitals	Maternity units, consultant contact; anaesthetic facilities	E & W	1966	[QRL 318]	4.1.4	S
General practitioner hospitals	Maternity beds available, proximity to consultant beds, separate GP unit	E & W; Hosp. Reg.	1968	[QRL 199]	(4.1.4) 4.3.6	L; Q
Health centres—named	Individual centres opened or planned, address, opening date, numbers of GPs and patients, LA/RHB services; type of surgery	UK; Stand. Reg., Cos, LHAs	1972	[QRL 98]	4.1.5	S
Health centres—named	Individual centres opened or planned, address, number of GPs, estimated completion date	NI; H&SS Boards	Ann. from 1974	[QRL 502]	(4.1.5) 4	VS
Health centres and clinics	Health centres, number; places provided for GPs; percentage of GPs in health centres	E & W; Hosp. Reg., RHAs, AHAs	1964–5, 1971–5	[QRL 728]	(4.1.5)	S
Health centres and clinics	Number of health centres, gross and net expenditures, income	E & W; LAs	Ann. to 1974	[QRL 348]	4.1.5	S
Health centres and clinics	Net expenditure per child under 5 in clinics and centres	E & W; LAs	Ann. to 1974	[QRL 348]	4.1.5	VL
Health centres and clinics	Types and numbers of premises used for maternity and child care	E & W	1964, 1971–4	[QRL 728]	(4.1.5)	L

Medical and dental manpower

All grades of hospital doctors	Grade, specialty 1972; WTE, born overseas 1972; changes 1963–70; pay scales 1973; workload/ region staff ratios 1971	E & W	1963–73	[QRL 334]	(4.2) 4.2.5	L
All grades of hospital doctors	Scottish graduates 1962, posts held, training, specialty	Scot.	1973	[QRL 428]	(4.2) 4.2.5	S
All grades of hospital doctors	Grade, whole/part time; specialty	NI; named hosps	Ann. to 1974	[QRL 503]	(4.2) 4	M
All grades of hospital doctors	Hospital appointments of consultants, registrars and senior registrars by specialty	NI	Ann. from 1974	[QRL 502]	(4.2) 4	VS
All grades of hospital doctors—for children	Paediatrics, paediatric surgery, mental illness in children, grade, numbers, WTE rates	E & W; (Hosp. Reg., RHAs)	1964, 1969, 1974	[QRL 728]	(4.2)	M
All grades of hospital doctors—for children	Paediatric academic staff, status	GB	1970–3	[QRL 728]	(4.2)	VS

Topic and type of data	Detail of analysis	Area	Year	Publication (see QRL key)	Text reference	Remarks
Resources—*contd.*						
Medical and dental manpower—contd.						
All grades of hospital doctors—gynaecology and obstetrics	Gynaecology and obstetrics combined, grade, number, WTE, indices	GB; E & W, Scot.	1963, 1968–71	[QRL 385]	(4.2)	M
All grades of hospital doctors—gynaecology and obstetrics	Gynaecology staff in post, additional staff needed for abortion work	GB; Hosp. Reg.	1972	[QRL 385]	(4.2)	M; Q
All grades of hospital doctors—gynaecology and obstetrics	Gynaecology and obstetrics combined, grade, numbers, WTE	E & W; Hosp. Reg., Teaching Hosps	1968	[QRL 199]	(4.2) 4.3.6	M
Community doctors	LHA posts in clinical work, number, WTE, rate per population 0–14 years	E & W; Hosp. Reg.	1966, 1971–3	[QRL 728]	(4.2.1)	M
Community doctors	Community health medical staff, grade and nature of contract	E & W	1975	[QRL 728]	(4.2.1)	L
Community doctors	All grades, part time GPs, hospital specialists, type of authority; sex, age	E	1967	[QRL 690]	4.2.1	M
Community doctors	Transferred officers, aspirations, training needs	E	1974	[QRL 5]	4.2.1	S
Community physicians	MOsH; distribution, duties, personal/professional details, type of authority; 'part-timers'; starting salaries	E	1965	[QRL 689]	4.2.1	S
Community physicians	DCPs; time allocations, committees, support facilities, problems	E	1974	[QRL 207]	4.2.1	VS
Community physicians	Medical officers; distribution, personal/professional details	Scot.	1966	[QRL 716]	4.2.1	S
Community physicians	Appointments	NI	Ann. from 1974	[QRL 502]	(4.2.1)	VS
Consultants	Numbers; specialty, age (tables for various years)	GB; E & W, Scot.	1949–59	[QRL 479]	(4.2.2) 4.2.5	L

Consultants	Dental WTE	E & W; Hosp. Reg., Teaching Hosps	1962	[QRL 161]	(4.2.2) 4.2.3	VS
Consultants	Hours of work weekly by activity and grouped specialties; workload; desired staffing levels	E & W	1972	[QRL 334]	4.2.2	S; Q
Consultants	Vacancies by specialty 1971; annual appointments and recruits qualified overseas 1968–72	E & W	1968–72	[QRL 334]	4.2.2	S
Consultants	Medical schools; regions of student and present residence	E; Stand. Reg.	1966	[QRL 386]	4.2.2	S; Q
Consultants	Distinction awards	NI	Ann. to 1974	[QRL 503]	(4.2.2) 4	S
Dental practitioners	Distribution, NHS/private practice, changes; money spent	UK; Stand. Reg., ECs	1952, 1962–3	[QRL 161]	4.2.3	L
Dental practitioners	Professional details; practice size and organization; treatments	UK	1970	[QRL 612]	(4.2.3) 5.2.2	M
Dental practitioners	Number and status; number of children 5–14 years per dentist; rate per 10,000 population 0–14 years	E & W; RHAs, (AHAs)	1974	[QRL 728]	(4.2.3)	L
Dental practitioners	Dentists, type of practice (previous 10 years)	NI	Ann. from 1974	[QRL 502]	(4.2.3) 4	S
Dental practitioners	Attendances at refresher courses; complaints against	NI	Ann. from 1974	[QRL 502]	(4.2.3) 4	S
General practitioners	Obstetric qualifications; current involvement in obstetric care; rural doctors	UK	1974	[QRL 709]	(4.2.4)	S
General practitioners	Professional details; type of practice; practice size and organization; access to hospital facilities; other appointments and interests	GB (E & W, Scot.)	1969	[QRL 349]	(4.2.4) 5.1.2.1	S
General practitioners	Professional details; practice size and organization; access to hospital facilities; hospital appointments	E & W; 12 Parl. Const.	1964	[QRL 127]	(4.2.4) 5.1.2.1	M; Q
General practitioners	Vocational trainers receiving allowances; trainees	E & W	1962–70	[QRL 191]	4.2.4	S, S
General practitioners	New unrestricted principals and assistants, personal details; hospital experience, specialty; other experience	E & W; (Stand. Reg.)	1969	[QRL 191]	4.2.4	M; Q
General practitioners	New unrestricted principals 1969–70, experience, place of training	E & W	1970	[QRL 458]	4.2.4	S

Topic and type of data	Detail of analysis	Area	Year	Publication (see QRL key)	Text reference	Remarks
Resources—*contd.*						
Medical and dental manpower—contd.						
General practitioners	New unrestricted principals 1969–70, mobility over 2–3 years, sex, age	E & W	1972	[QRL 703]	4.2.4	S
General practitioners	Unrestricted principals in group practice	E & W; Stand. Reg.	1971–4	[QRL 728]	(4.2.4)	L
General practitioners	Percentage in health centres; average list sizes; rate per 10,000 population 0–14 years	E & W; RHAs, (AHAs)	1974	[QRL 728]	(4.2.4)	L
General practitioners	Medical schools; regions of student and present residence	E; Stand. Reg.	1966	[QRL 386]	4.2.4	M; Q
General practitioners	Influences on practice location; type of practice area; mobility; personal/professional details; practice organization; access to other services; other activities	E; (Stand. Reg., ECs)	1969	[QRL 108]	4.2.4	M; Q
General practitioners	Scottish graduates 1962, time spent in general practice	Scot.	1973	[QRL 428]	(4.2.4) 4.2.5	S
General practitioners	Personal lists, experience, partnership sizes, urban/rural; employment of assistants; practice organization; access to other services; other activities	NI; HAs	1970	[QRL 482]	(4.2.4) 5.1.2.1	S; Q
General practitioners	Hospital appointments, access to hospital beds, working in hospitals	NI; HAs	1970	[QRL 482]	(4.2.4) 5.1.2.1	S; Q
General practitioners	Principals, list size, partnership size, variations in doctors' lists	NI; H&SS Boards	Ann. from 1974	[QRL 502]	(4.2.4) 4	S
General practitioners	Attendances at post-graduate courses; complaints against	NI	Ann. from 1974	[QRL 502]	(4.2.4) 4	S
General practitioners	All doctors providing medical services, type of practice, 1965–74; dispensing doctors	NI	Ann. from 1974	[QRL 502]	(4.2.4) 4	S
Junior hospital dentists	Duty and off-duty hours weekly, specialty, grade, whole/part-time, residence	GB	1975	[QRL 194]	4.2.5	M
Junior hospital doctors	Academic record, hospital training, career choice	UK and abroad	1966	[QRL 388]	4.2.5	M

Junior hospital doctors	Career preferences	UK and abroad	1966	[QRL 389]	4.2.5	M; Q
Junior hospital doctors	Men's and women's career preferences; qualifications; training status; specialty preferences; employment status	UK and abroad	1966	[QRL 626]	4.2.5	M; Q
Junior hospital doctors	Career preferences and location; personal, examination and employment details; seniority, responsibility, hours with patients	UK and abroad	1966, 1969	[QRL 387]	4.2.5	M, M
Junior hospital doctors	Career preferences 1974 graduates, country of birth; specialties, sex, medical school	UK	1975	[QRL 524]	4.2.5	M
Junior hospital doctors	Grade, personal/professional details, specialties, experience, region, vacancies, doctors from overseas	GB	1949–59, 1960	[QRL 479]	4.2.5	L
Junior hospital doctors	Senior registrars—specialty, training posts, age	GB; E & W, Scot.	1958–60	[QRL 479]	4.2.5	M
Junior hospital doctors	SHMOs—specialty, age	GB; E & W, Scot.	1953, 1958	[QRL 479]	4.2.5	M
Junior hospital doctors	Duty and off-duty hours weekly, specialty, grade, whole/part-time, residence	GB	1975	[QRL 194]	4.2.5	M
Junior hospital doctors	Consultants' satisfactions with staffing levels; views on requirements for all grades	E & W	1972	[QRL 334]	4.2.5	S; Q
Junior hospital doctors	Senior registrars—vacancies by specialty 1971; in training 1968–72	E & W	1968–72	[QRL 334]	4.2.5	M
Medical migration	Doctors qualified in Br. Isles, registration periods, places of birth, training, residence, sex; employment	UK and abroad	1962	[QRL 3]	4.2.6	M; Q
Medical migration	Residents abroad who qualified in Br. Isles; registration periods; places of birth, training, residence; sex; year leaving GB, last hospital grade; current occupation; intentions to return	UK and abroad	1962	[QRL 3]	4.2.6	S; Q
Medical migration	Doctors born and qualified in Br. Isles; countries of involvement; occupation; hospital type E & W, grade	UK and abroad	1962–6	[QRL 267]	4.2.6	M
Medical migration	Foreign-born doctors in GB; countries of birth and qualifications; age, occupation, experience; emigration; hospital type E & W, grade	UK and abroad	1962–7	[QRL 267]	4.2.6	L

Topic and type of data	Detail of analysis	Area	Year	Publication (see QRL key)	Text reference	Remarks
Resources—*contd.*						
Medical and dental manpower—contd.						
Student doctors	Final years 1961, 1966, first years 1966; region; personal details; schooling; pre-medical study; grants, living and studying arrangements; current courses; career aspirations	UK	1966, 1961	[QRL 581]	4.2.7	L
Student doctors	Manpower projections; costs; organization of medical education, results; results from specialists' colleges; overseas students (tables are for various years)	UK	1960–95	[QRL 581]	4.2.7	VL
Women doctors	Professional/personal/family details; current appointment; experience; region; employment aspirations; husband's attitude	UK	1962–3	[QRL 353]	4.2.8	M
Women doctors	Career preferences; academic qualifications; training status; specialty preferences; employment status	UK and abroad	1966	[QRL 626]	4.2.8	S; Q
Women doctors	Career preferences	UK	1975	[QRL 524]	(4.2.8) 4.2.5	S
Nursing and midwifery manpower						
Note: See entries in the QRL on EVALUATION (Chapter 6) for views about the work of nurses						
All nurses and midwives	Postal survey; morale; community post-qualifications; age; hours of work; prospects	GB	1971	[QRL 190]	4.3.1	L; Q
All nurses and midwives	Staffing levels, grade, sex, hospital types, type of LA; trained district nurses; trainees and wastage rates; LA attachment levels	GB; Hosp. Reg., Teaching Hosps.	1966–71	[QRL 190]	4.3.1	VL
All nurses and midwives	Interviews; working conditions, SC, age; teaching and training courses; nurse relationships	GB	1971	[QRL 190]	4.3.1	M; Q
All nurses and midwives	Earnings and hours worked on average monthly, and composition by grade, sex; special payments	GB; Health Reg.	1974	[QRL 193]	4.3.1	VL
All nurses and midwives	Earnings indices compared with other occupations	GB	1970–4	[QRL 193]	4.3.1	VL
All nurses and midwives	Hospital manpower, grade (WTE), 1966–73; psychiatric manpower 1960–73	GB; E & W, Scot.	1960–73	[QRL 193]	4.3.1	VL

All nurses and midwives	Numbers on duty at different times by type of staff, London teaching/other hospitals; shift systems	GB	1974	[QRL 193]	4.3.1	VL
All nurses and midwives	Mental illness hospitals, psychiatric units; nursing staff, grade, sex, whole/part-time	E & W	1966	[QRL 477]	(4.3.1)	VL
All nurses and midwives—from overseas	Area of origin; personal and nursing details; experience in Br.	GB	1971	[QRL 644]	4.3.1	S
All nurses and midwives—from overseas	Mental hospital staffs' fluency in English, grade, sex; origin	2 Met. RHBs	1965	[QRL 477]	(4.3.1)	M
All nurses and midwives—reserves	Estimates of qualified females, age; current nursing employment; future employment intentions	GB	1971	[QRL 589]	4.3.1	S; Q
All nurses and midwives—reserves	Ex-nurses' personal and family details, qualifications, experience; desire for refresher courses	GB	1971	[QRL 589]	4.3.1	S; Q
Community nurses of all types	Practice teams of HVs, DNs, GPs; reports about team liaison and selection, organization of clinics and domiciliary work, responsibility for immunizations, etc., contacts with other agencies	GB	1970–1	[QRL 265]	4.3.2	S
Community nurses of all types	Three health centre teams; content of nurses' work	GB	1971–2	[QRL 265]	4.3.2	VS
Community nurses of all types	Administrative grades, health and tuberculosis visitors, home nurses, midwives, school nursing, other; WTE; rates per 10,000 population of selected sex and age	E & W; RHAs, (AHAs)	1974	[QRL 728]	(4.3.2)	VL
Community nurses of all types—attachment schemes	Numbers of attachments, health visitors, population rates	E; LHAs	1963	[QRL 45]	4.3.2	VS
Community nurses of all types—attachment schemes	Types of general practices with attachments, nature of involvement	E	1963	[QRL 45]	4.3.2	S
Community nurses of all types—attachment schemes	Type, type of LHAs; levels of staff participation; initiators; proposed schemes; success factors	E & W	1967–8	[QRL 1]	4.3.2	VS; Q
Community nurses of all types—attachment schemes	Implications re appointments, costs, staff travelling time and workload; administrative organization	E & W	1967–8	[QRL 1]	4.3.2	VS; Q

Resources—*contd.*

Nursing and midwifery manpower—*contd.*

Topic and type of data	Detail of analysis	Area	Year	Publication (see QRL key)	Text reference	Remarks
Community nurses of all types—attachment schemes	GPs' involvement and terms of agreement with LHAs	E & W	1967–8	[QRL 1]	4.3.2	VS; Q
Community nurses of all types—attachment schemes	Type of nurse, type of LHAs	E & W	1969	[QRL 23]	4.3.2	L
Health visitors	Diary recordings; people served, personal/health details; type of borough, place of contact; time spent; HVs' experience; topics covered; techniques	GLC	1969	[QRL 446]	4.3.3	L; Q
Health visitors	Experience and working arrangements; type of borough	GLC	1969	[QRL 446]	4.3.3	S; Q
Health visitors	Home-visit recordings; households visited, type, purpose; source of referrals; visit lengths, outcome, topics covered; contacts with other agencies; clients' and GPs' roles; personal/qualification details	Berkshire	1969	[QRL 144]	4.3.3	M; Q
Home nurses	Workload recordings, patients' personal/medical details, estimated usage rates, time on books, outcome on discharge, treatments received, mobility; patients off books; primary conditions of hospital discharges; persons referring patients; type of area	Scot.	1964	[QRL 122]	4.3.4	M; Q
Home nurses	Nurses' time allocations, type of travel, procedures performed; types of areas and nurses	Scot.	1964	[QRL 122]	4.3.4	VS; Q
Home nurses	Numbers by type of duties; type of area; marital status; qualifications; population ratios	Scot.	1964	[QRL 122]	4.3.4	M
Home nurses	Workload recordings; sex, age of patients; diagnostic groups; items of care	E; 6 LHAs	1967	[QRL 323]	4.3.4	M
Home nurses	Nurses' qualifications, types of work undertaken	E; 6 LHAs	1967	[QRL 323]	4.3.4	S

Home nurses—deployment of SENs	SENs, SRNs, HVs—personal/qualification details, experience; transport methods; refresher courses attended; views on career choices and changes	UK	1971	[QRL 325]	4.3.4	M
Home nurses—deployment of SENs	Workload recordings, contacts, place, nursing activities; patients' personal/medical details; off-duty days	UK	1971	[QRL 325]	4.3.4	L; Q
Home nurses—deployment of SENs	GPs' practice sizes, attached nursing staff	UK	1971	[QRL 325]	4.3.4	S
Hospital nurses	Children's wards and segregated beds in adult wards (non-psychiatric hospitals), grade, number, WTE; training; student nurses	E & W	1975	[QRL 728]	(4.3.5)	M
Hospital nurses	Numbers	NI; named hosps	Ann. to 1974	[QRL 503]	(4.3.5) 4:	L
Hospital nurses—gynaecology departments	Grade, types of duty, ratios to beds; additional staff needed for abortion work	GB; Hosp. Reg.	1972	[QRL 385]	(4.3.5)	L; Q
Hospital nurses—senior nurses	Grade; type of hospital; personal and qualification details; experience; responsibilities for maternity departments and training schools	GB; E & W, Scot.	1964	[QRL 480]	4.3.5	VL
Midwives	Midwifery nursing staff and state certified midwives in obstetrics and gynaecology	GB; E & W, Scot.	1963, 1968–71	[QRL 385]	(4.3.6)	L
Midwives	Numbers on midwives' roll 1957–68; domiciliary and hospital staff (WTE) 1959–68; age distribution 1965–8; division of work between the services 1959–68	E & W	1957–68	[QRL 199]	4.3.6	L
Midwives—domiciliary	Midwives and administrative/supervisory staff, whole/part-time; type of LAs	E & W	1968	[QRL 199]	4.3.6	L
Midwives—domiciliary	Vacancies, wastage, part-time workers, LA part II training; changes in deployment; type of LAs	E & W	1967	[QRL 199]	4.3.6	S; Q
Midwives—domiciliary	Involvement in hospitals	E & W	1968	[QRL 199]	4.3.6	L; Q
Midwives—hospital	Special duties, vacancies	E & W	1968	[QRL 199]	4.3.6	M; Q
Midwives—hospital	Training schools and places	E & W; Hosp. Reg.	1968	[QRL 199]	4.3.6	L; Q
Midwives—of overseas origin	Country of origin, present location	UK	(1967)	[QRL 267]	4.3.6	M

Topic and type of data	Detail of analysis	Area	Year	Publication (see QRL key)	Text reference	Remarks
Resources—*contd.*						
Nursing and midwifery manpower—*contd.*						
Nurses—general practice	Nurses employed, hours worked; practices employing nurses; type of premises, employed/attached nurses	E	1974	[QRL 557]	4.3.7	L
Professional and technical manpower						
Chiropodists	Current registrations 1968–74; manpower in NHS hospitals and LAs 1964–73; grade	GB	1964–74	[QRL 195]	4.4	M
Chiropodists	Department sizes, London teaching/other hospitals, non-weekday staffing	GB	1974	[QRL 195]	4.4	S
Chiropodists	Earnings average monthly, composition, sex, grade	GB; E & W, Scot.	1974	[QRL 195]	4.4	M
Chiropodists	Training school, NHS/other, annual intake	E & W	1974	[QRL 195]	4.4	VS
Dental technicians	Type of employment, age; hospital grade	E & W	1967	[QRL 478]	(4.4)	S
Dietitians	Current registration 1968–74; manpower in NHS hospitals 1964–73; grade	GB	1964–74	[QRL 195]	4.4	M
Dietitians	Department sizes, London teaching/other hospitals, non-weekday staffing	GB	1974	[QRL 195]	4.4	S
Dietitians	Earnings average monthly, composition, sex, grade	GB; E & W, Scot.	1974	[QRL 195]	4.4	S
Dietitians	Qualified members, schooling, personal/family details, experience	E & W	1964–5	[QRL 451]	4.4	S; Q
Dietitians	Students, schooling, personal details; training requirements	E & W	1964–5	[QRL 451]	4.4	VS; Q
Dietitians	Training schools, annual intake	E & W	1974	[QRL 195]	4.4	VS
Dietitians	Number by grade (WTE), teaching/other hospitals	E; Hosp. Reg.	1972	[QRL 183]	4.4	S
Helpers	Earnings average monthly, composition, sex, grade	GB; E & W, Scot.	1974	[QRL 195]	4.4	M
Occupational therapists	Current registration 1968–74; manpower in NHS hospitals 1964–73; grade	GB	1964–74	[QRL 195]	4.4	M
Occupational therapists	Department sizes, London teaching/other hospitals	GB	1974	[QRL 195]	4.4	S

Occupational therapists	Earnings average monthly, composition, sex, grade	GB; E & W, Scot.	1974	[QRL 195]	4.4	M
Occupational therapists	Qualified members, schooling, personal/family details, experience	E & W	1964–5	[QRL 451]	4.4	S; Q
Occupational therapists	Students, schooling, personal details; training requirements	E & W	1964–5	[QRL 451]	4.4	VS; Q
Occupational therapists	Training schools, NHS/other, annual intake	E & W	1974	[QRL 195]	4.4	S
Ophthalmic personnel	Medical practitioners, opticians, dispensing opticians, 1965–74; opticians attending refresher courses	NI; H&SS Boards	Ann. from 1974	[QRL 502]	(4.4) 4:	VS
Orthoptists	Current registration 1968–74; manpower in NHS hospitals 1964–73; grade	GB	1964–74	[QRL 195]	4.4	S
Orthoptists	Department sizes, London teaching/other hospitals	GB	1974	[QRL 195]	4.4	S
Orthoptists	Earnings average monthly, composition, sex, grade	GB; E & W, Scot.	1974	[QRL 195]	4.4	S
Orthoptists	Qualified members, schooling, personal/family details, experience	E & W	1964–5	[QRL 451]	4.4	S; Q
Orthoptists	Students, schooling, personal details; training requirements	E & W	1964–5	[QRL 451]	4.4	VS; Q
Orthoptists	Training schools, annual intake	E & W	1974	[QRL 195]	4.4	VS
Pharmaceutical staff	Hospital pharmacists, pharmaceutical students, pharmacy technicians, student technicians— grade, sex, number, WTE, part-time	GB	1968	[QRL 197]	4.4	M
Pharmaceutical staff	Schools of pharmacy, output	GB	1960–9	[QRL 197]	4.4	S
Pharmacists	General practice pharmacists, premises	NI; H&SS Boards	Ann. from 1974	[QRL 502]	(4.4) 4:	S
Pharmacists	Appliance contractors, premises	NI; H&SS Boards	Ann. from 1974	[QRL 502]	(4.4) 4:	VS
Physiotherapists	Current registration 1968–74; manpower in NHS hospitals 1964–73; grade	GB	1964–74	[QRL 195]	4.4	L
Physiotherapists	Department sizes, London teaching/other hospitals; non-weekday staffing	GB	1974	[QRL 195]	4.4	S
Physiotherapists	Earnings average monthly, composition, sex, grade; emergency-duty payments	GB; E & W, Scot.	1974	[QRL 195]	4.4	L
Physiotherapists	Qualified members, schooling, personal/family details, experience	E & W	1964–5	[QRL 451]	4.4	S; Q

Topic and type of data	Detail of analysis	Area	Year	Publication (see QRL key)	Text reference	Remarks
Resources—*contd.*						
Professional and technical manpower—contd.						
Physiotherapists	Students, schooling, personal details; training requirements	E & W	1964–5	[QRL 451]	4.4	S; Q
Physiotherapists	Training schools, NHS/other, annual intake	E & W	1974	[QRL 195]	4.4	S
Radiographers	Current registration 1968–74; manpower in NHS hospitals 1964–73; grade	GB	1964–74	[QRL 195]	4.4	L
Radiographers	Department sizes, London teaching/other hospitals; non-weekday staffing	GB	1974	[QRL 195]	4.4	S
Radiographers	Earnings average monthly, composition, sex, grade; emergency-duty payments	GB; E & W, Scot.	1974	[QRL 195]	4.4	L
Radiographers	Qualified members, schooling, personal/family details, experience	E & W	1964–5	[QRL 451]	4.4	S; Q
Radiographers	Students, schooling, personal details; training requirements	E & W	1964–5	[QRL 451]	4.4	S; Q
Radiographers	Training schools, annual intake	E & W	1974	[QRL 195]	4.4	M
Remedial gymnasts	Current registration 1968–74; manpower in NHS hospitals 1964–73; grade	GB	1964–74	[QRL 195]	4.4	S
Remedial gymnasts	Department sizes, London teaching/other hospitals, non-weekday staffing	GB	1974	[QRL 195]	4.4	S
Remedial gymnasts	Earnings average monthly, composition, sex, grade; emergency-duty payments	GB; E & W, Scot.	1974	[QRL 195]	4.4	S
Remedial gymnasts	Training schools, annual intake	E & W	1974	[QRL 195]	4.4	VS
Speech therapists	Current registration 1968–74; manpower in NHS hospitals 1964–73; grade	GB	1964–74	[QRL 195]	4.4	M
Speech therapists	Department sizes, London teaching/other hospitals	GB	1974	[QRL 195]	4.4	S
Speech therapists	Earnings average monthly, composition, sex, grade	GB; E & W, Scot.	1974	[QRL 195]	4.4	M
Speech therapists	Training schools, NHS/other, annual intake	GB	1974	[QRL 195]	4.4	S

Other resources

Prescribing costs	Prescription numbers, net ingredient costs, therapeutic groups; seasonal variations; indexes of quantities and prices; proprietary drugs, year of introduction	GB; Stand. Reg.	1961–2	[QRL 471]	4.5.1	VL
Prescribing costs	Doctors' age, practice category, list size, EC cost category	E & W	1961–2	[QRL 471]	4.5.1	M
Prescribing costs	Prescription numbers, net ingredient costs, therapeutic groups; seasonal variations; indexes of quantities and prices; proprietary drugs; year of introduction; regional variations	GB; Stand. Reg.	1962–3	[QRL 473]	4.5.1	VL
Prescribing costs	Gross costs and frequencies per person of prescriptions dispensed	NI; H&SS Boards	Ann. from 1974	[QRL 502]	(4.5.1) 4	VL
Prescribing costs	Prescription numbers, net ingredient costs, therapeutic groups	NI	Ann. from 1974	[QRL 502]	(4.5.1) 4	VL
Radiography costs	Mass radiography, costs per cases detected, 100 patients examined, cases avoided	E & W	1950–8	[QRL 305]	(4.5.1) 5.5.1	VL
Radiography costs	Mass miniature radiography service, rates of cases found per unit; costs	Scot.	1949–69	[QRL 124]	(4.5.1) 5.5.1	VL

Use of services

General practitioner services

All inclusive GP attitudinal studies	Practice type and size; premises and equipment; ancillary help; appointment systems	GB; (E & W, Scot.)	1969	[QRL 349]	5.1.2.1	S
All inclusive GP attitudinal studies	Access to hospital diagnostic facilities	GB	1969	[QRL 349]	5.1.2.1	S
All inclusive GP attitudinal studies	Qualifications; type of appointments, special interests; investments in premises	GB	1969	[QRL 349]	5.1.2.1	S
All inclusive GP attitudinal studies	Practice size; periods on call; appointment systems; ancillary help	E & W	1964	[QRL 127]	5.1.2.1	S; Q
All inclusive GP attitudinal studies	Access to hospital beds and diagnostic facilities	E & W	1964	[QRL 127]	5.1.2.1	S; Q

Topic and type of data	Detail of analysis	Area	Year	Publication (see QRL key)	Text reference	Remarks
Use of services—*contd.*						
General practitioner services—*contd.*						
All inclusive GP attitudinal studies	Professional attributes; hospital appointments	E & W	1964	[QRL 127]	5.1.2.1	S; Q
All inclusive GP attitudinal studies	List sizes, appointment systems, working time usage, off duty provisions	E & W	1972	[QRL 458]	(5.1.2.1) 5.1.2.8	S
All inclusive GP attitudinal studies	Type of practice area; practice size; ancillary help; nights on call	E; (Stand. Reg., ECs)	1969	[QRL 108]	5.1.2.1	M; Q
All inclusive GP attitudinal studies	Access to hospital beds; communications about discharged in-patients; type of practice area	E	1969	[QRL 108]	5.1.2.1	M; Q
All inclusive GP attitudinal studies	Professional and social characteristics; appointments held; influences on location of practice; post-graduate opportunities; type of practice area	E; (Stand. Reg., ECs)	1969	[QRL 108]	5.1.2.1	M; Q
All inclusive GP attitudinal studies	Practice type and size; premises; assistant doctors; ancillary help; appointment systems; age/sex registers	NI; HAs	1970	[QRL 482]	5.1.2.1	S; Q
All inclusive GP attitudinal studies	Access to hospital diagnostic facilities and beds	NI; HAs	1970	[QRL 482]	5.1.2.1	S; Q
All inclusive GP attitudinal studies	GPs' experience; LA clinics taken; hospital appointments and sessions; attitudes to hospital involvement	NI; HAs	1970	[QRL 482]	5.1.2.1	S; Q
All inclusive GP attitudinal studies	Practice size and organization; procedures and special interests, other medical work, personal details	Camden	1968	[QRL 611]	5.1.2.1	VS
All inclusive GP workload studies	Patients consulting, consultation numbers and rates by sex and age; illness episodes	E & W; Stand. Reg.	1970–1	[QRL 511]	5.1.2.1	VL; Q
All inclusive GP workload studies	Diagnosed conditions; diagnostic amendments; consultations for reasons other than illness	E & W; Stand. Reg.	1970–1	[QRL 511]	5.1.2.1	VL; Q
All inclusive GP workload studies	Referrals and type, urban/rural; home visits	E & W; Stand. Reg.	1970–1	[QRL 511]	5.1.2.1	VL; Q
All inclusive GP workload studies	Practice type, partnership and list sizes; arrivals/departures from practices	E & W; Stand. Reg.	1970–1	[QRL 511]	5.1.2.1	VL; Q

All inclusive GP workload studies	Direct and indirect consultations, home visits; patients' age, sex, social group, type of condition; daily workload	SW Engl.	1964–5	[QRL 726]	5.1.2.1	VL
All inclusive GP workload studies	Access to diagnostic facilities; rates of referral	SW Engl.	1964–5	[QRL 726]	5.1.2.1	M
All inclusive GP workload studies	Practice details; appointment systems; equipment; range of procedures done; ancillary staff	SW Engl.	1964–5	[QRL 726]	5.1.2.1	VS
All inclusive GP workload studies	GPs' details, additional functions	SW Engl.	1964–5	[QRL 726]	5.1.2.1	VS
All inclusive GP workload studies	Direct consultations and type; home visits; morbidity; severity of condition; sex, age	S Wales	1965–6	[QRL 713]	5.1.2.1	VL
All inclusive GP workload studies	Referral rates; out-patient arrangements; access to beds	S Wales	1965–6	[QRL 713]	5.1.2.1	L
All inclusive GP workload studies	Practice type; range of procedures done; ancillary staff	S Wales	1965–6	[QRL 713]	5.1.2.1	VS
All inclusive GP workload studies	Hospital appointments; other work and leisure activities	S Wales	1965–6	[QRL 713]	5.1.2.1	VS
All inclusive GP workload studies	Average yearly patient contacts, surgery attendance and home visit rates by age/sex	Exeter	1966–7	[QRL 37]	5.1.2.1	VL; Q
All inclusive GP workload studies	Principal diagnostic categories by age/sex	Exeter	1966–7	[QRL 37]	5.1.2.1	VL; Q
All inclusive GP workload studies	Referrals and certifications by age/sex	Exeter	1966–7	[QRL 37]	5.1.2.1	VL; Q
All inclusive GP workload studies	Direct consultations, patients' age; consultation site; disease category	NE Scot.	1969–70	[QRL 572]	5.1.2.1	VL
All inclusive GP workload studies	GPs' age, experience; variability; ancillary staff	NE Scot.	1969–70	[QRL 572]	5.1.2.1	VS
Allocation of consultation time	Surgery and home consultations, activities, average time taken; common procedures; examinations; diagnostic investigations	Scot.	1970	[QRL 103]	5.1.2.2	M
Allocation of consultation time	Disease groups; special conditions	Scot.	1970	[QRL 103]	5.1.2.2	M
Allocation of consultation time	Patient contacts' age, SC	Scot.	1970	[QRL 103]	5.1.2.2	M
Allocation of working time	Time spent over 1 week, patients seen; GPs' details	Merseyside & N Wales	1964–5	[QRL 224]	5.1.2.2	VL; Q
Appointment systems	Types of practices using systems; types and operation of systems; effects; unsuccessful systems	GB	1963–5	[QRL 64]	5.1.2.3	S; Q
Appointment systems	GPs' reported usage	GB	1963–5	[QRL 64]	5.1.2.3	S; Q
Appointment systems	Practices' patient survey; SC, home telephones	GB	1963–5	[QRL 64]	5.1.2.3	S; Q

Topic and type of data	Detail of analysis	Area	Year	Publication (see QRL key)	Text reference	Remarks
Use of services—*contd.*						
General practitioner services—*contd.*						
Appointment systems	General patient survey; SC, use of systems, home telephones, travel time	GB	1963–5	[QRL 64]	5.1.2.3	M; Q
Appointment systems	Workloads of experimental practices before and after system; patient punctuality; persons in waiting areas; lengths of consultations	10 practices	1963–5	[QRL 64]	5.1.2.3	VL; Q
Assessments of use by all individuals	Consultations in last 12 months, adults/sex, children; usage of prescribed and non-prescribed medicines, symptoms; categories of prescribed medicines	GB	1969	[QRL 220]	(5.1.1) 5.1.2.8	M; Q
Assessments of use by all individuals	Contacts with GPs over 2 weeks, sex, age, site of consultation; MS; socio-economic groups; diagnostic groups 1971	GB; Stand. Reg.	1971, 1972 & 1973	[QRL 510, 512, 513]	5.1.1	VL; Q
Assessments of use by all individuals	Consultations, average number per year, sex, age, MS; socio-economic groups 1971	GB; Stand. Reg., E & W, Scot.	1971, 1972 & 1973	[QRL 510, 512, 513]	5.1.1	VL; Q
Assessments of use by all individuals	Comparisons between GHS 1971 and NMS 1970–1 consultation rates, age, sex; diagnostic groups; quarterly data	E & W	1972	[QRL 512]	5.1.1	VL; Q
Assessments of use by all individuals	GP consultations in last 12 months, age, sex, SC, frequency; conditions	E & W	1964	[QRL 127]	5.1.1	M; Q
Assessments of use by all individuals	Home visits received; conditions	E & W	1964	[QRL 127]	5.1.1	M; Q
Assessments of use by all individuals	Action taken for selected conditions and cut leg	E & W	1964	[QRL 127]	5.1.1	M; Q
Assessments of use by all individuals	Check-up examinations and X-rays, place	E & W	1964	[QRL 127]	5.1.1	M; Q
Assessments of use by all individuals	Children's attendances at clinics, type, age	E & W	1964	[QRL 127]	5.1.1	M; Q
Assessments of use by all individuals	Older patients' use of services, chronic conditions, family circumstances	E & W	1964	[QRL 127]	5.1.1	M; Q
Assessments of use by individuals aged 16	Consultations over past year; reasons	GB	1973–4	[QRL 241]	(5.1.1) 2.5.10.1	L

Assessments of use by individuals aged 21 and over	Visited a family doctor and/or was visited in past 14 days; period since last consulted GP	Bermondsey & Southwark	1962–3	[QRL 669]	5.1.1	M
Assessments of use by individuals aged 21 and over	Diagnoses made by doctor/other person	Bermondsey & Southwark	1962–3	[QRL 669]	5.1.1	M
Assessments of use by individuals aged 21 and over	Medications medically and lay prescribed	Bermondsey & Southwark	1962–3	[QRL 669]	5.1.1	M
Assessments of use by individuals dying	Consultations over last year, symptoms, nature of restrictions; bereaved persons' contact with GP	E & W	1969	[QRL 130]	5.1.1	S
Assessments of use by individuals impaired and handicapped	Regular GP attendances and frequency, period since GP last seen, age, degree of handicap	GB; Stand. Reg.	1968–9	[QRL 297]	5.1.1	L; Q
Assessments of use by individuals impaired and handicapped	Drug usage and estimated weekly cost, age, degree of handicap	GB	1968–9	[QRL 297]	5.1.1	VL; Q
Assessments of use by individuals impaired and handicapped	Registered blind mature persons, contacts with GP, sex, age	Greater London	1968–70	[QRL 2]	(5.1.1)	S
Assessments of use by individuals with long-standing illness	Consulted a doctor over 2 weeks, sex, age	E & W	1971	[QRL 510]	5.1.1	VL; Q
Assessments of use by individuals with long-standing illness	Frequency of contacts with GP by period off sick (1, 3, 6 and 12 months); duration of last NI Certificate	E	1972–3	[QRL 450]	5.1.1	M; Q
Assessments of use by individuals with long-standing illness	Costs and methods of payment for prescribed medicines, other expenses by period off sick; period of time before doctor said what was wrong	E & W	1972–3	[QRL 450]	5.1.1	M; Q
Assessments of use by individuals with restricted activity	Consulted a doctor over 2 weeks, age, sex, reason	E & W	1971	[QRL 510]	5.1.1	VL; Q
Assessments of use of GP family planning services	Abortion patients; consultations with GPs and other doctors	GB	1971	[QRL 131]	(5.1.1) 2.5.1	S; Q
Assessments of use of GP family planning services	Mothers; advice sought from GP, family size, SC; GP as first prescriber of pill or fitter of other methods, examination done, length of first prescription	E & W	1967–8	[QRL 128]	(5.1.1) 5.1.2.5	M

Use of services—*contd.*

General practitioner services—*contd.*

Topic and type of data	Detail of analysis	Area	Year	Publication (see QRL key)	Text reference	Remarks
Assessments of use of GP family planning services	Fathers; discussion with GP	E & W	1967–8	[QRL 128]	(5.1.1) 5.1.2.5	S
Assessments of use of GP family planning services	Mothers; discussions with GP and others	E & W	1970	[QRL 128]	(5.1.1) 5.1.2.5	S
Assessments of use of GP family planning services	Mothers; discussion with GP	E & W	1967–8, 1973	[QRL 129]	(5.1.1) 5.1.2.5	M
Assessments of use of GP family planning services	Women aged 16–40; use of GP and clinic services by marital status, fecundity, age of marriage, SC, parity, religion	E & W	1970	[QRL 76]	(5.1.1) 5.1.2.5	M; Q
Deputizing services	GPs using services, age, list and practice sizes; type of practices	E & W; Stand. Reg.	1972	[QRL 712]	5.1.2.4	L
Family planning and abortion	GPs; methods advised; views on contraceptive methods, abortion, sterilization, information sources; personal/practice details; influence of religion; north/south variations; HVs; advice given to patients; caseloads	E & W	1967–8	[QRL 128]	5.1.2.5	S, S
Family planning and abortion	Abortion referrals made and refused by GPs; attitudes to abortion, contraception and NHS services; GPs' personal details, religion	E & W (Hosp. Reg.)	1970–1	[QRL 133]	5.1.2.5	S; Q
Family planning and abortion	Contraceptive methods advised by GPs; referrals to clinics, etc.; attitudes to birth-control services and sterilization; GPs' personal details, religion; north/south variations; changes since 1967–8	E & W	1970–1	[QRL 134]	5.1.2.5	S; Q
Home visiting	Visit types (urban/rural), disease categories, age; timing of requests; inappropriate visits; hospital admissions; GPs' experience	NE Engl.	1969	[QRL 448]	5.1.2.6	VL
Home visiting— patient transportation schemes	Organization, usage rates and costs of schemes; users' disease categories, age	GB; 5 practices	1968–70	[QRL 384]	5.1.2.6	L

Home visiting—patient transportation schemes	Practices' consultation rates, GPs' use of time, and mileages before and after schemes	GB; 5–9 practices	1968–70	[QRL 384]	5.1.2.6	VL
Investigations (recorded by GPs)	Referral rates per 1000 population	E & W; Stand. Reg., urban/rural	1970–1	[QRL 511]	5.1.2.7	VL; Q
Investigations (recorded by GPs)	Referral rate; test types, diagnostic/screening, results; reports waiting times; actions taken	Leicester	1970	[QRL 531]	5.1.2.7	M
Investigations (recorded in hospital depts.)	Use of direct access facilities, type of practice	Barrow	1957–8	[QRL 243]	(5.1.2.7) 4.1.2	VL
Investigations (recorded in hospital depts.)	Practices' laboratory and X-ray requests as rates; type and size of practices	Edinburgh	1962	[QRL 599]	(5.1.2.7) 5.4.3.1	VL
Investigations—pathology (recorded in hospital depts)	GP requests as proportion of total pathology workload, laboratory divisions; types of tests requested; test requests per patient referred, age group	Unnamed Co. Hosp. Group	1966	[QRL 577]	5.1.2.7	VL
Investigations—pathology (recorded in hospital depts)	Range of requests per GP; qualifications; distance surgery to laboratory; rates of requests for three towns	Unnamed Co. Hosp. Group	1966	[QRL 577]	5.1.2.7	VL
Investigations—pathology (recorded in hospital depts)	Correlation between GPs' laboratory tests by type and referrals to six specialties	NE Scot.	1962	[QRL 44]	(5.1.2.7) 5.4.3.1	VL
Investigations—pathology (recorded in hospital depts)	GP tests performed, type, for selected years between 1959–71; range of specimen numbers per practice and doctor, urban/rural	NE Scot.	1959–71	[QRL 547]	5.1.2.7	VL
Investigations—radiology (recorded in hospital depts)	Type of X-ray, abnormal findings, referral rates per 1000 patients, type of practice	Aberdeen	1973	[QRL 444]	5.1.2.7	VL
Investigations—radiology (recorded in hospital depts.)	Patients referred; type of X-ray, source, results	Guy's Hosp.	1964–7	[QRL 22]	5.1.2.7	M
Investigations—radiology (recorded in hospital depts.)	Patients referred; type of X-ray, results	Middlesex Hosp.	1964–5	[QRL 162]	5.1.2.7	M
Maternity medical claims	Claims paid to GP obstetricians and other GPs; types of services, numbers of cases attended	E & W	1968	[QRL 199]	(5.1.2)	VL
Medical records	Information recorded; adequacy of envelope system, qualification period; ancillary staff as an influence on recording practices; records taken when visiting	Scot.	1969	[QRL 165]	5.1.2	S; Q

Topic and type of data	Detail of analysis	Area	Year	Publication (see QRL key)	Text reference	Remarks
Use of services—*contd.*						
General practitioner services—contd.						
Medical records	Items GPs consider essential and non-essential	Scot.	1975	[QRL 570]	5.1.2	S
Prescribing	Main sources of new product information; usefulness of drug firms' literature, representatives and meetings	GB	1966	[QRL 651]	5.1.2.8	S; Q
Prescribing	Journals, etc., looked at regularly; attendances at medical bodies' meetings; participation in clinical trials	GB	1966	[QRL 651]	5.1.2.8	S; Q
Prescribing	Initial prescribing of preparations; four particular products, five illness situations, brand name products	GB	1966	[QRL 651]	5.1.2.8	S; Q
Prescribing	GPs' age, partnership sizes; average prescription costs	GB	1966	[QRL 651]	5.1.2.8	S; Q
Prescribing	Self-treatable illness situations; proportion of consultations which are self-treatable in GPs' opinion	GB	1970	[QRL 220]	5.1.2.8	S; Q
Prescribing	Sources of information about new drugs	GB	1970	[QRL 220]	5.1.2.8	S; Q
Prescribing	GPs' age, practice size, prescribing patterns and average costs	GB	1970	[QRL 220]	5.1.2.8	S; Q
Prescribing	Advertisements of drugs, direct mail and periodicals, therapeutic classes; citing of references	E & W	1974–5	[QRL 458]	5.1.2.8	L
Prescribing	Rates per 1000 patients for 1 month, site of action/therapeutic type; single-handed GPs, prescribing patterns	3 unnamed towns	1961	[QRL 396]	5.1.2.8	VL
Prescribing	Details of GPs, practices; prescriptions by type of drug; prescribing rate; cost	3 unnamed towns	1961	[QRL 395]	5.1.2.8	VL
Prescribing	Mean numbers of prescriptions issued 1 month, practice characteristics	3 unnamed towns	1961	[QRL 363]	5.1.2.8	VL
Prescribing— by new principals	Use of proprietary preparations; period prior to use, year of qualifying	E & W	1969–71, 1972	[QRL 458]	5.1.2.8	S
Prescribing— by new principals	High-cost prescriptions	E & W	1969–73	[QRL 458]	5.1.2.8	M

Prescribing— by new principals	Sources of information, meetings attended, views on sources and training	E & W	1972	[QRL 458]	5.1.2.8	S
Prescribing— by new principals	Therapeutic classes, proprietary and non-proprietary, usage by national and survey GPs	E	1970–1	[QRL 458]	5.1.2.8	VL
Prescribing— by new principals	Patients 0–14, 15–65, 65 and over, sex, therapeutic classes, proprietary and non-proprietary	E	1970–1	[QRL 458]	5.1.2.8	VL
Prescribing— by new principals	Prescribing patterns of holders of DCH, therapeutic classes	Lancashire, Cheshire	1972–3	[QRL 458]	5.1.2.8	L
Prescribing— by new principals	Scripts written by ancillaries, therapeutic groups, patients' age, sex	E	1970–1	[QRL 458]	5.1.2.8	VL
Prescribing— selected drugs	Amphetamines, practice numbers and sizes, units	NI; Cos	1966, 1971	[QRL 668]	5.1.2.8	VL
Prescribing— selected drugs	Insulin/oral hypoglycaemics prescribed; details of patients, 1967, 1970	NI; Cos	1966–71	[QRL 667]	5.1.2.8	VL
Prescribing— selected drugs	Chloramphenicol, rates per 1000 patients; educational, consultant, personal interview indices; practice characteristics	Several Engl. towns	1961	[QRL 455]	5.1.2.8	VL
Prescribing— selected drugs	Steroids, diseases, length of treatment, type of steroid, side-effects	Wessex	1967	[QRL 616]	5.1.2.8	VL
Prescribing— selected drugs	Steroids, diseases, sex, side-effects, dosage	NE Engl.	1970	[QRL 340]	5.1.2.8	VL
Prescribing— selected drugs	Psychotropic drugs, prescriptions issued, treatments, individual drugs, oral contraceptive agents; patients' age and sex, disorders; interpractice variations	Midland city	1967–8	[QRL 522]	5.1.2.8	L, VL
Prescribing— selected drugs	Psychotropic drugs, therapeutic subgroups of tranquillizer and anti-depressant drugs	E & W	1963–8	[QRL 522]	5.1.2.8	VL
Referrals (recorded by GPs)	Rates for in-patients, out-patients, investigations, LA, death, multiple, other, urban/rural	E & W; Stand. Reg.	1970–1	[QRL 511]	5.1.2.9	VL; Q
Referrals (recorded by GPs)	Rates of referral; access to diagnostic facilities	SW Engl.	1964–5	[QRL 726]	5.1.2.9	VL
Referrals (recorded by GPs)	Referral rates; OP arrangements; access to beds	S Wales	1965–6	[QRL 713]	5.1.2.9	VL
Referrals (recorded by GPs)	Rate per 1000 patient contacts by sex and age	Exeter	1966–7	[QRL 37]	5.1.2.9	VL; Q
Referrals (recorded by GPs)	Type of hospital service; GPs' referral reasons; patients' reasons for private care; receipt of reports; out-patient waiting times	Leicester	1970	[QRL 248]	5.1.2.9	M

Topic and type of data	Detail of analysis	Area	Year	Publication (see QRL key)	Text reference	Remarks
Use of services—*contd.*						
General practitioner services—contd.						
Referrals (recorded in out-patient depts)	Specific out-patient referral rates to acute specialties per 1000 population by sex/age	E; 5 CBs	1962	[QRL 244]	(5.1.2.9) 5.4.3.1	VL
Referrals (recorded in out-patient depts)	GP referrals as proportion of all out-patient referrals, six specialties; crude annual referral rates per 1000 population; correlation between GPs' referrals and laboratory tests	NE Scot.	1962	[QRL 44]	(5.1.2.9) 5.4.3.1	M
Referrals (recorded in out-patient depts)	Level of diagnosis in referral letter; diagnostic categories	NE Scot.	1962	[QRL 44]	(5.1.2.9) 5.4.3.1	M
Referrals (recorded in out-patient depts)	Reasons in letters for out-patient referrals; GP referrals as proportion of all referrals	2 SE Engl. Hosp. Groups & Guy's Hosp.	1962–3	[QRL 140]	(5.1.2.9) 5.4.3.1	M
Referrals (recorded in out-patient depts)	Patients' distance from GP related to rates of referral for common diagnoses; reasons for referral	Scottish Border Cos.	1969	[QRL 285]	(5.1.2.9) 5.4.3.3	M
Referrals to psychiatric services	Psychiatric facilities available to GPs; preferred methods of socio-medical management	Greater London	1961–2	[QRL 610]	5.1.2.9	VS; Q
Referrals to psychiatric services	Social details of practice populations and consulting psychiatric patients	Greater London	1961–2	[QRL 610]	5.1.2.9	L; Q
Referrals to psychiatric services	Practice workloads; psychiatric morbidity; treatment and management, interpractice variations	Greater London	1961–2	[QRL 610]	5.1.2.9	L; Q
Sickness certification	Rate per 1000 patient contacts by age/sex	Exeter	1966–7	[QRL 37]	5.1.2.10	VL; Q
Dental practitioner services						
Assessments of children's use	Dental attendance pattern, dental condition, age	E & W	1973	[QRL 650]	5.2.1	M; Q
Assessments of children's use	Dental services chosen for child, age, reasons; mother's dental attendance pattern, SC	E & W	1973	[QRL 650]	5.2.1	M; Q

Assessments of children's use	School dental inspections, period since last inspection, age	E & W; Stand. Reg.	1973	[QRL 650]	5.2.1	M; Q
Assessments of children's use	General dental services, age started, reasons, treatments received; orthodontic treatments	E & W	1973	[QRL 650]	5.2.1	M; Q
Assessments of use by individuals aged 16 and over	Current dental attendance pattern, length of time since last visit, age; condition of teeth	E & W; Stand. Reg.	1968	[QRL 282]	5.2.1	M; Q
Assessments of use by individuals aged 16 and over	Major type of treatment last course, number of visits, X-ray taken	E & W; Stand. Reg.	1968	[QRL 282]	5.2.1	M; Q
Assessments of use by individuals aged 16 and over	Treatment through the School Dental Service	E & W; Stand. Reg.	1968	[QRL 282]	5.2.1	M; Q
Assessments of use by individuals aged 16 and over	Current dental attendance pattern, length of time since last visit, condition of natural teeth, sex, age, SC	Scot.	1972	[QRL 652]	5.2.1	M; Q
Assessments of use by individuals aged 16 and over	Major type of treatment last visit	Scot.	1972	[QRL 652]	5.2.1	M; Q
Assessments of use by individuals aged 21 and over	Visited a GP dentist in last 14 days	Bermondsey & Southwark	1962–3	[QRL 669]	(5.2.1) 5.1.1	M
Assessments of use by individuals aged 21 and over	Visits to dentist, period, frequency, age, SC, denture status; use of NHS/private practice	Salisbury & Darlington	1963	[QRL 105]	5.2.1	S; Q
Assessments of use by individuals aged 21 and over	Reasons for last visit, choice of dentist; views on charges, fluoridation, self-care	Salisbury & Darlington	1963	[QRL 105]	5.2.1	S; Q
Dental practitioner surveys	NHS/private practice; practice size; patients under 12; dentists' status, half-days worked; year of qualification	UK	1971	[QRL 612]	5.2.2	M
Dental practitioner surveys	Time spent on treatments other than restorative/ prosthetic dentistry	UK	1971	[QRL 612]	5.2.2	M
Dental practitioner surveys	Dental hygienists distribution, half-day sessions worked	UK	1971	[QRL 612]	5.2.2	M
Dental practitioner surveys	Dental surgery assistants distribution, half-days worked, dentists' year of qualification; chairside working patterns	UK	1971	[QRL 613]	5.2.2	M
Dental practitioner surveys	Employment of hygienists; dentists' attitudes to practice, hygienists, oral hygiene, smoking by north/south Engl.	6 unnamed towns	1975	[QRL 167]	5.2.2	S

Topic and type of data	Detail of analysis	Area	Year	Publication (see QRL key)	Text reference	Remarks
Use of services—*contd.*						
Dental practitioner services—contd.						
Dental practitioner workload statistics— all treatments	Number of courses approved for payment, fees authorized, patients' contributions, average cost of treatment courses (for previous 10 years); replacement of dentures and orthodontic appliances; patients examined by dental officers	NI	Ann. from 1974	[QRL 502]	(5.2.2) 5.6.6.	VL
Dental practitioner workload statistics— orthodontic treatments	Dental practices doing orthodontics, patients, rate of patients per dentist; age of patients; type of malocclusion; treatment patterns and duration	E & W; Stand. Reg.	1965	[QRL 607]	5.2.2	L, VL
Dental practitioner workload statistics— orthodontic treatments	Treatments by active appliances, rate of discontinued cases, age, 1964–71; reasons for discontinuation 1969–71	Scot.	1964–71	[QRL 303]	5.2.2	L
Community health services						
Annual and *ad hoc* statistics	Ambulances; numbers of persons carried; costs per person carried and vehicle mile	E & W; LAs	Ann. to 1974	[QRL 348]	5.3	VL
Annual and *ad hoc* statistics	Chiropody; treatments through voluntary organizations, by LA; average cost per LA treatment	E & W; LAs	Ann. to 1974	[QRL 348]	5.3	VL
Annual and *ad hoc* statistics	Child health centres, attendances, sessions held by type of staff	E & W	1964, 1971–4	[QRL 728]	(5.3)	VL
Annual and *ad hoc* statistics	Clinics and centres; net expenditure per child under 5	E & W; LAs	Ann. to 1974	[QRL 348]	5.3	VL
Annual and *ad hoc* statistics	Dental services; children under 5 inspected and treated	E & W	1966–74	[QRL 728]	(5.3)	VL
Annual and *ad hoc* statistics	Domiciliary midwifery; division of work between hospitals and domiciliary services	E & W	1959–68	[QRL 199]	(5.3) 4.3.6	VL; Q
Annual and *ad hoc* statistics	Domiciliary deliveries attended; discharged hospital cases visited, type of LHAs	E & W	1967	[QRL 199]	(5.3) 4.3.6	VL; Q
Annual and *ad hoc* statistics	Domiciliary midwifery; number of confinements; cost per confinement of employees, other expenses, total	E & W; LAs	Ann. to 1974	[QRL 348]	5.3	VL

Annual and *ad hoc* statistics	Family planning clinic provision, staffing and attendance rates, session scheduling	E & W; 12 Regist. Districts	1967	[QRL 128]	(5.3) 5.1.2.5	S
Annual and *ad hoc* statistics	Family planning clinic types and location attended by mothers; accessibility; SC and usage	E & W; 12 Regist. Districts	1967–8	[QRL 128]	(5.3) 5.1.2.5	M
Annual and *ad hoc* statistics	Family planning services; rates per 1000 population of net expenditure through voluntary bodies, gross expenditure, income and net expenditure by LA	E & W; LAs	Ann. to 1974	[QRL 348]	5.3	VL
Annual and *ad hoc* statistics	Health centres; number of centres, gross expenditure, income, net expenditure	E & W; LAs	Ann. to 1974	[QRL 348]	5.3	S
Annual and *ad hoc* statistics	Health centres, number; places provided for GPs; percentage of GPs in health centres; premises used for maternity and child health	E & W; Hosp. Reg., RHAs, (AHAs)	1964–5, 1971–5	[QRL 728]	(5.3)	S
Annual and *ad hoc* statistics	Health centres, planned or opened, address, numbers of GPs and patients; LA/RHB services; surgery types	UK; Stand. Reg., LHAs	1972	[QRL 98]	(5.3)	S
Annual and *ad hoc* statistics	Health centres, planned or opened, address, number of GPs	NI; H&SS Boards	Ann. from 1974	[QRL 502]	(5.3)	VS
Annual and *ad hoc* statistics	Health visiting; number of cases visited, cost per case visited, number of visits, cost per visit	E & W; LAs	Ann. to 1974	[QRL 348]	5.3	VL
Annual and *ad hoc* statistics	Home nursing; number of visits and attendances, cost per visit or attendance	E & W; LAs	Ann. to 1974	[QRL 348]	5.3	VL
Assessments of use by all individuals	Community health services (14) used over 1 month, source of referral; domiciliary services (6), age, gross weekly household income of persons over 64	E & W	1971	[QRL 510]	5.3.1	VL; Q
Assessments of use by individuals aged 21 and over	Have visited chiropodist, an antenatal clinic, seen a clinic doctor, been visited by a HV in last 14 days	Bermondsey & Southwark	1962–3	[QRL 669]	(5.3.1) 5.1.1	M; Q
Assessments of use by individuals dying	District nurse visits over last year, type of help given; help from other community services	E & W	1969	[QRL 130]	5.3.1	S
Assessments of use by individuals impaired and handicapped	Health and welfare services received, degree of handicap, LA registration	GB	1968–9	[QRL 297]	5.3.1	L; Q

Use of services—*contd.*

Community health services—contd.

Topic and type of data	Detail of analysis	Area	Year	Publication (see QRL key)	Text reference	Remarks
Assessments of use by individuals with long-standing illness	Visits from six domiciliary services over 1 month, age, sex	E & W	1971	[QRL 510]	5.3.1	VL; Q
	Help or advice from district nurse, HV, by period off sick (1, 3, 6 and 12 months)	E & W	1972–3	[QRL 450]	5.3.1	M; Q
Assessments of use of chiropody services	Foot consultations in past 4 weeks and past 6 months; type of professional; conditions treated by chiropodist	E & W	1966	[QRL 146]	5.3.1	M; Q
Assessments of use of family planning clinics by mothers	Advice sought, family size, SC; clinic doctor as first prescriber of pill or fitter of other methods; attendance patterns; methods used	E & W	1967–8	[QRL 128]	(5.3.1) 5.1.2.5	M
Assessments of use of family planning clinics by mothers	Advantages/disadvantages of clinic compared with GP; reasons for not going to clinic	E & W	1967–8	[QRL 128]	(5.3.1) 5.1.2.5	M
Assessments of use of family planning clinics by mothers	Type and location of clinics attended; accessibility; SC and usage	E & W	1967–8	[QRL 128]	(5.3.1) 5.1.2.5	M
	Discussions held	E & W	1967–8, 1973	[QRL 129]	(5.3.1) 5.1.2.5	M
Assessments of use of family planning clinics by women aged 16–40	Clinic and GP services used by marital status, fecundity, age of marriage, SC, parity, religion; domiciliary visits	E & W	1970	[QRL 76]	5.3.1	M; Q
Assessments of use of school dental service	School dental inspections, period since last inspection, age	E & W; Stand. Reg.	1973	[QRL 650]	5.3.1	M; Q
Referrals by doctors	GPs' responses to four case histories; services used in past month; contacts with HV; information sources	2 Cos	1964–5	[QRL 24]	5.3.2	S
Referrals by doctors	Referral rates per 1000 population to LA agencies, urban/rural	E & W; Stand. Reg.	1970–1	[QRL 511]	5.3.2	VL; Q
School dental service	Pupils inspected and treated in maintained schools	E & W	1966–74	[QRL 728]	5.3.3	VL

School health service	Costs per 1000 population from total net rate and grant-borne expenditure	E & W; LAs	Ann. to 1974	[QRL 347]	5.3.3	VL
School health service	Selective examination schemes, number of authorities; dates introduced; pupil numbers; team membership; information sources	E & W	1967	[QRL 418]	5.3.3	VL
School health service	Pupils inspected, defects treated in maintained schools	E & W	1964–74	[QRL 728]	5.3.3	VL
School health services—child guidance	LA clinics, hospital departments of child psychiatry; attendances, staff; source of referral; waiting lists; provisions for special groups; LA back-up facilities	E & W; Grouped Cos	1969	[QRL 143]	5.3.3	VS; Q
School health services—child guidance	Psychiatric social workers, grade; qualification details; salaries; caseloads, content; teaching/supervisory roles, students; various administrative responsibilities	E & W; Grouped Cos	1969	[QRL 143]	5.3.3	VS; Q
School health services—child guidance	Psychiatrists, psychotherapists, educational and clinical psychologists; numbers, sessions, place of training, workloads	E & W; Grouped Cos	1969	[QRL 143]	5.3.3	VS; Q

Hospital A & E and out-patient services

Assessments of use by all individuals	Attendances at 'out-patients' over 3 months, age, sex; marital status (1971)	GB; Stand. Reg. GB; E & W, Scot.	1971, 1972 & 1973	[QRL 510, 512, 513]	5.4.1	VL; Q
Assessments of use by all individuals	Combined results 1971–2; socio-economic groups	GB; Stand. Reg.	1972	[QRL 512]	5.4.1	VL; Q
Assessments of use by individuals aged 15 and over	Has been to any kind of hospital as an out-patient or casualty (over about 6 months), age/sex, SC, St. Thomas's Group/ other; reclassified estimates after records check	N Lambeth	1966	[QRL 521]	5.4.1	L
Assessments of use by individuals aged 21 and over	Number of out-patient attendances in previous 12 months; length of episodes; conditions	E & W	1964	[QRL 127]	5.4.1	M; Q
Assessments of use by individuals aged 21 and over	Experienced hospital out-patient treatment, visited hospital casualty, visited hospital dentist, in last 14 days	Bermondsey & Southwark	1962–3	[QRL 669]	(5.4.1) 5.1.1	M
Assessments of use by individuals with long-standing illness/disability	Has attended casualty or out-patient dept. during 3 months, age, sex	E & W	1971	[QRL 510]	5.4.1	VL; Q
	Visits to see consultant, to have tests, to have treatment, by period off sick (1, 3, 6 and 12 months); waiting times for first appointment, tests and treatment	E & W	1972–3	[QRL 450]	(5.4.1) 5.1.1	M; Q

Use of services—*contd.*

Hospital A & E and out-patient services—contd.

Topic and type of data	Detail of analysis	Area	Year	Publication (see QRL key)	Text reference	Remarks
Assessments of use by individuals with long-standing illness/disability	Registered blind mature persons, contacts with out-patients, age, sex	Greater London	1968–70	[QRL 2]	(5.4.1) 2.5.17	S; Q
A & E services	A & E depts, number, planned provision 1973; adequacy of premises; closures; attendance figures	E & W Hosp. Reg.	1970	[QRL 336]	5.4.2	S
A & E services	Consultants in charge of major depts, sessions worked; specialty; times when 'on call'; supporting medical staff	E & W Hosp. Reg.	1970	[QRL 336]	5.4.2	S
A & E services	Accident centres/casualty depts, with/without beds, population served, Platt standards	E & W Hosp. Reg.	1970	[QRL 598]	5.4.2	S; Q
A & E services	Workload, new and total cases, non-GP referred admissions	E & W; Hosp. Reg.	1970	[QRL 598]	5.4.2	S; Q
A & E services	Staffing, grades, costs, weekly hours	E & W	1970	[QRL 598]	5.4.2	S; Q
A & E services	Consultants, specialty, sessional allowances, projected requirements	E & W	1970	[QRL 598]	5.4.2	S; Q
A & E services	Employment of GPs in A & E depts	E & W; Hosp. Reg.	1970	[QRL 598]	5.4.2	S; Q
A & E services	Casualty depts, annual attendances, staffing; accident centres annual admissions, staffing	E & W; named hosps	1970	[QRL 598]	5.4.2	S; Q
A & E services	New and total casualty attendances	NI	Ann. to 1974	[QRL 503]	(5.4.2) 5.6.6	VL
A & E services	New patients in hospital and survey returns, individual hospitals; area of origin	Tees-side	1957–8	[QRL 11]	(5.4.2) 4.1.2	VL
A & E services	Casual attenders; SC; medical care required; procedures, final diagnosis	Newcastle	1970	[QRL 486]	5.4.2	S
A & E services	Children; age, nature of injury	3 hosps	1973–4	[QRL 728]	(5.4.2)	VL
Out-patient services— *ad hoc* studies	New patients seen age/sex by specialty; civil status	E & W	1962	[QRL 244]	5.4.3.1	L
Out-patient services— *ad hoc* studies	Referral rates, age; three specialties	E & W; 11 Hosp. Groups	1962	[QRL 244]	5.4.3.1	L

Out-patient services— *ad hoc* studies	Investigations done, selected diagnoses; treatments and cross referrals, specialty	E & W	1962	[QRL 244]	5.4.3.1	L
Out-patient services— *ad hoc* studies	Outcome after 6 months, specialty; final diagnoses	E & W	1962	[QRL 244]	5.4.3.1	L
Out-patient services— *ad hoc* studies	New patients, sex/age, source of referral; specialty	Edinburgh	1961–2	[QRL 599]	5.4.3.1	M; Q
Out-patient services— *ad hoc* studies	Diagnosis at first visit; disposal at visit, specialty	Edinburgh	1961–2	[QRL 599]	5.4.3.1	M; Q
Out-patient services— *ad hoc* studies	New patients, age/sex; six specialties, source of referral, referral rates	NE Scot.	1962	[QRL 44]	5.4.3.1	M
Out-patient services— *ad hoc* studies	GP and hospital diagnoses; immediate disposal, subsequent appointments	NE Scot.	1962	[QRL 44]	5.4.3.1	M
Out-patient services— *ad hoc* studies	Out-patient facilities available, catchment areas, distance; non-attenders	NE Scot.; individual hosps	1962	[QRL 44]	5.4.3.1	M
Out-patient services— *ad hoc* studies	New patients, age/SC; source and reason for referral, specialties; distance to patients' homes	2 SE Engl. Hosp. Groups & Guy's Hosp.	1962	[QRL 140]	5.4.3.1	M
Out-patient services— *ad hoc* studies	Hospital diagnostic groups, immediate disposal, outcome at 6 months	2 SE Engl. Hosp. Groups & Guy's Hosp.	1962	[QRL 140]	5.4.3.1	M
Out-patient services— *ad hoc* studies	New patients, age/sex, distance; source and reasons for referral, specialties	Guy's Hosp.	1962	[QRL 112]	5.4.3.1	M
Out-patient services— *ad hoc* studies	GP and hospital diagnoses, disposal	Guy's Hosp.	1962	[QRL 112]	5.4.3.1	M
Out-patient services— *ad hoc* studies	Rates of total attendances, principal diagnostic categories by age/sex	Exeter	1966–7	[QRL 37]	(5.4.3.1) 5.1.2.1	VL
Out-patient services— chest clinics	Attendances, size of clinics, source of referral; diagnostic groups; type of attendances, age/sex; investigations ordered, type; disposal; caseload per session by grade of staff	Scot.	1970	[QRL 602]	(5.4.3.1) 5.5.1	VL
Out-patient services— chest clinics	Sessions held, total and average attendances	Scot.; 20 clinics	1970	[QRL 602]	(5.4.3.1) 5.5.1	VL
Out-patient services— chest clinics	Consultants with respiratory interests, medical assistants and SHMOs, age; caseload per session	Scot.; Hosp. Reg.	1970	[QRL 602]	(5.4.3.1) 5.5.1	S
Out-patient services— Northern Ireland	New and total out-patient attendances	NI	Ann. to 1974	[QRL 503]	(5.4.3) 5.6.6	VL
Out-patient services— organization	See entries in the QRL on Unmet Demand (Chapter 3)					

Topic and type of data	Detail of analysis	Area	Year	Publication (see QRL key)	Text reference	Remarks
Use of services—*contd.*						
Hospital A & E and out-patient services—contd.						
Out-patient services— peripheral clinics	Health centres in which RHB clinics were held, specialty	UK; named centres	1972	[QRL 98]	(5.4.3.3) 4.1.5	S
Out-patient services— peripheral clinics	New patients, clinic types and sites, specialty; rates of referral; reasons for referral; status of doctor seeing patient	Scottish Border Cos.	1969	[QRL 285]	5.4.3.3	M
Out-patient services— peripheral clinics	Diagnostic groups, level of confidence; disposal after first consultation	Scottish Border Cos.	1969	[QRL 285]	5.4.3.3	M
Out-patient services— peripheral clinics	Patients' distance from GP related to rates of referral for common diagnoses, level of diagnosis, disposal; distance travelled to Edinburgh	Scottish Border Cos.	1969	[QRL 285]	5.4.3.3	M
Out-patient services— peripheral clinics	Demographic data, hospital facilities	Scottish Border Cos.	1969	[QRL 285]	5.4.3.3	M
Out-patient services— peripheral clinics	Follow-up study; death, age/sex; hospital/ discharge status; specialty, return visits, purpose; doctor signing discharge letter	Scottish Border Cos.	1970	[QRL 285]	5.4.3.3	M
Hospital diagnostic services						
Pathology services	Laboratory technicians per 100,000 in-patients	E & W; Hosp. Reg.	1968	[QRL 403]	(5.5.1) 4.1.2	VL
Pathology services	Ranges of units used per hospital, selected diagnoses	8 DGHs, SE Engl.	1969	[QRL 41]	5.5.1	M
Pathology services	Referral source, patient and request numbers, age; laboratory division	Co. Hosp. Group	1966	[QRL 577]	5.5.1	VL
Pathology services	GP referrals; rates of requests, type of test, GPs' year of qualifying, distance from surgery to laboratory; referral rates for three towns	Co. Hosp. Group	1966	[QRL 577]	5.5.1	VL

Pathology services	Hospital specialty, in-patient and out-patient requests per patient, laboratory division; complexity of requests	Co. Hosp. Group	1966	[QRL 577]	5.5.1	VL
Pathology services	Demographic details of the survey area; costs in one region	Co. Hosp. Group	1966	[QRL 577]	5.5.1	VL
Pathology services	Specimens examined by laboratory services, type	NI; named labs	Ann. to 1974	[QRL 503]	(5.5.1) 5.6.6	VL
Pathology services— sputum cytology	Numbers of laboratories, specimens examined; source; categories of results	E & W; (Hosp. Reg.)	1972–3	[QRL 519]	5.5.1	VL
Pathology services— sputum cytology	Staffing, grade, time spent on laboratory procedures	E & W	1972–3	[QRL 519]	5.5.1	M
Radiology services	Radiology units and radiographers as rates	E & W; Hosp. Reg.	1968	[QRL 403]	(5.5.1) 4.1.2	VL
Radiology services	Chest services; X-rays ordered, diagnostic groups, clinic sizes	Scot.	1970	[QRL 602]	5.5.1	VL
Radiology services	Mass radiography, rates of patients examined; cases detected, avoided; costs; estimated probability of secondary cases	E & W	1950–8	[QRL 305]	5.5.1	VL
Radiology services	Mass miniature radiography service, rates of cases found per unit; costs	Scot.	1949–69	[QRL 124]	5.5.1	VL
Radiology services	Mass miniature radiography service; number of units, examinations performed, results	Scot.	1969	[QRL 602]	5.5.1	VL
Radiology services	Mass radiography; mobile unit, GP, results	NI	Ann. to 1974	[QRL 503]	(5.5.1) 5.6.6	VL
Radiology services	Units of X-ray service	NI; HMCs, named hosps	Ann. to 1974	[QRL 503]	(5.5.1) 5.6.6	VL
Radiology services	Ranges of units used per hospital, selected diagnoses; RHB variations 1968	8 DGHs, SE Engl.	1969	[QRL 41]	5.5.1	M

Hospital in-patient services

Assessments of use by all individuals	Medical or surgical in-patient spells during 3 months, age, sex	GB; E & W E & W; GB	1971, 1972 & 1973	[QRL 510, 512, 513]	5.6.1	VL; Q
Assessments of use by individuals aged 15 and over	Has been a patient in a ward of any kind of hospital (over about 6 months), age/sex, SC, St. Thomas's Group/other; reclassified estimates after records check	N Lambeth	1966	[QRL 521]	5.6.1	L

Use of services—*contd.*

Hospital in-patient services—*contd.*

Topic and type of data	Detail of analysis	Area	Year	Publication (see QRL key)	Text reference	Remarks
Assessments of use by individuals aged 15 and over	Persons aged 16; operations in lifetime	GB	1973–4	[QRL 241]	(5.6.1) 2.5.10.1	L
Assessments of use by individuals aged 21 and over	Ex-patients; length of stay; period between initial GP contact and referral, and OP visit and admission; GP's part in admission	E & W	1960–1	[QRL 126]	5.6.1	S; Q
Assessments of use by individuals aged 21 and over	Hospital in-patient in last 14 days	Bermondsey & Southwark	1962–3	[QRL 669]	(5.6.1) 5.1.1	M
Assessments of use by individuals aged 21 and over	Individuals' reports of experiencing four surgical conditions in past year; desire for surgery	Warrington	1967–8	[QRL 403]	(5.6.1) 4.1.2	S
Assessments of use by individuals dying	Length of time in hospital/institution over last year, place of death; type of institution, help needed; clinical, personal and household characteristics	E & W	1969	[QRL 130]	(5.6.1) 2.5.32	S
Assessments of use by individuals with long standing illness	Has been an in-patient (non-maternity) during 3 months, age, sex	E & W	1971	[QRL 510]	5.6.1	VL; Q
Assessments of use by individuals with long standing illness	In-patient experience by period off sick (1, 3, 6 and 12 months); length of wait for admission	E & W	1972–3	[QRL 450]	(5.6.1) 5.1.1	M; Q
Assessments of use by individuals with long standing illness	Registered blind mature persons; in-patient admissions in last 3 years, age, sex	Greater London	1968–70	[QRL 2]	(5.6.1) 2.5.17	S; Q
Ad hoc studies— acute services	Admission rates surgical and medical; waiting times for admission, specialty; mean lengths of stay surgical and medical; below-average throughput, general medicine; standardized mortality ratios (tables relate to various years)	E & W; Hosp. Reg.	1963–9	[QRL 403]	(5.6.2) 4.1.1	VL
Ad hoc studies— acute services	Operating theatres, selected regions	E	1966	[QRL 403]	(5.6.2) 4.1.1	S

Ad hoc studies—acute services	Areal use of in-patient services, social factors, births	Tees-side	1957–8	[QRL 11]	(5.6.2) 4.1.1	VL
Ad hoc studies—acute services	Admission rates, various conditions, type of GP practices	Barrow	1957–8	[QRL 243]	(5.6.2) 4.1.1	VL
Ad hoc studies—acute services	Bed days, sex, age, diagnoses; projected use of hospitals by 1977	Barrow	1957–8	[QRL 243]	(5.6.2) 4.1.1	VL
Ad hoc studies—acute services	Clinical necessity, sex, medicine, surgery, paediatrics	Barrow	1957–8	[QRL 243]	(5.6.2) 4.1.1	VL
Ad hoc studies—acute services	Admission rates; mean lengths of stay, selected surgical conditions, coronary heart disease, SC; operations, frequency; throughput; redundant bed days (tables relate to various years)	Liverpool RHB; (HMCs, individual hosps)	1963–9	[QRL 403]	(5.6.2) 4.1.1	VL
Ad hoc studies—acute services	Hospital discharge rates per 1000 pop., type of hospital, type of catchment area, age; long stay admissions; occupied bed days; GP beds, eventide and welfare places	NE RHB (Scot.)	1965	[QRL 633]	5.6.2	L
Ad hoc studies—acute services	Diagnostic indices and groups, type of hospital, age	NE RHB (Scot.)	1965	[QRL 633]	5.6.2	L
Ad hoc studies—acute services	Readmission rates, types of catchment areas and discharges, age; fatality rates	NE RHB (Scot.)	1965	[QRL 633]	5.6.2	L
Ad hoc studies—acute services	Acute medical wards, duration of stay, occupied bed days; emergency and waiting list admissions, sex, season, day of week	Aberdeen hosps	1967	[QRL 633]	5.6.2	L
Ad hoc studies—acute services	Rates of admission, principal diagnostic categories, duration of stay by age/sex	Exeter	1966–7	[QRL 37]	(5.6.2) 5.1.2.1	VL
Ad hoc studies—children and adolescents	Numbers in NHS non-psychiatric wards, age/sex, specialties of patients	E & W; (Hosp. Reg.)	1964 & 1965	[QRL 474]	5.6.2	L; Q
Ad hoc studies—children and adolescents	Type and specialties of wards; occupancy rates; levels of separation; RSCNs on regular staff	E & W; (Hosp. Reg.)	1964 & 1965	[QRL 474]	5.6.2	L; Q
Ad hoc studies—children and adolescents	Parents staying overnight, facilities; tuition not received	E & W	1964 & 1965	[QRL 474]	5.6.2	L; Q
Ad hoc studies—children and adolescents	Patients in 2 DGHs, estimates of distances travelled and costs, redeployment of paediatric units; holiday resort admissions; facilities in A & E units	Wales	1971	[QRL 707]	5.6.2	VS
Ad hoc studies—children and adolescents	Patients in psychiatric/other long-stay units, journey length to hospital, visiting frequency	Wales	1971	[QRL 707]	5.6.2	VS

Use of services—*contd.*

Hospital in-patient services—*contd.*

Topic and type of data	Detail of analysis	Area	Year	Publication (see QRL key)	Text reference	Remarks
Ad hoc studies— long-stay patients in acute beds	Nursing dependency of patients, specialty, type of hospital, medical category, age	Scot.	1966–7	[QRL 459]	5.6.2	M
	Referrals to MSW, reasons, sites of admission from and discharge to	Scot.	1966–7	[QRL 459]	5.6.2	S; Q
Ad hoc studies— long-stay patients in acute beds	Doctors' opinions of need for care by patients' age/sex, marital status, principal conditions on admission, prognoses, needs for medical services and care	Liverpool RHB; indi- vidual hosps	1967–8	[QRL 109]	5.6.2	M; Q
Ad hoc studies— long-stay patients in acute beds	Length of stay; services needed and arrangements for discharge assessed by social workers and nurses	Liverpool RHB	1967–8	[QRL 109]	5.6.2	M; Q
Ad hoc studies— long-stay patients in acute beds	Method of discharge, sex, age, marital status; type of admission; diagnostic groups; type of catchment area	Aberdeen	1967	[QRL 633]	5.6.2	S
Ad hoc studies— long-stay patients in acute beds	Ward activity, short and long-stay patients over 65, diagnosis, duration of stay, method of discharge	Aberdeen	1968	[QRL 633]	5.6.2	S
Emergency bed services	Direct and medical referee admissions, patients referred back to GPs, sex/age, commonest diagnoses, time of referral	Greater London	1965–6	[QRL 691]	5.6.3	VL
General practitioner hospital services	(See Subsections 5.6.4 and 4.1.4)					
Gynaecology services	Statistics on abortion and other work	GB; Hosp. Reg.	1962–71	[QRL 385]	(5.6)	VL
Gynaecology services	Daily bed occupancy over 1 week; operations	GB; Hosp. Reg.	1972	[QRL 385]	(5.6)	L; Q
Gynaecology services	Abortion operations; admissions for abortion complications; separation of case types; follow-up of abortion patients; catchment areas for abortions; other departments doing abortion work	GB; Hosp. Reg.	1972	[QRL 385]	(5.6)	M; Q
Maternity services	Live and stillbirths in obstetric units, GP maternity units	E & W; Hosp. Reg.	1966–73	[QRL 728]	(5.6)	VL

Mental handicap and mental illness services	Mentally ill patient numbers, admissions, discharges/deaths, transfers, regradings; bed complement	NI; named hosps	Ann. to 1974	[QRL 503]	(5.6.5) 5.6.6	L
	Categories of mentally ill, and special-care patients by sex	NI	Ann. to 1974	[QRL 503]	(5.6.5) 5.6.6	L
Mental handicap and mental illness services—for children and adolescents	Children with mental illness; available beds, discharges and deaths, waiting lists	E & W; Hosp. Reg., RHAs	1964, 1971–4	[QRL 728]	(5.6.5)	M
	Child admissions to mental illness hospitals and units; number, rates, age	E & W	1964 1970–4	[QRL 728]	(5.6.5)	VL
	Child admissions to mental handicap hospitals and units; number, rates, age	E & W	1964, 1970–4	[QRL 728]	(5.6.5)	L
Mental handicap and mental illness services—for children and adolescents	Children resident in mental handicap hospitals and units; number, rates, sex, age	E & W; Hosp. Reg., RHAs	1963, 1974	[QRL 728]	(5.6.5)	L
	Adolescents with mental illness; available beds, discharges and deaths, waiting lists	E & W; Hosp. Reg., RHAs	1972–4	[QRL 728]	(5.6.5)	S
Mental handicap services—censuses	Patients, age, sex, length of stay; type of hospital; diagnosis	E & W; (Hosp. Reg.)	1963	[QRL 97]	5.6.5.1	VL
Mental handicap services—censuses	Patients, age/sex; mental category; degree of mental handicap, period since last assessed; intelligence level; legal status; prevalence of incapacities	E & W	1970	[QRL 188]	5.6.5.1	VL; Q
Mental handicap services—censuses	Type of hospital; time spent in continuous hospital residence; resident/short leave; education, training, employment; extent of visiting, age	E & W	1970	[QRL 188]	5.6.5.1	VL; Q
Mental handicap services—censuses	Severely, mildly and all handicapped patients, sex/age specific rates	E & W; Hosp. Reg.	1970	[QRL 188]	5.6.5.1	VL; Q
Mental handicap services—censuses	Known area of residence, degree of mental handicap, number and rate	E & W; LAs	1970	[QRL 188]	5.6.5.1	VL; Q
Mental handicap services—censuses	Comparisons in age/sex, and time spent in current hospital or unit, 1954, 1963, 1970	E & W	1970	[QRL 188]	5.6.5.1	VL; Q
Mental illness services—censuses	Patients, age, sex, length of stay; type of hospital; diagnosis	E & W; (Hosp. Reg.)	1963	[QRL 97]	5.6.5.2	VL
Mental illness services—censuses	Resident patients, sex/age, marital status; mental category, order of admission, legal status, diagnosis	E & W	1971	[QRL 201]	5.6.5.2	VL; Q
Mental illness services—censuses	Type of hospital/unit; special units or wards; time spent in hospital; hospital occupation	E & W	1971	[QRL 201]	5.6.5.2	VL; Q
Mental illness services—censuses	Resident patients, age/sex specific rates; time spent continuously in hospital	E & W; Hosp. Reg.	1971	[QRL 201]	5.6.5.2	VL; Q

Topic and type of data	Detail of analysis	Area	Year	Publication (see QRL key)	Text reference	Remarks
Use of services—*contd.*						
Hospital in-patient services—contd.						
Mental illness services—censuses	Known area of residence, age; time spent continuously in hospital; disparities	E & W; LAs	1971	[QRL 201]	5.6.5.2	VL; Q
Mental illness services—censuses	Comparisons in age/sex, time spent in current hospital 1954, 1963, 1971	E & W	1971	[QRL 201]	5.6.5.2	VL; Q
Mental illness services—industrial therapy	Working patients, sex, type of work; first employment after discharge	E & W	1967	[QRL 685]	5.6.5.2	VL; Q
Mental illness services—industrial therapy	Sizes of industrial units, type of accommodation; working conditions, type of machinery; patient throughput, methods of payment, sex	E & W	1967	[QRL 685]	5.6.5.2	VS; Q
Mental illness services—industrial therapy	Type of staff, 1967 salary scales; patients as supervisors	E & W	1967	[QRL 685]	5.6.5.2	VS; Q
	Unit numbers; staff/patient ratios; availability of work; nature of work	E & W; Hosp. Reg.	1967	[QRL 685]	5.6.5.2	VS; Q
Mental illness services—industrial therapy	Patients' average productivity, hours and income	E & W; named hosps	1967	[QRL 685]	5.6.5.2	VL; Q
Northern Ireland routine in-patient statistics	Admissions, discharges/deaths (general, psychiatric); waiting lists for admission, specialty	NI; HMCs, named hosps	Ann. to 1974	[QRL 503]	5.6.6	VL
Day hospital services						
Geriatric day hospitals	Patients, age, marital status, SC; domestic composition; urinary incontinence, source of referral; diagnostic groups; reasons for attendance	SE Met. RHB; 5 Day Hosps	1968	[QRL 95]	5.7.1	S
Geriatric day hospitals	Patients attending over 6 years, age, diagnosis; attendances, reasons, frequency, duration; manner of discharge; outcome	Lennard Day Hosp	1963–8	[QRL 95]	5.7.1	S
Psychiatric day hospitals—census	Day patients, sex/age, marital status, diagnostic group; source of referral, previous psychiatric in-patient care	E & W	1972	[QRL 201]	5.7.2	L; Q

Psychiatric day hospitals—census	Type of hospital, day hospitals, day places; duration of current spell and frequency of attendance; comparisons with in-patients	E & W	1972	[QRL 201]	5.7.2	L; Q
Psychiatric day hospitals—census	Day patients, sex/age; type of hospital	E & W; Hosp. Reg.	1972	[QRL 201]	5.7.2	L; Q
Psychiatric day hospitals—census	Known area of residence, age; duration of current attendance spell; disparities	E & W; LAs	1972	[QRL 201]	5.7.2	L; Q

Other hospital services

Appliances and hearing aids	Type of appliance, numbers ordered and supplied	NI	Ann. to 1974	[QRL 503]	(5.8) 5.6.6	VL
	Variety of hearing aids, numbers supplied, repairs; waiting list	NI; named hosps	Ann. to 1974	[QRL 503]	(5.8) 5.6.6	L
Blood-transfusion service	Nature of work carried out	NI	Ann. to 1974	[QRL 503]	(5.8) 5.6.6	VL
Domiciliary consultations	Number of domiciliary and hospital consultations, specialty	NI	Ann. to 1974	[QRL 503]	(5.8) 5.6.6	L
Emergency obstetric services	Calls received in 1967, type of case, domiciliary/GP unit; journey times and distances; personnel involved	E & W	1968	[QRL 199]	(5.8) 4.3.6	VS; Q
Limb-fitting centres	New patients, site of amputation, cause, sex, age; all patients on books, site of amputation 1969	E	1969–70	[QRL 200]	5.8	VL
Limb-fitting centres	New patients, adults/children, arms/legs, WP/NHS	Scot.; named centres	1966–9	[QRL 601]	5.8	L
Operations	Numbers performed	NI; HMCs, named hosps	Ann. to 1974	[QRL 503]	(5.8) 5.6.6	VL
Physiotherapy	Units	NI; HMCs, named hosps	Ann. to 1974	[QRL 503]	(5.8) 5.6.6	VL
Rehabilitation— in hospitals	Hospitals with 200 or more beds, persons responsible; sessions weekly; resettlement clinics, staff, attenders	E & W	1969	[QRL 200]	5.8	S; Q
Rehabilitation— in hospitals	Consultants in physical medicine and rheumatology	E & W; Hosp. Reg.	1949–71	[QRL 200]	5.8	VS
Rehabilitation— in industrial centres	Rehabilitation courses, completed and terminated; outcome of completed courses, reason for termination by medical group; sources of recruitment; categories of disability	GB (named units)	1970	[QRL 200]	5.8	L
Rehabilitation— in industrial centres	Government training centres, number of places, opening date	GB; named units	1970	[QRL 200]	5.8	L

Topic and type of data	Detail of analysis	Area	Year	Publication (see QRL key)	Text reference	Remarks
Evaluation						
Evaluation of general practice						
Ancillary staff— district nurse— views of nurses	Nurse satisfaction by area, type of work, housing, working relationships	S	1964	[QRL 122]	(6.2.5.3) 4.3.4	S
Ancillary staff— district nurse— views of nurses	Proportion of workload suitable for delegation to (a) nursing assistants, (b) other helpers; time spent travelling; professional isolation; interest in attachment	Six areas in E & W	1965	[QRL 322]	(6.2.5.3) 4.3.2	VS; Q
Ancillary staff— district nurse— views of GP	Training of district nurses; combination of duties with health visitor and midwife; difficulty in contacting DN; suitability of male nurses	6 areas in E & W	1965	[QRL 322]	(6.2.5.3) 4.3.2	S; Q
Ancillary staff— district nurse— views of nurses	Assessment of workload in relation to hours worked and whether attached; contact with hospital staff	6 areas in E & W	1967	[QRL 323]	(6.2.5.3) 4.3.4	S; Q
Ancillary staff— district nurse— attachment to hospital	Patients' views on length of stay and arrangements for post-operative care; age	1 area in E	1968–9	[QRL 324]	(6.2.5.3)	VS
Ancillary staff— district nurse— attachment to GP	Contact with GPs; assessment of skills needed	6 LAs in E & W	1968–9	[QRL 113]	(6.2.5.3)	S; Q
Ancillary staff— health visitor	Effect on speed of work, acceptance by patients; type of partnership	GB	1963	[QRL 45]	(6.2.4) 4.3.2	S
Ancillary staff— practice nurse	Doctors' method of working (patient contacts, diagnostic tests, actions and referrals) before and after attachment	Edinburgh	1968	[QRL 427]	(6.2.4)	VS
Ancillary staff— practice nurse	Patients' views of importance of nurse to doctor and to patient; SC, contact with nurse	London	1971	[QRL 176]	(6.2.5.3)	S
Ancillary staff— State Enrolled Nurse— views of GP	Training of nurse; most suitable worker for four situations	E & W	1971	[QRL 325]	(6.2.5.3) 4.3.4	S

Ancillary staff— views of nurse	Career changes, need for night service, preference for type of work and patient, most suitable worker for selected situations	E & W	1971	[QRL 325]	(6.2.5.3) 4.3.4	M; Q
Ancillary staff— social worker	Index of psychiatric abnormality and social adjustment before and after contact	London	1973	[QRL 163]	(6.2.4.2)	S
Appointment systems— views of GP	Effect upon planning time, distributing workload, influencing strain on GP, creating barrier for patient	E & W	1963–5	[QRL 64]	6.2.5.3 5.1.2.3	S; Q
Appointment systems— views of patients	Patients' views of system, barrier it creates, and impact upon waiting time	E & W	1963–5	[QRL 64]	6.2.5.3 5.1.2.3	M; Q
Appointments systems— effect on practice	Alteration in proportion of home visits; number of patients failing to attend; number arriving late	E & W	1963–5	[QRL 64]	(6.2.4) 5.1.2.3	S; Q
Compliance with drug therapy	Diagnosis, frequency duration and type of medication; compliance	Camberley	1966–9	[QRL 546]	6.2.3	S
Compliance with drug therapy	Dosage and duration of medication, compliance	Liverpool	1967	[QRL 259]	(6.2.3)	VS
Compliance with drug therapy	Iron in pregnancy: proportion patients taking drug; original haemoglobin	Glasgow	1968	[QRL 77]	6.2.3	VS
Direct-access investigation	Numbers, reason, type of investigation: rate/ list size; age doctor, higher qualifications	Cardiff	1961	[QRL 317]	(6.2.4.1)	L
Direct-access investigation	Mean usage; type of practice, list size	Edinburgh	1962	[QRL 599]	(6.2.4) 5.4.3.1	M
Direct-access investigation	Usage; referrals to OP	NE Scot.	1962–3	[QRL 44]	(6.2.4.1) 5.4.3.1	M
Direct-access investigation	Urban/rural practice; type of request; request rate; OP referral rate	Portsmouth	1962	[QRL 178]	6.2.4.1	VL
Direct-access investigation	Requests, month, type of investigation; findings (positive, indeterminate, negative)	SE London	1964–7	[QRL 22]	6.2.4.1	M
Direct-access investigation	Requests, reason, type of investigation, per cent abnormal	London	1964–5	[QRL 162]	(6.2.4.1)	M
Direct-access investigation	Adequacy of X-ray (plain and contrast), routine and diagnostic pathology, bacteriology, clinical chemistry, and ECG	SW Engl.	1964–5	[QRL 726]	(6.2.4.1) 2.2.2.2	VS
Direct-access investigation	Impact of health centre X-ray upon refusal and re-examination rates	Edinburgh	1971–2	[QRL 337]	(6.2.4.1)	M
Home visiting	Timing of requests; inappropriate visits; disease categories, age	NE Engl.	1969	[QRL 448]	(6.2.4) 5.1.2.6	VL

Topic and type of data	Detail of analysis	Area	Year	Publication (see QRL key)	Text reference	Remarks
Evaluation—*contd.*						
Evaluation of general practice—*contd.*						
Introduction of a transport service	Effect of service upon consultation rates by place of consultation; patients' views of service and home visits; impact of service on patients' views of their GP, mothers' and elderly patients' action if ill	5 locations in E, S, W	1968–70	[QRL 384]	(6.2.6) 5.1.2.6	M
Night calls	Doctors' views of necessity for call	Midlothian	1955–7	[QRL 99]	(6.2.5.3)	S
Overall functioning	Age, sex of doctors; structure of practice, procedures undertaken, use of hospital, contact with other professionals, appointments, attitudes and opinions, interviewers' assessments	Camden	1968	[QRL 611]	6.2.6 5.1.2.1	VS
Prescribing	Number of prescriptions, net ingredient cost, therapeutic group, quarter of year; age of doctor, single-handed/partnership, list size	E & W; Reg.	1961–2	[QRL 471]	(6.2.4.2) 4.5.1	VL
Prescribing—diabetic treatment	Use of oral drugs and insulin/1000 list size; age and subsequent mortality	NI	1966–70	[QRL 667]	(6.2.4.2)	S
Prescribing—vitamin B12	National prescribing, estimated requirements	E & W	1966	[QRL 154]	(6.2.4.2)	VL
Prescribing	Characteristics of GPs and their practices; prescription by type of drug; prescribing rate; cost	Unspecified	1961	[QRL 395]	(6.2.4.2)	VL
Prescribing	Duration of prescription, system being treated; CNS stimulants	Unspecified	1961	[QRL 702]	(6.2.4.2)	VL
Prescribing	Characteristics of GPs and their practices; use of CNS stimulants, sedatives, other drugs, other services	Unspecified	1961	[QRL 396]	(6.2.4.2)	VL
Prescribing	Mean no. prescriptions, indications for use; anti-depressant and amphetamine usage; practice organization, list size, workload, distribution of diagnoses, attitude to patients	Unspecified	1961	[QRL 363]	(6.2.4.2)	VL
Prescribing—chloramphenicol	Use of 'hazardous' drug, doctors' education, experience, 'quality' of performance	Unspecified	1961	[QRL 455]	(6.2.4.2)	S

Topic	Description	Place	Year	Ref	Section	Type
Prescribing—rheumatoid arthritis	Initial treatments used compared with accepted 'standard' treatment	Glasgow	1973	[QRL 398]	(6.2.4.2)	VS
Prescribing—knowledge of GPs	Drug interactions: per cent doctors aware of and experiencing interactions	NE Scot.	1971–2	[QRL 536]	(6.2.4.2)	S
Prescribing—knowledge of GPs	Effective treatment for arthritis	Glasgow	1973	[QRL 398]	6.2.4.2	S
Views of community nurses	Attachment schemes: level of staff participation; success factors	E & W	1967–8	[QRL 1]	(6.2.5.3) 4.3.2	VS; Q
Views of health visitors	Attitudes to work	Berkshire	1969	[QRL 144]	(6.2.5.3) 4.3.3	VS; Q
Views of patients	Impact of NHS upon attention received from GP	E & W	1952	[QRL 280]	(6.2.5.3)	L
Views of patients	Approachability of DR; waiting, examination procedures, equipment, referral habits; preference for single-handed doctor, or referral to hospital; beliefs of GPs' prestige	E & W	1964	[QRL 127]	(6.2.5.3) 5.1.1	M; Q
Views of patients	Overall satisfaction, treatment received, doctors willingness to visit, appointment systems, treatment and visiting by nurse, availability of 'personal doctor'	Newcastle	1974	[QRL 364, 447]	(6.2.5.3) 5.1.2.1	S
Views of GPs	Enjoyment; trivial consultations; late calls; pay; desire for hospital appointment; desire for access to beds; usual action for specific problems; age; qualifications and practice organization	E & W	1964	[QRL 127]	(6.2.5.3) 5.1.1	S; Q
Views of community nurses	Attitudes to work; communication between team	GB	1970–1	[QRL 265]	(6.2.5.3) 4.3.2	S

Evaluation of general practice/hospital links

Topic	Description	Place	Year	Ref	Section	Type
Communication—GP—consultant	Frequency and location of meetings, delay and problems with discharge letter; topics of interest to consultant in referral letter not included	SE Engl.	1973	[QRL 410]	(6.2.4)	VS
Communication—GP—consultant	Proportion of letters mentioning various items and omitting possible relevant information; no. referrals to OP; action taken at OP	Oxford Reg.	1958	[QRL 439]	(6.2.4)	L
Communication—GP—consultant	Length and content of referral letter; length, content, delay and proportion consultants' letters per visit	E & W	1962	[QRL 244]	(6.2.4) 5.4.3.1	L

Topic and type of data	Detail of analysis	Area	Year	Publication (see QRL key)	Text reference	Remarks
Evaluation—*contd.*						
Evaluation of general practice/hospital links—contd.						
Communication— GP—consultant	Consultants' opinion of usual faults and essential items; frequency of mention of various items in letters	NW London	1963	[QRL 14]	(6.2.4)	S
Communication— consultant—GP	GPs' opinion of value; details of information given to patient, warning of impending operation; delay to receipt	NW London	1954–9	[QRL 13]	(6.2.4)	S
Communication— consultant—GP	Delay in consultants' letters after OP appt.	Edinburgh	1962–3	[QRL 599]	(6.2.4) 5.4.3.1	S
Communication— consultant—GP	Delay in consultants' letters after OP appt.	SE Engl.	1963	[QRL 140]	(6.2.4) 5.4.3.1	M
Communication— consultant—GP	'Discharge' letters: category of hospital care, per cent reports received by GP; delay; content of preliminary report	E Midlands	1970–1	[QRL 248]	(6.2.4)	M
Direct-access investigation	Diagnostic and screening tests: delay to receipt of report; assessment of impact upon management of patient	E Midlands	1973	[QRL 531]	(6.2.4.1)	M
General practice— hospital links	Per cent GPs desiring hospital appointments, hospital beds, and work as member of consultant team; type of practice, list size, experience	NI; Health authorities	1970	[QRL 482]	(6.2.4) 5.1.2.1	M; Q
Referral to out-patients	Teaching/non-teaching hospital, decision by GP or patient, referral to consultants by name, valuing investigation or opinion; use of direct-access investigation; method of obtaining emergency admission; qualification pre/post-1940	SE London	1962	[QRL 6]	(6.2.4.1)	VS
Evaluation of out-patients						
Ambulance transport	Delay during journey and impact on patient	NW London	1972	[QRL 59]	(6.2.4)	
Communication doctor/patient	Items of information given by doctor; items retained by patient	London	1968	[QRL 362]	6.2.5.3	VS

Compliance with drug therapy (psychiatric OP)	Diagnosis; medication; compliance	E London	1965	[QRL 565]	(6.2.3)	VS
Compliance with drug therapy (psychiatric OP)	Diagnosis; medication, side effects, compliance	S London	1965	[QRL 710]	(6.2.3)	VS
Consultants' views	Preference for IP/OP work; controlling flow of out-patients, tracing non-attenders; support from junior staff	E & W	1962	[QRL 244]	(6.2.5.3) 5.4.3.1	L
Non-attenders	Attenders/non-attenders: reason for referral; distance from clinic; reason given for non-attendance	Manchester	1964	[QRL 326]	6.2.3	S
Out-patient referrals	Disposal after first visit; hospital status after 6 months; specialty	SE Engl.	1963	[QRL 140]	(6.2.5) 5.4.3.1	M
Out-patient referrals	Disposal after first visit; subsequent management; specialty	NE Scot.	1962–3	[QRL 44]	(6.2.5) 5.4.3.1	M
Out-patient referrals	Status DR seeing new patients; disposal after first visit, distance travelled, age, hospital status after 1 year	Scottish Borders	1969–70	[QRL 285]	(6.2.6) 5.4.3.3.	M
Out-patient surgery	Hernia repairs: complications, readmission, patients' views	Edinburgh	1950–5	[QRL 235]	(6.2.5)	S
Out-patient surgery	Operations performed, views of patients	Aberdeen	1960	[QRL 628]	(6.2.5.3)	VS
Out-patient/early discharge surgery	Operation, bed savings, complications, GP and patient satisfaction	Edinburgh	1967–70	[QRL 582]	(6.2.5)	S
Out-patient/early discharge surgery	Varicose veins: costs of treatments and loss of earnings from sickness absence	Cardiff	1967–71	[QRL 538]	(6.2.5)	S
Out-patient/early discharge surgery	Varicose veins: follow-up results	Cardiff	1967–71	[QRL 142]	(6.2.5)	S
Out-patient/surgery—children	Diagnosis	Southampton	1969–73	[QRL 43]	(6.2.3)	M
Out-patient surgery	Diagnosis; complications	Edinburgh	1970–3	[QRL 583]	(6.2.5)	S
Patients' views	Loss of working time and income, cost of journey, preference for place of care	6 areas in E & W	1967	[QRL 323]	(6.2.5.3) 4.3.4	M; Q

Evaluation of in-patient care

Emergency admission—acute coronary	Medical intervals of delay onset/admission; influence of time of day	Edinburgh	1967–8	[QRL 28]	(6.2.4.1)	M
Emergency ambulance calls	Diagnosis, management	Nottingham	1974	[QRL 119]	(6.2.4)	S
Need for admission	Age, type of hospital, facilities required	Birmingham	1958–9	[QRL 434]	(6.2.4.3)	L

Topic and type of data	Detail of analysis	Area	Year	Publication (see QRL key)	Text reference	Remarks
Evaluation—*contd.*						
Evaluation of in-patient care—contd.						
Need for emergency admission	Source of referral, GP/hospital view on need for consultant care; age, main reason for care	Dundee	1971	[QRL 655]	(6.2.4.3)	S
Need for admission	Alternatives to admission, delay from investigations, earlier discharge feasible	Oxford	1969	[QRL 412]	(6.2.4.3)	S
Need for admission	Elderly admitted to geriatric/psychiatric hospitals: proportion misplaced; outcome	Belfast	1960–1	[QRL 373]	(6.2.4.3)	S
Patients admitted to teaching hospital	Comparison of in-patients with regional and national data: age, sex, SC, diagnosis	London	1964	[QRL 61]	(6.2.4.3)	L
Reason for admission— psychiatric patients	Admitted and not-admitted patients: treatment required, protection required, community aspects	Camberwell	1970	[QRL 271]	(6.2.4.3)	VS
Alternative location of care	Age, severity of illness, other care suitable	Birmingham	1952–4	[QRL 172]	(6.2.4.3)	M
Alternative location of care	Obstetric patients: relationship birth rate in localities and proportion of mothers admitted to hospital	Tees-side	1957–8	[QRL 11]	(6.2.4.3) 4.1.2	M
Alternative location of care	Patients not requiring or requiring admission or retention on medical grounds; type of hospital, services needed, home circumstances	Birmingham	1958–9	[QRL 435]	(6.2.4.3)	M
Alternative location of care	Admission considered not required on medical grounds: specialty, sex, season	Barrow	1958	[QRL 243]	(6.2.4.3) 4.1.2	S
Alternative location of care	Age; numbers 'stuck' in acute wards; facilities required for home discharge, arrangements recommended, weeks' stay after recommendation	Leeds	1965–7	[QRL 441]	(6.2.4.3)	M
Alternative location of care	Patients with four surgical conditions: daily nursing dependency; proportion of days fit for home care	Liverpool	1966	[QRL 403]	(6.2.4.3) 4.1.2	VS
Alternative location of care	Myocardial infarction: mortality of patients, elective or random place of care, age, history of disease	SW Engl.	1966–9	[QRL 453]	(6.2.4.3)	M

Alternative location of care	Myocardial infarction: mortality up to 330 days: males, elective or random allocation home/hospital, age, previous medical history, interval onset to treatment, initial hypotension	SW Engl.	1966–70	[QRL 454]	(6.2.4.3) M
Alternative location of care	In-patients considered suitable for other care: sex, age, specialty; alternative care appropriate	Scot.	1966–7	[QRL 459]	(6.2.4.3) 5.6.2 M
Alternative location of care	DR's opinion of need for care, type of hospital, month interview, diagnosis, change in condition during admission, prognosis, nursing dependency, sex, age, MS, ability for self-care, attitudes to discharge, services required, discharge arrangements, availability of services	Liverpool R	1967–8	[QRL 109]	(6.2.4.3) 5.6.2 M
Alternative location of care	Patients staying in hospital more than 30 days: medical staff views on appropriate location and other types of care needed; medical services and nursing dependency	Liverpool	1967–8	[QRL 403]	(6.2.4.3) 4.1.2 M
Alternative location of care	Potential saving in bed days; specialty, alternative care appropriate	Oxford	1968	[QRL 412]	(6.2.4.3) S
Investigations	Requested: results present in notes	Aberdeen	1971	[QRL 584]	(6.2.4.1) M
Long-stay geriatric patients	Length of stay, age, sex, home background, diagnosis; disabilities; reasons for long stay	London	1965–7	[QRL 578]	(6.2.4.3) VS
Length of stay— haemorrhoids	Operation age, sex, symptoms; time in hospital; return to work; complications	Manchester	1971–3	[QRL 26]	(6.2.4.3) VS
Length of stay— hernia	Length of stay, complications, duration of convalescence, workload of GPs	Mansfield	1966	[QRL 489]	(6.2.4.3) VS
Length of stay— hernia and VVs	Operations performed, complications, home circumstances, number out-patient visits	Worcestershire	1967–9	[QRL 209]	(6.2.4.3) S
Length of stay— maternity	Length of stay; complications	Bradford	1958–9	[QRL 641]	(6.2.4.3) M
Length of stay— maternity	Length of stay; perinatal mortality; infant readmission by cause; breast feeding	Bradford	1959–65	[QRL 32]	(6.2.4.3) L
Length of stay— maternity	Reasons for short/long stay; complications	London	1961–3	[QRL 540]	(6.2.4.3) S
Length of stay— maternity	Length of stay; readmission; complications treated at home	Wolverhampton	1962–3	[QRL 423]	(6.2.4.3) M
Length of stay— maternity	Age, parity, length of stay, complications at delivery	Bradford	1965–6	[QRL 168]	(6.2.4.3) L

Evaluation—*contd.*

Evaluation of in-patient care—*contd.*

Topic and type of data	Detail of analysis	Area	Year	Publication (see QRL key)	Text reference	Remarks
Length of stay—maternity	Early discharge patients: SC, parity, complications treated at home, views of experience	Newcastle	1966	[QRL 587]	(6.2.4.3)	S
Length of stay—medical patients	Diagnosis, age, sex, home circumstances, reasons for long stay	NE Scot.	1967–8	[QRL 633]	(6.2.4.3)	S
Length of stay—myocardial infarct	Age, sex, initial comparability; length of stay; complications; return to work	Chelmsford	1968–70	[QRL 294]	(6.2.4.3)	S
Length of stay—myocardial infarct	Length of stay; age, sex, severity of condition, complications	Belfast	1970–2	[QRL 79]	(6.2.4.3)	S
Length of stay—myocardial infarct	Initial comparability; mortality; complications	Glasgow	1970–3	[QRL 80]	(6.2.4.3)	S
Length of stay—myocardial infarct	Initial comparability; complications, readmission	Nottingham	1972–3	[QRL 302]	(6.2.4.3)	VS
Length of stay—myocardial infarct	Deaths in initial admission, after discharge, upon readmission; age, previous medical history	Stoke	1974–5	[QRL 261]	(6.2.4.3)	S
Length of stay—ophthalmology	Usual length of stay reported by surgeons, operation	GB	1973	[QRL 264]	(6.2.4.3)	S
Length of stay—prostatecotomy	Operation; financial considerations	London, Liverpool, Portsmouth	1968–73	[QRL 27]	(6.2.4.3)	S
Length of stay—psychiatric patients	Diagnosis, number of admissions, length of history, stay, year of admission	London	1930–51	[QRL 295]	(6.2.4.3)	S
Length of stay—psychiatric patients	Age, sex, marital status, diagnosis, number of admissions	E & W	1954–5	[QRL 96]	(6.2.4.3)	VL
Length of stay—psychiatric patients	Discharges, deaths; admissions, sex, age; bed requirements	E & W	1955–9	[QRL 653]	(6.2.4.3)	VL
Length of stay—psychiatric patients	Age, sex, type of hospital, region, diagnosis	E & W	1963	[QRL 97]	(6.2.4.3)	VL
Length of stay—psychiatric patients	Discharges in year of admission; projected discharges; age, sex, length of stay	NE Scot.	1963–6	[QRL 46]	(6.2.4.3)	L
Length of stay—psychiatric patients	Length of stay, age, sex; projected run down	E & W	1963–73	[QRL 221]	(6.2.4.3)	VL

Length of stay—psychiatric patients	Number of long stay, age, sex, diagnosis	Camberwell	1965–70	[QRL 719]	(6.2.4.3)	M
Length of stay—psychiatric patients	Projected discharges by sex	Wessex	1967–70	[QRL 18]	(6.2.4.3)	VL
Length of stay—psychiatric patients	Type of accommodation required, sex, diagnosis	Camberwell	1969–70	[QRL 445]	(6.2.4.3)	VS
Length of stay—psychiatric patients	Likelihood of discharge, age, sex, diagnosis, employment status, outcome	S London	1973–5	[QRL 66]	(6.2.4.3)	M
Miscellaneous—feeding unconscious patient	Discrepancies between recommended diet and actual content of nutrients administered; observer error in measuring fluid balance	12 selected hospitals E & W	1974	[QRL 360]	(6.2.4.1)	S
Miscellaneous—obstetric anaesthesia	Grade of staff and facilities; assistance available; techniques for emergency Caesarean; complications	Birmingham Reg.	1972–3	[QRL 516]	6.2.2	VS
Miscellaneous—ophthalmology	Beds available, consultant staff, nursing, waiting lists, bed usage, 'clinical' productivity, diagnosis	E & W	1972	[QRL 517]	6.2.2	VS
Mortality from surgical condition	Case fatality of appendicitis, perforated ulcer, prostrate hyperplasia; sex, age, severity; teaching/non-teaching hospital	E & W	1951–4	[QRL 397]	6.2.5.1	L
Mortality from prostatic hyperplasia	Mortality in hospital and on follow-up: age, unfavourable social and medical factors, mode of admission, operation, teaching/non-teaching hospital	Unspecified	1964–9	[QRL 40]	6.2.5.1	M
Mortality of discharged in-patients	Deaths following hospital care; proportion unrecorded in notes; cause of death, relationship to treated disease; age patient	Oxford	1963–4	[QRL 552]	6.2.5.1	S
Morbidity in discharged in-patients	*Note*: relevant references are indexed under Rehabilitation in Chapter 2, NEED					
Nursing dependency	Assessment of nursing dependency of in-patients and those nursed at home	Essex	1970	[QRL 529]	(6.2.4.3)	S
Patients' views—general	Time of wakening, nursing staff, other patients, privacy, size of ward, communication, medical treatment, contact with surgical staff, visiting by general practitioner; maternity patients—isolation in labour, presence of husband in labour, privacy, sex, age, SC, type of hospital	12 areas in E & W	1961	[QRL 126]	(6.2.5.3) 5.6.1	S; Q
Patients' views—general	Satisfaction with the ward, sanitary accommodation, meals, activities, care	28 hospitals in E & W	1966–71	[QRL 553]	6.2.5.3	L

Topic and type of data	Detail of analysis	Area	Year	Publication (see QRL key)	Text reference	Remarks
Evaluation—*contd.*						
Evaluation of in-patient care—contd.						
Patients' views—general	Preference for place of care, length of stay, progress with treatment, needs after discharge	6 areas E & W	1967	[QRL 323]	(6.2.5.3) 4.3.4	S; Q
Patients' views—admission	Patients' anxiety and degree of worry, opinions of nursing quality, knowledge about ward	4 locations in E & W	1973	[QRL 246]	6.2.5.2	VS
Patients' views—maternity	Patients' criticisms of communication in hospitals and other aspects of care; distribution of responses before and after changes in communication	3 selected hospitals in E	1964–6	[QRL 335]	(6.2.5.3)	S
Patients' views—noise	Proportion of patients reporting distress from noise, by source	E & W	1957–60	[QRL 316]	6.2.5.3	M
Patients' views—nursing attention	Patients' satisfaction and views of nurses; nurses' expectations, satisfaction, relationships; doctors' views of nurses and nursing	3 hospitals in E & W	1970	[QRL 21]	(6.2.5.3)	S
Patients' views—nursing attention	Nurses' views of contact and communication with popular and unpopular patients; patients' views of contact with nurses	4 selected hospitals in E & W	1971	[QRL 632]	(6.2.5.3)	S
Patients' views—psychiatric hospitals	Patient satisfaction: general, the ward, patient care, life in the hospital	9 hospitals in E & W	1969–71	[QRL 554]	6.2.5.3	L
Patients' views—satisfaction and complaints	Level of satisfaction, topics raised by patients, discussions with staff; improving communication; suggested complaints procedure; type of hospital	S	1967	[QRL 123]	6.2.5.3	M
Patients' views—suggestions and complaints	Proportion making written complaint, oral complaint or suggestion, having suggestion or complaint but not reporting this; reason for not voicing complaint	E & W	1971	[QRL 181]	6.2.5.3	S
Patients' views—voluntary staff	Patients' satisfaction with voluntary workers	13 hospitals in E & W	1967	[QRL 576]	6.2.5.3	S
Discharged in-patients	Notification of intention to discharge—when sent; promptness of GP's visit; GP's knowledge of local authority services	NE England	1967	[QRL 263]	6.2.6	VS

Prescribing—drug administration	Errors of administration; no. of drugs being given, frequency of administration; type of error	London	1963	[QRL 666]	6.2.3	L
Prescribing—drug administration	Errors in prescribing, administration, and recording of IP medication	London	1966	[QRL 313]	(6.2.4.2)	S
Consultant staff	Satisfaction with senior and junior staffing levels; views on requirements	E & W	1972	[QRL 334]	(6.2.5.3) 4.2.5	S; Q
Nurses and midwives	Morale; wastage rates; views on working conditions	GB	1971	[QRL 190]	(6.2.6) 4.3.1	L; Q
Nurses and midwives from overseas	Views on nursing in GB; advice to others	GB	1971	[QRL 644]	(6.2.5.3) 4.3.1	S
Nurses and midwives—reserves	Work intentions; attitudes to work	GB	1971	[QRL 589]	(6.2.5.3) 4.3.1	S; Q
Waiting lists	Failure to respond to call-up; age of patient, length time on waiting list, specialty, site of operation, holiday periods, notice given	Mansfield	1967	[QRL 488]	(6.2.4.1)	M

Evaluation of day care

Geriatric day hospital	Discharged in-patients: sex; age; days attendance/patient: physical and mental health, social adjustment on follow-up; additional support required; cost	Sunderland	1960–1	[QRL 724]	(6.2.5)	S
Geriatric day hospital	Diagnostic category, duration of attendance, outcome after initial course of treatment, second and subsequent periods of attendance	SE Engl.	1963–8	[QRL 95]	(6.2.5) 5.7.1	S

Evaluation of residential care

Homes for the elderly	Proportion of houses with good standard for range of facilities; type of home	Scot.	1969	[QRL 125]	(6.2.2)	S; Q

Evaluation of specific medical problems

Abortion	Attitude of GP and other DR; MS, consultation/ operation delay	E & W	1969–72	[QRL 385]	6.2.4.2	M
Abortion	Referral by GPs; action on NHS consultant refusal; views on appropriate care; age, sex, religion of GP	E & W; Region	1970–1	[QRL 133]	6.2.6 5.1.2.5	S; Q

Topic and type of data	Detail of analysis	Area	Year	Publication (see QRL key)	Text reference	Remarks
Evaluation—*contd.*						
Evaluation of specific medical problems—contd.						
Abortion	Action taken by doctors; delay; patients' views of care received	E & W	1972	[QRL 131]	(6.2.6)	S; Q
Abortion	Mental state 6 months after abortion, outcome of pregnancy when abortion refused: age, MS, parity, stress at conception, emotional support	London	1961–7	[QRL 145]	(6.2.5)	S
Abortion	Contraceptive use before and 3 months after abortion	S London	1972–3	[QRL 58]	(6.2.4.2)	S
Abortion	Numbers requesting abortion—refused by GP, referred to NHS or private care; miscarriage and continuing pregnancy	Somerset	1972	[QRL 527]	(6.2.6)	VS
Abortion—subsequent pregnancy	Foetal loss	Bristol	1975	[QRL 573]	(6.2.5.1)	S
Addiction—alcohol	Age specific hospital discharge rate: doctors other SC I males	Scot.	1963–72	[QRL 497]	(6.2.5.2)	S
Adverse drug reactions	Selected extracts from register of adverse reactions: reaction; place of action of drug, class of drug, specific drug	E & W	1964–73	[QRL 192]	6.2.5.2 2.5.4	VL
Adverse drug reactions	Reported deaths; drug used; deaths/million prescriptions	UK	1964–71	[QRL 266]	(6.2.5.2)	M
Adverse drug reactions	Prescribing of drugs with known serious reactions; secular trend in relation to official warnings; specific drugs; use/1000 list size	NI	1966–71	[QRL 668]	(6.2.5.2)	S
Adverse drug reactions	Reported adverse reactions; source of report, severity of reaction, assessment of causal drug relationship	E & W	1971	[QRL 345]	(6.2.5.2)	VL
Adverse drug reactions	Teratogenicity following prescribed/self-administered drugs	E & W	1969	[QRL 173]	(6.2.5.2)	L
Adverse drug reactions	Jaundice after Halothane anaesthetic; frequency anaesthetic, year, diagnosis, age	UK	1964–72	[QRL 344]	6.2.5.2	VS

Adverse drug reactions	Observed reactions; specialty, age, length of stay, number of drugs given, type of reaction, drugs used	Belfast	1965–6	[QRL 341]	(6.2.5.2)	M
Adverse drug reactions	α-methyldopa: adverse effects identified, during hospital stay and on follow-up; haematological values; other adverse effects	Aberdeen	1969	[QRL 166]	(6.2.5.2)	S
Adverse drug reactions	Amitriptyline: sudden unexpected death; arrythmia induced by anaesthesia; other drugs prescribed	Aberdeen	1968–71	[QRL 484]	(6.2.5.2)	S
Adverse drug reactions	Pentazocine: perceptual disturbances	Aberdeen	1972	[QRL 722]	(6.2.5.2)	S
Alimentary disease— Crohn's disease	Mortality by cause: initial age, site of lesion, treatment	Birmingham	1931–68	[QRL 549]	(6.2.5.1)	S
Alimentary disease— peptic ulcer	Patients following surgery—symptom grading, patients' assessment	Yorkshire	1944–74	[QRL 288]	(6.2.5.3)	VS
Alimentary disease— duodenal ulcer	5–8-year post-operative symptoms, and recurrent ulceration; initial treatment	Yorkshire	1960–7	[QRL 275]	(6.2.5.3)	S
Alimentary disease— duodenal ulcer	5–8-year post-operative symptoms and recurrent ulceration; initial treatment	Yorkshire	1960–71	[QRL 276]	(6.2.5.3)	S
Alimentary disease— dyspepsia	Subsequent peptic ulceration; age, initial duration of symptoms	Cardiff	1964–70	[QRL 283]	(6.2.5.2)	S
Peptic ulcer— gastrointestinal haemorrhage	Further haemorrhage and case fatality; sex, age, previous history, site and severity of bleeding	NE Scot.	1967–9	[QRL 358]	(6.2.5)	S
Peptic ulcer— surgery	Symptom grading, 'quality of life'	Edinburgh & Dumfries	1974	[QRL 138]	(6.2.5.3)	VS
Blood diseases— anaemia	Subsequent mortality: sex, miners/non-miners; initial serum iron and PCV	S Wales	1958–68	[QRL 697]	(6.2.5.1) 2.2.2.2	S
Blood diseases— anaemia	Subsequent mortality by cause in women; age, smoking, initial haematocrit	S Wales	1964–72	[QRL 228]	(6.2.5.1) 2.2.2.2	L
Cancer: delay in seeking care	Length of delay, reasons, IQ	Manchester	1954	[QRL 12]	6.2.3	S
Cancer: delay	Diagnosis, age, SC; patient delay in months	Manchester Region	1962–3	[QRL 17]	6.2.3	M
Cancer: delay	Symptoms, stage; patient/GP/hospital delay	London	1963–4	[QRL 580]	6.2.3	S
Cancer: delay	MS, length education, anxiety, domestic responsibility; patient/GP/hospital delay	London	1966	[QRL 118]	6.2.3	VS
Cancer	5-year survival: site, sex, age, treatment	Birmingham Region	1960–2	[QRL 692]	6.2.5.1 2.5.8	VL
Cancer	5-year survival: site, sex, stage, treatment, age corrected	Manchester Region	1932–64	[QRL 222]	6.2.5.1 2.5.8	L

Topic and type of data	Detail of analysis	Area	Year	Publication (see QRL key)	Text reference	Remarks
Evaluation—*contd.*						
Evaluation of specific medical problems—contd.						
Cancer—leukaemia	Age, treatment; survival, infections, 'quality of life'	London	1969–75	[QRL 106]	(6.2.5)	VS
Cancer—rectal	Quality of life: colostomy actions daily, dietary restriction, medication, sexual activity, psychological and social grading, contact with health services	London	1962–70	[QRL 203]	(6.2.5.3)	VS
Cardiovascular disease—IHD	15-year survival in 'population' sample of men; mode of presentation, cause of death	UK	1940–54	[QRL 492]	(6.2.5.1)	S
Cardiovascular disease—IHD	12-year survival in women: presentation, risk factors at presentation	Edinburgh	1953–70	[QRL 515]	(6.2.5.1)	VS
Cardiovascular disease—IHD	Age, sex, duration until death, place of death	Belfast	1965–6	[QRL 440]	(6.2.5.1)	S
Cardiovascular disease—IHD	1-month survival in 'population' sample; previous history, presentation, place of treatment	SW Engl.	1966–9	[QRL 453]	(6.2.5.1)	M
Cardiovascular disease—IHD	1-month survival in 'population' sample; mode of presentation	Oxford	1966–7	[QRL 378]	(6.2.5.1)	S
Cardiovascular disease—IHD	Deaths in first 4 weeks; age, sex, diagnosis, first/subsequent attack	Edinburgh	1967–8	[QRL 28]	(6.2.5.1)	M
Cardiovascular disease—IHD	1-year survival in 'population' sample, mode of presentation, sex, previous history	Edinburgh	1967–8	[QRL 257]	(6.2.5.1)	M
Cardiovascular disease—angina	Outcome at 6 months and complications; history, treatment	Edinburgh	1970–3	[QRL 217]	(6.2.5)	S
Cardiovascular disease—hypertension	Subsequent health; initial pressure, age, influence of treatment	Blackpool	1955–70	[QRL 630]	(6.2.5.2)	VS
Cardiovascular disease—hypertension	Subsequent pressures and general health; sex, treatment/control	London	1967–70	[QRL 55]	(6.2.5.2)	S
Cardiovascular disease—hypertension	Mortality and complications; sex, age, initial pressure	S London	1949–69	[QRL 254]	(6.2.5)	S

Topic	Description	Region	Years	Ref	Section	Type
Cardiovascular disease—hypertension	Subsequent blood pressure and requirement of treatment	S Wales	1968–73	[QRL 298]	(6.2.5.2)	S
Cardiovascular disease—stroke	Death rates; sex, BP	NI	1948–65	[QRL 460]	(6.2.5.1)	S
Cardiovascular disease—stroke	Fatality and grade recovery: sex, age, diagnosis, speed of onset	W London	1951–4	[QRL 272]	(6.2.5)	S
Cerebrovascular accident	Intracerebral haemorrhage: sex, age, other illness; BP, clinical features; treatment; survival	S London	1959–60	[QRL 436]	(6.2.5.1)	VS
Cerebrovascular accident	Thrombosis/embolism: sex, age, previous illness; BP, clinical features; life table survival, cause of death	W London	1959–60	[QRL 449]	(6.2.5.1)	VS
Cerebrovascular accident	Ruptured intracranial aneurysm, sex; mortality within 6 months	S London, N Surrey	1962–3	[QRL 170]	(6.2.5.1)	VS
Childhood—post-neonatal deaths	Cause of death, age, duration illness; maternal age, parity, SC, previous pregnancy history, country of birth	E	1964–6	[QRL 187]	6.2.3	S; Q
Childhood—sudden death	Sex, age, month death, illness in preceding fortnight, type of bedding	E	1954–63	[QRL 472]	(6.2.5.1)	S; Q
Childhood—pulmonary collapse	Age, length of history, site of lung affected, aetiology; resolution	W London	1945–55	[QRL 352]	(6.2.5.2)	S
Congenital abnormality—spina bifida	Live births by calendar year; survival until 5	E & W	1954–72	[QRL 701]	6.2.5.2	VL
Congenital abnormality—spina bifida	Survival; place residence; schooling	E & W	1965–71	[QRL 700]	6.2.5.2	S
Congenital abnormality—spina bifida	Survival and residual disability; age, diagnosis, adverse factors at treatment, treatment	Sheffield	1962–71	[QRL 411]	(6.2.5.2)	S
Congenital abnormality—spina bifida	Sensory level, overall and specific disability, predictive features	Cambridge	1963–72	[QRL 339]	(6.2.5.2)	VS
Congenital abnormality—spina bifida	Disability, hydrocephalus in treated; adverse factors and age death untreated	Sheffield	1971–3	[QRL 411]	(6.2.5.2)	VS
Dental disease—dentures	Use, difficulty with dentures, type of denture: sex, SC	E & W	1968	[QRL 282]	(6.2.5.3) 2.5.12	M; Q
Dental disease—dentures	Use, difficulty with dentures	S	1972	[QRL 652]	(6.2.5.3) 2.5.12	M; Q

Topic and type of data	Detail of analysis	Area	Year	Publication (see QRL key)	Text reference	Remarks
Evaluation—*contd.*						
Evaluation of specific medical problems—*contd.*						
Diabetes	Degree of dietary control of diabetics living at home	Leeds	1948	[QRL 661]	(6.2.3)	VS
Diabetics— hyperglycaemia	Age, sex, treatment, blood sugar, vascular events	Bedford	1962–7	[QRL 367]	(6.2.5.2)	S
Diabetics— hyperglycaemia	Untreated patients: age, secular change in glucose tolerance, incidence diabetes	Aberdeen	1964–73	[QRL 409]	(6.2.5.2)	VS
Eye disease— registered blind	Sex, age, MS, SC; cause of blindness; patients' attitude to GP's action and treatment of condition by all agencies	GLC	1968–70	[QRL 2]	(6.2.5.3)	S
Family planning	Parents' knowledge, views of advice from GP, HV and FPA clinic	E & W	1968–70	[QRL 128]	6.2.3 2.5.18	M
Family planning	GP attitudes to contraception, initiation of action	E & W	1970–1	[QRL 134]	(6.2.5.3) 5.1.2.5	
Family planning— women	MS; type of contraceptive used, acceptability, opinion of services available	E & W	1970	[QRL 76]	(6.2.5.3) 2.5.18	M; Q
Family planning	Plans for 'family building', subsequent action and intentions; SC, family size, method of contraception	E & W	1972–5	[QRL 135]	(6.2.5.3)	M
Family planning— vasectomy	Number performed, type hospital, indication, adequacy of NHS facilities, delegation, out-patient surgery, complications	E & W	1971	[QRL 674]	(6.2.6)	S
Family planning— health visitors' advice	Predicted action; influence of age, MS, religion	E & W	1970–1	[QRL 672]	(6.2.5.3)	S
Family planning— midwives' advice	Predicted action; influence of age, MS, religion	E & W	1970–1	[QRL 673]	(6.2.5.3)	S
Family planning— morbidity in 'pill' takers	Relative risk of hospital death from DVT or pulmonary embolism in women on 'the pill'	London	1964–6	[QRL 205]	(6.2.5.2)	VS
Family planning— morbidity in 'pill' takers	Use of 'the pill' in women 20–40 dying from thrombo embolism	E & W	1966	[QRL 205]	(6.2.5.2)	VS

Family planning—morbidity in 'pill' takers	'Pill' takers/ex-takers/controls: morbidity by diagnoses; adjustment for confounding factors	UK	1968–72	[QRL 365]	(6.2.5.2) VL
Genito-urinary disease—renal transplants	Subsequent renal function: renal disease, duration dialysis, 'warm' time, units of blood transfused	London	1963–8	[QRL 543]	(6.2.5.2) VS
Genito-urinary disease—renal transplants	Results: renal disease, general condition, age, sex, other treatment	Edinburgh	1960–8	[QRL 725]	(6.2.5.2) VS
Genito-urinary disease—renal transplants	Sex, age, follow-up status	NI	1968–70	[QRL 424]	(6.2.5.2) VS
Genito-urinary disease—renal transplants	Tissue type, length of ischaemia; renal function, actuarial survival	Glasgow	1969–72	[QRL 60]	(6.2.5.2) VS
Haemorrhoids—Lord's procedure	Preoperative symptoms, symptoms after 5 years	Edinburgh	1969–74	[QRL 684]	(6.2.5.3) VS
Maternity—mortality	Cause of maternal death: maternal age, parity, MS, gestation; place delivery, booking arrangements, avoidable factors	E & W Reg.	1970–2	[QRL 31]	6.2.3 2.5.2.2 S
Maternity—perinatal mortality	Stillbirth and neonatal mortality rates; prematurity	GB	1946	[QRL 210]	(6.2.5.1) 2.5.10.1 L; Q
Maternity—stillbirth and infant mortality	Cause of death: maternal age, parity, SC, MS; place of residence; multiple births	E & W; Planning Reg.	1949–50	[QRL 304]	(6.2.5.1) 2.5.10.3 VL
Maternity—perinatal mortality	Cause of death; characteristics of mother, arrangements for delivery	GB; Planning Reg.	1958	[QRL 111]	6.2.5.1 2.5.10.1 VL; Q
Maternity—mortality and morbidity in children	FU to age 7: maternal SC, parity, smoking; disorders or pregnancy and delivery; perinatal risk factors	E & W	1958–65	[QRL 179]	(6.2.5) 2.5.10.1 L; Q
Maternity—stillbirth and infant mortality	Cause of death: maternal age, parity, SC, MS	E & W; Planning Reg.	1964–5	[QRL 624]	(6.2.5.1) 2.5.10.3 L
Maternity	Perinatal mortality rate: LAs classified by population structure, housing, voting patterns, SC and occupation, educational facilities, adult mortality; LAs with 'aberrant' results	E & W	1966–8	[QRL 38]	6.2.5.1 VL
Maternity	Abortion, stillbirth, first-week deaths, birth injury, and illness in first week: characteristics of mother, obstetric care received	UK	1970	[QRL 141]	(6.2.5) L; Q

Evaluation—*contd.*

Evaluation of specific medical problems—contd.

Topic and type of data	Detail of analysis	Area	Year	Publication (see QRL key)	Text reference	Remarks
Maternity—perinatal	Place delivery, risk group, booking arrangements, access to GP unit, distance to consultant unit	Oxford	1962	[QRL 319]	(6.2.5.1)	L
Maternity—perinatal mortality	Primips: place of booking and delivery; previous miscarriage, complications of pregnancy, method of delivery	Oxford	1962–4	[QRL 320]	(6.2.5.1)	L
Maternity—perinatal mortality	Local authority, population structure, death rates for degenerative diseases, health services available, health service usage	Birmingham and SW RHB	1966–8	[QRL 39]	6.2.5.1	VL
Maternity—perinatal mortality	Cause of death, booking, parity, maternal height	S Wales	1968	[QRL 664]	(6.2.5.1)	VS
Maternity—subsequent intelligence of child	Intelligence; obstetric factors—parity, gestation, illness in pregnancy, plurality, mode delivery, illness in neonate	Birmingham	1950–4	[QRL 50]	(6.2.5.2)	VL
Maternity—subsequent intelligence of child	Intelligence; sex, SC, gestation, mode of delivery, obstetric complications	Newcastle	1960–72	[QRL 500]	(6.2.5.2) 2.5.10.1	L
Maternity—place of delivery	Place of delivery, urban/rural, birth weight deaths in first month of life	E & W; Reg.	1956–65	[QRL 36]	(6.2.5.1)	VL
Maternity—patterns of care	Length of stay: age, MS, SC, source admission, parity, obstetric history, babies' weight	Oxford	1962	[QRL 4]	(6.2.4.3)	M
Maternity—place of confinement	Views of mothers, GPs and midwives to selection and risk factors; attitudes to early discharge	South Coast town	1965–6	[QRL 654]	(6.2.5.3)	S
Maternity—place of confinement	Age, parity, legitimacy, social conditions, house delivery	Glasgow	1967	[QRL 566]	(6.2.4.3)	S
Maternity—GP unit use	Age, parity, duration of stay; views of mothers and attendants of experience	Salford	1967–8	[QRL 555]	(6.2.4.3)	S
Maternity—late booking	Parity, MS, attitudes to obstetric care, view of pregnancy	12 locations in E & W	1968	[QRL 575]	(6.2.3)	S
Maternity—patterns of antenatal care	Classification of care: neonatal survivors, perinatal deaths, birth weight	Unspecified	1972–4	[QRL 240]	(6.2.4.3)	M
Maternity—economics	Type of hospital/unit, size of unit, staff, no. of deliveries, distance from consultant unit; cost to NHS for additional delivery; family cost	Devon	1970	[QRL 39]	(6.2.5.4)	M

Maternity—family costs	Items of cost, place delivery, SC	Exeter	1970	[QRL 239]	(6.2.5.4) S
Mental illness	Survival following hospital admission; sex, age, diagnosis	W Sussex	1948–51	[QRL 579]	(6.2.5.1) S
Mental illness—schizophrenia	Social drift: age, fathers' SC	E London	1958–60	[QRL 273]	(6.2.5.2) VS
Mental illness—schizophrenia	Relapse influenced by age, sex, family, work ability, previous history, severity of disease	S London	1966–8	[QRL 101]	(6.2.5.2) VS
Miscellaneous minor ailments	Long-term outcome and influence of treatment	Beckenham	1947–73	[QRL 254]	(6.2.5.2) L
Rehabilitation—time off work	Length of sickness absence, contact with health and welfare services, attitudes to return to work	E & W	1972–3	[QRL 450]	(6.2.5.2) L
Rehabilitation—psychiatric patients	Follow-up status—psychiatric illness, place of residence, mental state, behaviour, attitudes	Epsom	1959	[QRL 717]	(6.2.5.2) VS
Rehabilitation—time off work	Myocardial infarction: per cent returning to work by 3 months	N London	1961–3	[QRL 605]	(6.2.5.2) S
Rehabilitation—time off work	Myocardial infarction: work status at onset of illness, no. returning to work, days off work	Oxford	1966–7	[QRL 377]	6.2.5.2 S
Rehabilitation—psychiatric patients	Outcome; diagnosis, symptom severity, accommodation needs	Camberwell	1968–9	[QRL 721]	(6.2.5.2) VS
Rehabilitation—time off work	Herniorrhaphy patients: length of stay, patient characteristics, time off work, occupation, sick pay	Oxford area	1971–2	[QRL 603]	6.2.5.2 VS
Respiratory disease—chronic bronchitis	Mortality on 10-year follow-up, by cause of death; age, sex, breathlessness at diagnosis, length of history, initial and subsequent smoking	London	1951–63	[QRL 520]	(6.2.5.1) S
Terminal care	GPs' difficulty in admitting patients; GP, DN, HV views of community and hospital facilities required; GPs' view of DN; DNs' view of GP; relatives' views of communication	E & W	1969	[QRL 130]	(6.2.5.3) 2.5.32 S
Terminal care	Arrangements for care; no. requiring nursing support beyond home resources	Manchester	1969	[QRL 16]	(6.2.4.3) VS
Terminal care	Cause of death, duration illness, percentage experiencing anxiety, depression, pain, respiratory or physical distress	Mid Wales	1969–70	[QRL 559]	(6.2.6) VS
Terminal care	Cause of death, duration of illness; place of death; age, sex, symptoms	Sussex	1969–70	[QRL 116]	(6.2.6) VS

Topic and type of data	Detail of analysis	Area	Year	Publication (see QRL key)	Text reference	Remarks
Evaluation—*contd.*						
Evaluation of specific medical problems—contd.						
Terminal care	Place of death, duration of home nursing, support for home nursing, hospital procedures, preference for place of care	Sheffield	1971	[QRL 686]	(6.2.4.3)	S
Terminal care	Place of death; urban/rural residence; community attitude to optimum care	NE Engl.	1970	[QRL 260]	(6.2.4.3)	L
Terminal care—pelvic cancer	Place of death: reason for hospital admission	Newcastle	1960–3	[QRL 586]	(6.2.4.3)	VS
Terminal care—cancer	Diagnosis, nursing required, family support, home conditions	Sheffield	1963–4	[QRL 708]	(6.2.4.3)	S
Evaluation of preventive medicine						
Anti-smoking campaigns	Percentage change in smoking	Edinburgh	1958–9	[QRL 132]	(6.2.3)	M
Anti-smoking campaigns	Amount smoked, sex, campaign/control schools; subsequent occupation (boys)	SW Herts.	1959–66	[QRL 354]	(6.2.3)	S
Anti-smoking campaigns	Change in smoking, age, campaign/control schools	SE Engl.	1965–6	[QRL 329]	(6.2.3)	L
Anti-smoking campaigns	Change in smoking from group therapy; age, sex, MS, SC, referral, general health, smoking history	Dundee	1964–70	[QRL 237]	(6.2.3)	S
Anti-smoking campaigns	Conversion rate in school children: method of education, sex	Edinburgh	1964	[QRL 699]	(6.2.3)	S
Cervical cytology	Detection rate of *in situ* cancer, incidence of clinical cancer; age	Aberdeen	1958–67	[QRL 425]	6.2.3	VL
Cervical cytology	Incidence of clinical cancer, 5-year survival; age, stage, year of diagnosis	Aberdeen	1960–9	[QRL 426]	6.2.3	VL
Cervical cytology	Costs: source of smears; stage of cancer detected, items of expenditure	Aberdeen	1971	[QRL 647]	(6.2.5.4)	L
Cervical cytology: domiciliary testing	Response, prevalence *in situ* carcinoma, age, SC	Derby	1964–5	[QRL 518]	6.2.3	M

Cervical cytology: response	Computer assisted call-up; initial response; refusals after visits	W Sussex	1967–8	[QRL 592]	(6.2.3)	VL
Cervical cytology: response	'Do-it-yourself' pipette: response, SC, urban/rural residence	W Sussex	1970	[QRL 568]	(6.2.3)	L
Cervical cytology	Knowledge of purpose and availability, age, reasons for not attending	NW Engl.	1970	[QRL 182]	6.2.3	VS
Cervical cytology recall	Migration, response, reasons for non-response	Manchester RHB	1971	[QRL 590]	6.2.3	M
Cervical cytology recall	Response, SC, parity, outcome of health visitor	Derbyshire & West Riding	1972	[QRL 19]	(6.2.3)	M
Fluoridation	Study and control areas: age, average no. decayed/missing/filled teeth, per cent free dental decay	Anglesey, Ayr, Kilmarnock, Sutton, Watford	1955–67	[QRL 481, 198]	6.2.5.2	L
Immunization and vaccination	Percentage of infants protected each year against whooping cough; notification and deaths from whooping cough by year and age	Oxford	1940–66	[QRL 688]	(6.2.3)	L
Immunization and vaccination	Immunity indices by type; cost per completed procedure	W Sussex	1963–8	[QRL 591]	(6.5.2.4)	VL
Mass radiography	Cost/case detected and hundred persons examined; estimated probability of secondary cases; cost/case avoided	E & W	1950–68	[QRL 544]	(6.2.5.4)	VL
Lung cancer detection	Six-monthly X-ray: lung cancers detected, resectability, survival; age, smoking	N London	1965–7	[QRL 83]	(6.2.5.2)	VL
Lung cancer detection	Screening of employees versus conventional diagnosis: age, symptoms at diagnosis, 5-year survival	UK AEA	1962–7	[QRL 218]	(6.2.5)	VS

QUICK REFERENCE LIST KEY

[QRL 1] Abel, R. A. *Nursing Attachments to General Practice*. Department of Health and Social Security Social Science Research Unit Study No. 1. London, HMSO, 1969.

[QRL 2] Abel, R. A. *An Investigation into Some Aspects of Visual Handicap. Statistical and Research Report Series*, No. 14. London, HMSO, 1976.

[QRL 3] Abel-Smith, B. and Gales, K. 'British doctors at home and abroad.' *Occasional Papers on Social Administration*, No. 8. London, Bell, 1964.

[QRL 4] Acheson, E. D. and Feldstein, M. S. 'Duration of stay in hospital for normal maternity care.' *British Medical Journal*, **2**, 95 (1964).

[QRL 5] Acheson, R. M. 'An enquiry into the training needs of transferred officers.' *Public Health London*, **89**, 247 (1975).

[QRL 6] Acheson, R. M., Barker, D. J. P. and Butterfield, W. J. H. 'How general practitioners use out-patient services in two London boroughs.' *British Medical Journal*, **2**, 1315 (1962).

[QRL 7] Adams, G. F. and Cheeseman, E. A. *Old People in Northern Ireland*. Belfast, Northern Ireland Hospitals Authority, 1951.

[QRL 8] Adams, P., Davies, G. T. and Sweetnam, P. 'Osteoporosis and the effects of ageing on bone mass in elderly men and women.' *Quarterly Journal of Medicine*, **39**, 601 (1970).

[QRL 9] Adelstein, A. M. *et al*. 'Sequelae of virus infections in pregnancy.' In *Child Health: a Collection of Studies*, pp. 73–86. *Studies on Medical and Population Subjects*, No. 31. London, HMSO, 1976.

[QRL 10] Adler, M. W. *et al*. 'Assessment of medical care needs of individuals with chronic cardiorespiratory disease using subjective measures.' *International Journal of Epidemiology*, **2**, 73 (1973).

[QRL 11] Airth, A. D. and Newell, D. J. *The Demand for Hospital Beds. Results of an Enquiry on Tees-side*. Newcastle upon Tyne, University of Durham, Kings College, 1962.

[QRL 12] Aitken Swan, J. and Paterson, R. 'The cancer patient—delay in seeking advice.' *British Medical Journal*, **1**, 623 (1955).

[QRL 13] de Alarcon, R., Glanville, H. de and Hodson, J. M. 'Value of the specialist's report.' *British Medical Journal*, **2**, 1663 (1960).

[QRL 14] de Alarcon, R. and Hodson, J. M. 'Value of the general practitioners' letter.' *British Medical Journal*, **2**, 435 (1964).

[QRL 15] de Alarcon, R. and Rathod, N. H. 'Prevalence and early detection of heroin abuse.' *British Medical Journal*, **2**, 549 (1968).

[QRL 16] Alderson, M. R. 'Terminal care in malignant disease.' *British Journal of Preventive and Social Medicine*, **24**, 120 (1970).

[QRL 17] Alderson, M. R. and Nayak, R. 'Social class and delay in malignant disease.' *Medical Officer*, **124**, 313 (1970).

[QRL 18] Alderson, M. R. and Rushton, L. 'Long-stay mental patients and future planning.' *Health and Social Service Journal*, **85**, 2748 (1975).

[QRL 19] Allman, S. T., Chamberlain, J. and Harman, P. 'The national cervical cytology recall system: report of a pilot study.' *Health Trends*, **6**, 39 (1974).

[QRL 20] Amulree, Lord, Exton-Smith, A. N. and Crockett, E. S. 'Proper use of the hospital in the treatment of the aged sick.' *Lancet*, **1**, 123 (1951).

[QRL 21] Anderson, E. R. 'The role of the nurse—views of the patient, nurse and doctor in some general hospitals in England.' *The Study of Nursing Care Project Report Series 2*, No. 1. London, Royal College of Nursing, 1973.

[QRL 22] Anderson, J. A. D. 'Requests for X-ray examinations from general practitioners and hospital out-patients.' *Lancet*, **2**, 97 (1968).

[QRL 23] Anderson, J. A. D. *et al*. 'Attachment of community nurses to general practices. A follow-up study.' *British Medical Journal*, **4**, 103 (1970)

[QRL 24] Anderson, J. A. D. and Warren, E. A. 'Communications with general practitioners. II.' *Medical Officer*, **118**, 45 (1967).

[QRL 25]   Andrews, G. R., Cowan, N. R. and Ferguson Anderson, W. 'The practice of geriatric medicine in the community.' In *Problems and Progress in Medical Care*, 5th Series, ed. McLachlan, G., pp. 57–86. London, Oxford University Press for Nuffield Provincial Hospitals Trust, 1971.

[QRL 26]   Anscombe, A. R., Hancock, B. D. and Humphreys, W. V. 'A clinical trial of the treatment of haemorrhoids by operation and the Lord procedure.' *Lancet*, **2**, 250 (1974).

[QRL 27]   Argyroo, S. *et al*. 'Price of prostatectomy.' *British Medical Journal*, **3**, 511 (1974).

[QRL 28]   Armstrong, A. *et al*. 'Natural history of acute coronary heart attacks—a community study.' *British Heart Journal*, **34**, 67 (1972).

[QRL 29]   Arthure, H. *et al*. 'Report on confidential enquiries into maternal deaths in England and Wales, 1964–1966.' *Reports on Public Health and Medical Subjects*, No. 119. London, HMSO, 1969.

[QRL 30]   Arthure, H. *et al*. 'Report on confidential enquiries into maternal deaths in England and Wales, 1967–69.' *Department of Health and Social Security Reports on Health and Social Subjects*, No. 1. London, HMSO, 1972.

[QRL 31]   Arthure, H. *et al*. 'Report on confidential enquiries into maternal deaths in England and Wales, 1970–1972.' *Department of Health and Social Security Reports on Health and Social Subjects*, No. 11. London, HMSO, 1975.

[QRL 32]   Arthurton, M. W. and Bamford, F. N. 'Paediatric aspects of the early discharge of maternity patients.' *British Medical Journal*, **3**, 517 (1967).

[QRL 33]   Ashcroft, M. T. *et al*. 'Heights and weights of adults in rural and industrial areas of South Wales.' *British Journal of Preventive and Social Medicine*, **21**, 159 (1967).

[QRL 34]   Ashford, J. R. 'Smoking and the use of the health services.' *British Journal of Preventive and Social Medicine*, **27**, 8 (1973).

[QRL 35]   Ashford, J. R., Ferster, G. and Makuc, D. M. 'An approach to resource allocation in the reorganised National Health Service.' In *The Present and Future Indicatives*, ed. McLachlan, G., pp. 57–90. London, Oxford University Press for Nuffield Provincial Hospitals Trust, 1975.

[QRL 36]   Ashford, J. R. and Fryer, J. G. 'Perinatal mortality, birth weight, and place of confinement in England and Wales 1956–65.' In *In the Beginning*, ed. McLachlan, G. and Shegog, R., pp. 133–150. London, Oxford University Press for Nuffield Provincial Hospitals Trust, 1970.

[QRL 37]   Ashford, J. R. and Pearson, N. G. 'Who uses the health services and why?' *Journal of the Royal Statistical Society*, **133**, Series A, 295 (1970).

[QRL 38]   Ashford, J. R., Read, K. L. Q. and Riley, V. C. 'An analysis of variations in perinatal mortality amongst local authorities in England and Wales.' *International Journal of Epidemiology*, **2**, 31 (1973).

[QRL 39]   Ashford, J. and Riley, V. C. 'An approach to monitoring the quality of health care.' In *Measuring for Management*, ed. McLachlan, G., pp. 53–77. London, Oxford University Press for Nuffield Provincial Hospitals Trust, 1975.

[QRL 40]   Ashley, J. S. A., Howlett, A. and Morris, J. N. 'Case-fatality of hyperplasia of the prostate in two teaching and three regional board hospitals.' *Lancet*, **2**, 1308 (1971).

[QRL 41]   Ashley, J. S. A., Pasker, P. and Beresford, J. C. 'How much clinical investigation?' *Lancet*, **2**, 890 (1972).

[QRL 42]   Asscher, A. W. *et al*. 'Screening for asymptomatic urinary-tract infection in schoolgirls.' *Lancet*, **2**, 1, 1973.

[QRL 43]   Atwell, J. D. *et al*. 'Paediatric day-case surgery.' *Lancet*, **2**, 895 (1973).

[QRL 44]   Backett, E. M. *et al*. 'Studies of hospital outpatient services—hospitals in the North East Scottish region.' In *Problems and Progress in Medical Care*, 2nd Series, ed. McLachlan, G., pp. 79–122. London, Oxford University Press for Nuffield Provincial Hospitals Trust, 1966.

[QRL 45]   Baker, C. D. 'The extent in England of health visitor attachment to general practices.' *Journal of the Royal College of General Practitioners*, **8**, 171 (1964).

[QRL 46]   Baldwin, J. A. and Hall, D. J. 'Models of mental hospital function.' In *The Mental Hospital in the Psychiatric Service*, pp. 151–190. London, Oxford University Press for Nuffield Provincial Hospitals Trust, 1971.

[QRL 47]   Bamlett, R. and Milligan, H. C. 'Health and welfare services and the over 75's.' *Medical Officer*, **109**, 379 (1963).

[QRL 48]   Bankes, J. L. K. *et al*. 'Bedford glaucoma survey.' *British Medical Journal*, **1**, 791 (1968).

[QRL 49]   Banks, A. L. *et al*. 'A survey of handicapped persons.' *British Journal of Preventive and Social Medicine*, **11**, 22 (1957).

[QRL 50]   Barker, D. J. P. and Edwards, J. H. 'Obstetric complications and school performance.' *British Medical Journal*, **3**, 695 (1967).

[QRL 51]   Barker, D. J. P. and Gardner, M. J. 'Distribution of Paget's disease in England, Wales and Scotland.' *British Journal of Preventive and Social Medicine*, **28**, 226 (1974).

[QRL 52]   Barr, A. 'The population served by a hospital group.' *Lancet*, **2**, 1105 (1957).

[QRL 53] Barr, A. *Hospital Outpatients Services*. Oxford, Oxford Regional Hospital Board, 1962.
[QRL 54] Barr, A. *Is Waiting in Outpatients Really Necessary?* Oxford, Oxford Regional Hospital Board, 1967.
[QRL 55] Barraclough, M. *et al.* 'Control of moderately raised blood pressure.' *British Medical Journal*, 3, 434 (1973).
[QRL 56] Bateson, M. C. and Bouchier, I. A. D. 'Prevalence of gall stones in Dundee. A necropsy study.' *British Medical Journal*, 4, 427 (1975).
[QRL 57] Bax, M. and Whitmore, K. 'Neuro-developmental screening in the school-entrant medical examination.' *Lancet*, 2, 368 (1973).
[QRL 58] Beard, R. W. *et al.* 'King's termination study. II: contraceptive practice before and after outpatients termination of pregnancy.' *British Medical Journal*, 1, 418 (1974).
[QRL 59] Beer, T. C. *et al.* 'Can I have an ambulance, Doctor?' *British Medical Journal*, 1, 226 (1974).
[QRL 60] Bell, P. R. F. *et al.* 'Renal transplantation: an analysis of 33 cases.' *British Medical Journal*, 4, 408 (1972).
[QRL 61] Bennett, A. E. 'Case selection in a London teaching hospital.' *Medical Care*, 4, 138 (1966).
[QRL 62] Bennett, A. E., Garrad, J. and Halil, T. 'Chronic disease and disability in the community: A prevalence study.' *British Medical Journal*, 3, 762 (1970).
[QRL 63] Berry, R. J. and Muir, V. M. L. 'The natural history of man in Shetland.' *Journal of Biosocial Science*, 7, 319 (1975).
[QRL 64] Bevan, J. M. and Draper, G. J. *Appointment Systems in General Practice*. London, Oxford University Press for Nuffield Provincial Hospitals Trust, 1967.
[QRL 65] Bewley, T. H., Ben-Arie, O. and James, I. P., 'Morbidity and mortality from heroin dependence. I; survey of heroin addicts known to Home Office.' *British Medical Journal*, 1, 725 (1968).
[QRL 66] Bewley, T. H. *et al.* 'Census of mental hospital patients and life expectancy of those unlikely to be discharged.' *British Medical Journal*, 4, 671 (1975).
[QRL 67] Binnie, H. L. *The Attitudes to Drugs and Drug Takers of Students at the University and Colleges of Higher Education in an English Midland City*. Leicester, The University, Department of Education, 1969.
[QRL 68] Binnie, W. H. *et al.* 'Oral cancer in England and Wales—a national study of morbidity, mortality, curability and related factors.' *Studies on Medical and Population Subjects*, No. 23. London, HMSO, 1972.
[QRL 69] Birch, H. G. *et al. Mental Sub-normality in the Community*. Baltimore, Williams & Wilkins, 1970.
[QRL 70] Birmingham Diabetes Survey Working Party. 'A diabetes survey.' *British Medical Journal*, 1, 1499 (1962).
[QRL 71] Birmingham Diabetes Survey Working Party. 'Five-year follow-up report on the Birmingham diabetes survey of 1962.' *British Medical Journal*, 3, 310 (1970).
[QRL 72] Birmingham Diabetes Survey Working Party. 'Ten-year follow-up report on Birmingham diabetes survey of 1961.' *British Medical Journal*, 2, 35 (1976).
[QRL 73] Birmingham Pregnancy Advisory Service. *A Study of 2,814 Cases*, Birmingham, Birmingham Pregnancy Advisory Service, 1971.
[QRL 74] Blackwell, B. 'Why patients come to a casualty department.' *Lancet*, 1, 369 (1962).
[QRL 75] Blaxter, M. 'Hospital and community.' *Health Bulletin*, 34, 150 (1976).
[QRL 76] Bone, M. *Family Planning Services in England and Wales*. London, Social Survey Division OPCS, HMSO, 1973.
[QRL 77] Bonnar, J., Goldberg, A. and Smith, J. A. 'Do pregnant women take their iron?' *Lancet*, 1, 457 (1969).
[QRL 78] Boyle, C. M. 'Some factors affecting the smoking habits of a group of teenagers.' *Lancet*, 2, 1287 (1968).
[QRL 79] Boyle, D. McC. *et al.* 'Early mobilisation and discharge of patients with acute myocardial infarction.' *Lancet*, 2, 57 (1972).
[QRL 80] Boyle, J. A. *et al.* 'Early mobilisation after uncomplicated myocardial infarction.' *Lancet*, 2, 346 (1973).
[QRL 81] Bransby, E. R., Berry, W. T. C. and Taylor, D. M. 'Study of the Vitamin-D intakes of infants in 1960.' *British Medical Journal*, 1, 1661 (1964).
[QRL 82] Bransby, E. R. and Osborne, B. 'A social and food survey of the elderly, living alone or as married couples.' *British Journal of Nutrition*, 7, 160 (1953).
[QRL 83] Brett, G. Z. 'The value of lung cancer detection by six-monthly chest radiographs.' *Thorax*, 23, 414 (1968).
[QRL 84] Brimblecombe, F. S. W. *et al.* 'Family studies of respiratory infections.' *British Medical Journal*, 1, 117 (1958).

[QRL 85]   British Co-operative Clinical Group. 'Gonorrhoea study, 1966.' *British Journal of Venereal Diseases*, **44**, 55 (1968).

[QRL 86]   British Co-operative Clinical Group. 'Primary and secondary syphilis.' *British Journal of Venereal Diseases*, **44**, 167 (1968).

[QRL 87]   British Co-operative Clinical Group. 'Primary and secondary syphilis.' *British Journal of Venereal Diseases*, **44**, 307 (1968).

[QRL 88]   British Co-operative Clinical Group. 'Gonorrhoea study, 1968.' *British Journal of Venereal Diseases*, **46**, 62 (1970).

[QRL 89]   British Co-operative Clinical Group. 'Gonorrhoea study, 1969.' *British Journal of Venereal Diseases*, **46**, 470 (1970).

[QRL 90]   British Co-operative Clinical Group. 'Primary and secondary syphilis.' *British Journal of Venereal Diseases*, **46**, 477 (1970).

[QRL 91]   British Medical Association Committee. *The Rehabilitation and Resettlement of Disabled Persons*. (Chairman: R. E. Tunbridge.) London, British Medical Association, 1954.

[QRL 92]   British Medical Association Committee. *Accidents in the Home*. London, British Medical Association, 1964.

[QRL 93]   British Steel Corporation. *Annual Report, British Steel Medical Services, 1971*. London, British Steel Corporation, 1972.

[QRL 94]   Brockington, F. and Lempert, S. *The Social Needs of the Over-80's: the Stockport Survey*. Manchester, Manchester University Press, 1966.

[QRL 95]   Brocklehurst, J. C. *The Geriatric Day Hospital*. London, King Edward's Hospital Fund for London, 1970.

[QRL 96]   Brooke, E. M. 'A cohort study of patients first admitted to mental hospitals in 1954 and 1955.' *Studies on Medical and Population Subjects*, No. 18. London, HMSO, 1963.

[QRL 97]   Brooke, E. M. 'A census of patients in psychiatric beds, 1963.' *Ministry of Health Reports on Public Health and Medical Subjects*, No. 116. London, HMSO, 1967.

[QRL 98]   Brookes, B. *British Health Centres Directory 1973*. London, King Edward's Hospital Fund for London, 1973.

[QRL 99]   Brotherston, J. H. F. *et al*. 'Night calls; their frequency and nature in one general practice.' *British Medical Journal*, **2**, 1169 (1959).

[QRL 100] Brown, G. W., Bhrolchain, M. N. and Harris, T. 'Social class and psychiatric disturbance among women in an urban population.' *Sociology*, **9**, 225 (1975).

[QRL 101] Brown, G. W., Birley, J. L. T. and Wing, J. K. 'Influence of family life on the course of schizophrenic disorders: a replication.' *British Journal of Psychiatry*, **121**, 241 (1972).

[QRL 102] Brown, R. G., McKeown, T. and Whitfield, A. G. W. 'Observations on the medical condition of man in the seventh decade.' *British Medical Journal*, **1**, 555 (1958).

[QRL 103] Buchan, I. C. and Richardson, I. M. *Time Study of Consultations in General Practice. Scottish Health Service Studies*, No. 27. Edinburgh, Scottish Home and Health Department, 1973.

[QRL 104] Buckle, J. R. *Work and Housing of Impaired Persons in Great Britain, Part II, Handicapped and Impaired in Great Britain. Social Survey Report 418* (ii). London, HMSO, 1971.

[QRL 105] Bulman, J. S. *et al*. *Demand and Need for Dental Care*. London, Oxford University Press for Nuffield Provincial Hospitals Trust, 1968.

[QRL 106] Burge, D. *et al*. 'Quality and quantity of, survival in acute myeloid leukaemia.' *Lancet*, **2**, 621 (1975).

[QRL 107] Burn, J. L. 'A diabetic survey.' *Medical Officer*, **96**, 5 (1956).

[QRL 108] Butler, J. R., Bevan, J. M. and Taylor, R. C. *Family Doctors and Public Policy. A Study of Manpower Distribution*. London, Routledge & Kegan Paul, 1973.

[QRL 109] Butler, J. R. and Pearson, M. 'Who goes home? A study of long-stay patients in acute hospital care.' *Occasional Papers on Social Administration*, No. 34. London, Bell, 1970.

[QRL 110] Butler, N. R. and Alberman, E. D. *Perinatal Problems—the second report of the 1958 British Perinatal Mortality Survey*. Edinburgh, Livingstone, 1969.

[QRL 111] Butler, N. R. and Bonham, D. G. *Perinatal Mortality. First report of the British Perinatal Mortality Survey*. Edinburgh, Livingstone, 1963.

[QRL 112] Butterfield, W. J. and Wadsworth, M. E. J. 'Studies of hospital outpatient services—a London teaching hospital.' In *Problems and Progress in Medical Care*, 2nd Series, ed. McLachlan, G., pp. 125–152. London, Oxford University Press for Nuffield Provincial Hospitals Trust, 1966.

[QRL 113] Buttimore, A. 'Seven district nurse/general practice attachment schemes.' In *Co-operation in Patient Care*, ed. Hockey, L. London, Queen's Institute of District Nursing, 1970.

[QRL 114] Bynner, J. M. *Medical Students' Attitudes Towards Smoking. Government Social Survey Report 382*. London, HMSO, 1967.

[QRL 115] Bynner, J. M. *The Young Smoker: a study of smoking among schoolboys. Government Social Survey Report 383*. London, HMSO, 1969.

[QRL 116] Caldwell, J. R. 'One hundred deaths in practice.' *Journal of the Royal College of General Practitioners*, **21**, 460 (1971).
[QRL 117] Calnan, M. W. 'Accidental child poisoning.' *Community Health*, **6**, 91 (1974).
[QRL 118] Cameron, A. and Hinton, J. 'Delay in seeking treatment for mammary tumours.' *Cancer*, **21**, 1121 (1968).
[QRL 119] Cameron, M., Wilkinson, F. and Hampton, J. R. 'Follow-up of emergency ambulance calls in Nottingham.' *British Medical Journal*, **1**, 384 (1975).
[QRL 120] Carmichael, L. *et al.* 'Why are they waiting?' *British Medical Journal*, **1**, 736 (1963).
[QRL 121] Carstairs, G. M. and Brown, G. W. 'A census of psychiatric cases in two contrasting communities.' *Journal of Mental Sciences*, **104**, 72 (1958).
[QRL 122] Carstairs, V. *Home Nursing in Scotland. Scottish Health Service Studies*, No. 2. Edinburgh, Scottish Home and Health Department, 1966.
[QRL 123] Carstairs, V. *Channels of Communication. Scottish Health Service Studies*, No. 11. Edinburgh, Scottish Home and Health Department, 1970.
[QRL 124] Carstairs, V. and Howie, V. 'The mass miniature radiography service in Scotland.' *Health Bulletin*, **30**, 194 (1972).
[QRL 125] Carstairs, V. and Morrison, N. *The Elderly in Residential Care. Scottish Health Service Studies*, No. 19. Edinburgh, Scottish Home and Health Department, 1971.
[QRL 126] Cartwright, A. *Human Relations and Hospital Care*. London, Routledge & Kegan Paul, 1964.
[QRL 127] Cartwright, A. *Patients and Their Doctors. A Study of General Practice*. London, Routledge & Kegan Paul, 1967.
[QRL 128] Cartwright, A. *Parents and Family Planning Services*. London, Routledge & Kegan Paul, 1970.
[QRL 129] Cartwright, A. *How Many Children?* London, Routledge & Kegan Paul, 1976.
[QRL 130] Cartwright, A., Hockey, L. and Anderson, J. L. *Life before Death*. London, Routledge & Kegan Paul, 1973.
[QRL 131] Cartwright, A. and Lucas, S. 'Survey of abortion patients for the committee on the working of the Abortion Act.' *Report of the Committee on the Working of the Abortion Act*, Vol. III. London, HMSO, 1974.
[QRL 132] Cartwright, A., Martin, F. M. and Thomson, J. G. 'Efficacy of an anti-smoking campaign.' *Lancet*, **1**, 327 (1960).
[QRL 133] Cartwright, A. and Waite, M. 'General practitioners and abortion.' *Journal of the Royal College of General Practitioners*, **22**, Supplement No. 1 (1972).
[QRL 134] Cartwright, A. and Waite, M. 'General practitioners and contraception in 1970–71.' *Journal of the Royal College of General Practitioners*, **22**, Supplement No. 2 (1972).
[QRL 135] Cartwright, A. and Wilkins, W. *Changes in Family Building Plans. A follow up study to 'How many children?' Studies on Medical and Population Subjects*, No. 33. London, HMSO, 1976.
[QRL 136] Case, R. A. M. *et al. Serial Mortality Tables: Neoplastic Disease*. Vol. I: *England and Wales*. Vol. II: *Northern Ireland*. Vol. IV: *Scotland*. London, Institute of Cancer Research, 1976.
[QRL 137] Cassie, A. B. and Allan, W. R. 'Alcohol and road traffic accidents.' *British Medical Journal*, **2**, 1668 (1961).
[QRL 138] Cay, E. L. *et al.* 'Patients' assessment of the result of surgery for peptic ulcer.' *Lancet*, **1**, 29, 1975.
[QRL 139] Chalke, H. D. and Benjamin, B. 'The aged in their own homes.' *Lancet*, **1**, 588 (1953).
[QRL 140] Chamberlain, J. 'Studies of hospital outpatient services—two non-teaching hospitals in south-east England.' In *Problems and Progress in Medical Care*, 2nd Series, ed. McLachlan, G., pp. 45–76. London, Oxford University Press for Nuffield Provincial Hospitals Trust, 1966.
[QRL 141] Chamberlain, R. *et al. British Births, 1970*, Vol. 1: *The First Week of Life*. London, Heinemann Medical, 1976.
[QRL 142] Chant, A. D. B., Jones, H. O. and Weddell, J. M. 'Varicose veins: a comparison of surgery and injection/compression sclerotherapy.' *Lancet*, **2**, 1188 (1972).
[QRL 143] Child Guidance Special Interest Group. *The Child Guidance Service (Child Guidance Clinics and Departments of Child Psychiatry). Report of the 1969 Survey undertaken by Psychiatric Social Workers*. Birmingham, British Association of Social Workers, 1975.
[QRL 144] Clark, J. *A Family Visitor. A Descriptive Analysis of Health Visiting in Berkshire*. London, The Royal College of Nursing and National Council of Nurses of the United Kingdom, 1973.
[QRL 145] Clark, M. *et al.* 'Sequels of unwanted pregnancy.' *Lancet*, **2**, 502 (1968).
[QRL 146] Clarke, M. 'Trouble with feet.' *Occasional Papers on Social Administration*, No. 29. London, Bell, 1969.
[QRL 147] Clarke, M., Halil, T. and Salmon, N. 'Peptic ulceration in men.' *British Journal of Preventive and Social Medicine*, **30**, 115 (1976).
[QRL 148] Cochran, J. B., Clayson, C. and Fletcher, W. B. 'Pulmonary tuberculosis in a rural area in south Scotland.' *British Medical Journal*, **2**, 185 (1957).

[QRL 149] Cochrane, A. L. 'Rhondda Fach, South Wales.' *Millbank Memorial Fund Quarterly*, XLIII, 326 (1965).
[QRL 150] Cochrane, A. L. 'Relation between radiographic categories of coalworkers pneumoconiosis and expectation of life.' *British Medical Journal*, 2, 532 (1973).
[QRL 151] Cochrane, A. L., Glyn Cox, J. and Francis Jarman, T. 'Pulmonary tuberculosis in the Rhondda Fach.' *British Medical Journal*, 2, 843 (1952).
[QRL 152] Cochrane, A. L., Glyn Cox, J. and Francis Jarman, T. 'A follow-up chest X-ray survey in the Rhondda Fach.' *British Medical Journal*, 1, 371 (1955).
[QRL 153] Cochrane, A. L., Miall, W. E. and Clarke, W. G. 'Results of a chest X-ray survey in the vale of Glamorgan.' *Tubercle*, 37, 417 (1956).
[QRL 154] Cochrane, A. L. and Moore, F. 'Expected and observed values for the prescription of vitamin B_{12} in England and Wales.' *British Journal of Preventive and Social Medicine*, 25, 147 (1971).
[QRL 155] Colley, J. R. T. 'Respiratory symptoms in children and parental smoking and phlegm production.' *British Medical Journal*, 2, 210 (1974).
[QRL 156] Colley, J. R. T. 'Obesity in schoolchildren.' *British Journal of Preventive and Social Medicine*, 28, 221 (1974).
[QRL 157] Colley, J. R. T., Douglas, J. W. B. and Reid, D. D. 'Respiratory disease in young adults.' *British Medical Journal*, 3, 195 (1973).
[QRL 158] Colley, J. R. T. and Reid, D. D. 'Urban and social origins in childhood bronchitis in England and Wales.' *British Medical Journal*, 2, 213 (1970).
[QRL 159] Colling, A. *et al*. 'Teesside coronary survey.' *British Medical Journal*, 2, 1169 (1976).
[QRL 160] Commins, B. T. 'Polycyclic hydrocarbons in rural and urban air.' *International Journal of Air Pollution*, 1, 14 (1958).
[QRL 161] Cook, P. J. and Walker, R. O. 'The geographical distribution of dental care in the United Kingdom.' *British Dental Journal*, 122, 441 (1967).
[QRL 162] Cook, P. L. 'Experiences in the first year of an "open door" X-ray department.' *British Medical Journal*, 2, 351 (1966).
[QRL 163] Cooper, B. *et al*. 'An experiment in community mental health care.' *Lancet*, 2, 1356 (1974).
[QRL 164] Coppin, C. M. S. *The Slough Industrial Health Service—25th Annual Report*. Slough, Slough Industrial Health Service, 1976.
[QRL 165] Cormack, J. J. C. *The General Practitioner's Use of Medical Records. Scottish Health Service Studies*, No. 15. Edinburgh, Scottish Home and Health Department, 1971.
[QRL 166] Coull, D. C. *et al*. 'A method of monitoring drugs for adverse reactions, I. Methyldopa and haemolylic anaemia.' *European Journal of Clinical Pharmacology*, 3, 46 (1970).
[QRL 167] Craft, M. and Sheiham, A. 'Attitudes to prevention amongst dental practitioners. A comparison between north and south of England.' *British Dental Journal*, 141, 371 (1976).
[QRL 168] Craig, G. A. and Muirhead, J. M. B. 'Obstetric aspects of the early discharge of maternity patients.' *British Medical Journal*, 3, 520 (1967).
[QRL 169] Crawford, M. D., Gardner, M. J. and Morris, J. N. 'Changes in water hardness and local death-rates.' *Lancet*, 2, 327 (1971).
[QRL 170] Crawford, M. D. and Sarner, M. 'Ruptured intracranial aneurysm.' *Lancet*, 2, 1254 (1965).
[QRL 171] Crawford, T. and Crawford, M. D. 'Prevalence and pathological changes of ischaemic heart-disease in a hard-water and in a soft-water area.' *Lancet*, 2, 229 (1967).
[QRL 172] Crombie, D. L. and Cross, K. W. 'The care of seriously ill patients in hospital and general practice.' *Journal of the College of General Practitioners*, 4, 270 (1961).
[QRL 173] Crombie, D. L. *et al*. 'Teratogenic drugs; Royal College of General Practitioners survey.' *British Medical Journal*, 4, 178 (1970).
[QRL 174] Culpan, R. H., Davies, B. M. and Oppenheim, A. N. 'Incidence of psychiatric illness among hospital out-patients.' *British Medical Journal*, 1, 855 (1960).
[QRL 175] Culyer, A. J. and Cooper, J. G. 'Hospital waiting lists and the supply and demand of inpatient care.' *Social and Economic Administration*, 9, 13 (1975).
[QRL 176] Cunningham, D. J., Bevan, J. M. and Floyd, C. B. 'The role of the practice nurse from the patients' point of view.' *Community Medicine*, 127, 534 (1972).
[QRL 177] Curran, A. P. and Ferguson, T. 'Glasgow.' In *Further Studies in Hospital and Community*, pp. 15–72. London, Oxford University Press for Nuffield Provincial Hospitals Trust, 1962.
[QRL 178] Darmady, D. M. 'The changing pattern of pathology.' *Journal of Clinical Pathology*, 17, 477 (1964).
[QRL 179] Davie, R., Butler, N. and Goldstein, H. *From Birth to seven. The second report of the National Child Development Study*. London, Longmans, 1972.
[QRL 180] Davies, J. and Stacey, B. *Teenagers and Alcohol: a Developmental Study in Glasgow*. London, HMSO, 1972.

[QRL 181] Davies, Sir M. *Report of the Committee on Hospital Complaints Procedure*. Department of Health and Social Security and Welsh Office. London, HMSO, 1973.

[QRL 182] Davison, R. L. and Clements, J. E. 'Why don't they attend for a cytotest?' *Medical Officer*, **125**, 329 (1971).

[QRL 183] Dawes, K. S. 'Dietitians in the community and NHS.' *Health and Social Service Journal*, **70**, 2226 (1974).

[QRL 184] Dawson, B. *et al*. 'A survey of childhood asthma in Aberdeen.' *Lancet*, **1**, 827 (1969).

[QRL 185] Department of the Environment. *Drinking and Driving*. London, HMSO, 1976.

[QRL 186] Department of the Environment, Scottish Development Department, Welsh Department. *Road Accidents in Great Britain: Annual Report*. London, HMSO, Annual.

[QRL 187] Department of Health and Social Security. *Confidential Enquiry into Post Neonatal Deaths 1964–1966. Reports on Public Health and Medical Subjects*, No. 125. London, HMSO, 1970.

[QRL 188] Department of Health and Social Security. *Census of Mentally Handicapped Patients in Hospital in England and Wales at the end of 1970. Statistical and Research Report Series*, No. 3. London, HMSO, 1972.

[QRL 189] Department of Health and Social Security. *A Nutrition Survey of the Elderly—Report by the Panel on Nutrition of the Elderly. Report on Health and Social Subjects*, No. 3. London, HMSO, 1972.

[QRL 190] Department of Health and Social Security. *Report of the Committee on Nursing* (Chairman: Professor Asa Briggs), Cmnd. 5115. London, HMSO, 1972.

[QRL 191] Department of Health and Social Security. *Enquiry into the Previous Medical Experience of Doctors joining the General Medical Services for the first time as Unrestricted Principals or as Assistants (England and Wales). Reports on Health and Social Subjects*, No. 2. London, HMSO, 1972.

[QRL 192] Department of Health and Social Security. *Edited and Selected Extracts from Register of Adverse Reactions*, Vols. I, II, III. London, Department of Health and Social Security, 1973, 1974.

[QRL 193] Department of Health and Social Security. *Report of the Committee of Inquiry into the Pay and Related Conditions of Service of Nurses and Midwives* (Chairman: The Earl of Halsbury). London, HMSO, 1974.

[QRL 194] Department of Health and Social Security. *Review Body Doctors' and Dentists' Remuneration. Supplement to Fifth Report 1975* (Chairman: Sir Ernest Woodroofe), Cmnd. 6243. London, HMSO, 1975.

[QRL 195] Department of Health and Social Security. *Report of the Committee of Inquiry into the Pay and Related Conditions of Service of the Professions Supplementary to Medicine and Speech Therapists* (Chairman: The Earl of Halsbury). London, HMSO, 1975.

[QRL 196] Department of Health and Social Security. *A Nutrition Survey of Pre-school Children 1967–68. Report on Health and Social Subjects*, No. 10. London, HMSO, 1975.

[QRL 197] Department of Health and Social Security, Scottish Home and Health Department, Welsh Office. *Report of the Working Party on the Hospital Pharmaceutical Service*. London, HMSO, 1970.

[QRL 198] Department of Health and Social Security, Scottish Office, Welsh Office, Ministry of Housing and Local Government. *The Fluoridation Studies in the United Kingdom and the Results achieved after 11 years. Reports on Public Health and Medical Subjects*, No. 122. London, HMSO, 1969.

[QRL 199] Department of Health and Social Security, Welsh Office, Central Health Services Council. *Domiciliary Midwifery and Maternity Bed Needs. Report of the Sub-committee of the Standing Maternity and Midwifery Advisory Committee*. London, HMSO, 1970.

[QRL 200] Department of Health and Social Security, Welsh Office. *Rehabilitation. Report of a Sub-committee of the Standing Medical Advisory Committee* (Chairman: Sir Ronald Tunbridge). London, HMSO, 1972.

[QRL 201] Department of Health and Social Security, Welsh Office. *Censuses of A. Patients in Mental Illness Hospitals and Units in England and Wales at the end of 1971. B. Mental Illness Day Patients in England and Wales at April 1972. Statistical and Research Report Series*, No. 10. London, HMSO, 1975.

[QRL 202] Department of Industry. *National Survey of Air Pollution, 1961–1971*, Vols. 1–5. London, HMSO, 1974–6.

[QRL 203] Devlin, H. B., Plant, J. A. and Griffin, M. 'Aftermath of surgery for anorectal cancer.' *British Medical Journal*, **3**, 413 (1971).

[QRL 204] Diggory, P. L. C. 'Some experience of therapeutic abortion.' *Lancet*, **1**, 873 (1969).

[QRL 205] Doll, R. *et al*. 'Risk of thrombo-embolic disease in women taking oral contraceptives.' *British Medical Journal*, **2**, 355 (1967).

[QRL 206] Doll, R. and Peto, R. 'Mortality in relation to smoking: 20 years' observations on male British doctors.' *British Medical Journal*, **2**, 1525 (1976).

[QRL 207] Donaldson, R. J. 'A survey of district community physicians in England six months after N.H.S. reorganisation.' *Public Health London*, **89**, 253 (1975).

[QRL 208] Donaldson, R. J. 'The head louse in England.' *Royal Society of Health Journal*, **96**, 55 (1976).

[QRL 209] Doran, F. S. A., White, M. and Drury, M. 'The scope and safety of short-stay surgery in the treatment of groin herniae and varicose veins.' *British Journal of Surgery*, **59**, 333 (1972).

[QRL 210] Douglas, J. W. B. *Maternity in Great Britain. A Survey of Social and Economic Aspects of Pregnancy and Childbirth.* London, Oxford University Press, 1948.

[QRL 211] Douglas, J. W. B. *The Home and School. A Study of Ability and Attainment in the Primary School.* London, McGibbon & Key, 1964.

[QRL 212] Douglas, J. W. B. and Bloomfield, J. N. *Children Under 5.* London, Allen & Unwin, 1958.

[QRL 213] Douglas, J. W. B., Ross, J. M. and Simpson, H. R. *All Our Future.* London, Davies, 1968.

[QRL 214] Douglas, J. W. B. and Waller, R. E. 'Air pollution and respiratory infection in children.' *British Journal of Preventive and Social Medicine*, **20**, 1 (1966).

[QRL 215] Drillien, C. M. 'Studies in mental handicap: II. Some obstetric factors of possible aetiological significance.' *Archives of Diseases of Childhood*, **43**, 283 (1968).

[QRL 216] Drillien, C. M., Jameson, S. and Wilkinson, E. M. 'Studies in mental handicap: I. Prevalence and distribution by clinical type and severity of defect.' *Archives of Diseases of Childhood*, **41**, 528 (1966).

[QRL 217] Duncan, B. *et al.* 'Prognosis of new and worsening angina pectoris.' *British Medical Journal*, **1**, 981 (1976).

[QRL 218] Duncan, K. P. and Howell, R. W. 'Lung cancer prognosis and routine radiography.' *British Journal of Preventive and Social Medicine*, **22**, 110 (1968).

[QRL 219] Duncan, K. P. and Howell, R. W. 'Health of workers in the United Kingdom Atomic Energy Authority.' *Health Physics*, **19**, 285 (1970).

[QRL 220] Dunnell, K. and Cartwright, A. *Medicine Takers, Prescribers and Hoarders.* London, Routledge & Kegan Paul, 1972.

[QRL 221] Eason, R. J. and Grimes, J. A. 'In-patient care of the mentally ill: a statistical study of future provision.' *Health Trends*, **8**, 13 (1976).

[QRL 222] Easson, E. C. and Russell, M. H. *The Curability of Cancer*, London, Pitman, 1968.

[QRL 223] Edge, J. R. and Nelson, I. D. M. 'Survey of arrangements for the elderly in Barrow-in-Furness.' *Medical Care*, **1**, 202 and **2**, 7 (1963, 1964).

[QRL 224] Eimerl, T. S. and Pearson, R. J. C. 'Working-time in general practice. How general practitioners use their time.' *British Medical Journal*, **2**, 1549 (1966).

[QRL 225] Elwood, J. H. 'Major central nervous system malformations notified in Northern Ireland, 1964–68.' *Developmental Medicine and Child Neurology*, **14**, 731 (1972).

[QRL 226] Elwood, P. C. *et al.* 'Nutritional state of elderly Asian and English subjects in Coventry.' *Lancet*, **1**, 1224 (1972).

[QRL 227] Elwood, P. C. *et al.* 'Haemoglobin, vitamin B_{12} and folate levels in the elderly.' *British Journal of Haematology*, **21**, 557 (1971).

[QRL 228] Elwood, P. C. *et al.* 'Mortality and anaemia in women.' *Lancet*, **1**, 891 (1974).

[QRL 229] Elwood, P. C., Waters, W. E. and Greene, W. J. C. 'Evaluation of iron supplements in prevention of iron-deficiency anaemia.' *Lancet*, **2**, 175 (1970).

[QRL 230] Elwood, P. C. *et al.* 'Sucrose consumption and ischaemic heart-disease in the community.' *Lancet*, **1**, 1014 (1970).

[QRL 231] Elwood, P. C. and Wood, M. M. 'Effect of oral iron therapy on the symptoms of anaemia.' *British Journal of Preventive and Social Medicine*, **20**, 172 (1966).

[QRL 232] Exton-Smith, A. N. and Stanton, B. R. *Report of an Investigation into the Dietary of Elderly Women Living Alone.* London, King's Fund, 1965.

[QRL 233] Exton-Smith, A. N., Stanton, B. R. and Winsor, A. C. M. *Nutrition of Housebound Old People.* London, King's Fund, 1972.

[QRL 234] Fairbairn, A. S. and Reid, D. D. 'Air pollution and other local factors in respiratory disease.' *British Journal of Preventive and Social Medicine*, **12**, 94 (1958).

[QRL 235] Farquharson, E. L. 'Early ambulation: with special reference to herniorrhaphy as an out-patient procedure.' *Lancet*, **2**, 517 (1955).

[QRL 236] Fedrick, J. 'Epilepsy and pregnancy: a report from the Oxford Record Linkage Study.' *British Medical Journal*, **2**, 442 (1973).

[QRL 237] Fee, W. M. and Benson, C. 'Group therapy: a review of six years' experience in a Scottish anti-smoking clinic.' *Community Medicine*, **126**, 361 (1971).

[QRL 238] Ferguson, T. and MacPhail, A. N. *Hospital and Community.* London, Oxford University Press for Nuffield Provincial Hospitals Trust, 1954.

[QRL 239] Ferster, G., Cooper, J. A. and Makoc, D. M. 'Family costs of maternity care.' In *Measuring for Management*, ed. McLachlan, G., pp. 137–161. London, Oxford University Press for Nuffield Provincial Hospitals Trust, 1975.

[QRL 240] Ferster, G. and Jenkins, D. M. 'Patterns of antenatal care, perinatal mortality, and birth-weight in three consultant obstetric units.' *Lancet*, **2**, 727 (1976).

[QRL 241] Fogelman, K. *Britain's Sixteen-year Olds. Preliminary Findings from the Third Follow-up of the National Child Development Study (1958 Cohort)*. London, National Children's Bureau, 1976.

[QRL 242] Forrest, J. A. H. and Jarala, R. A. 'Abuse of drugs for kicks: a review of 252 admissions.' *British Medical Journal*, **4**, 136 (1973).

[QRL 243] Forsyth, G. and Logan, R. F. L. *The Demand for Medical Care. A Study of the Case-load in the Barrow and Furness Group of Hospitals*. London, Oxford University Press for Nuffield Provincial Hospitals Trust, 1960.

[QRL 244] Forsyth, G. and Logan, R. F. L. *Gateway or Dividing Line?* London, Oxford University Press for Nuffield Provincial Hospitals Trust, 1968.

[QRL 245] Forsyth, G., Thomas, R. G. and Jones, S. P. 'Planning in practice: a half-term report.' In *Problems and Progress in Medical Care*, 4th Series, ed. McLachlan, G., pp. 1–28. London, Oxford University Press for Nuffield Provincial Hospitals Trust, 1970.

[QRL 246] Franklin, B. L. *Patient Anxiety on Admission to Hospital. The Study of Nursing Care*, Series 1, No. 5. London, Royal College of Nursing, 1974.

[QRL 247] Fraser, G. R. 'The causes of profound deafness in childhood.' In *Sensorineural Hearing Loss—CIBA Symposium*, ed. Wolstenholme, G. London, CIBA Foundation, 1970.

[QRL 248] Fraser, R. C., Patterson, H. R. and Peacock, E. 'Referrals to hospitals in an East Midlands city—a medical audit.' *Journal of the Royal College of General Practitioners*, **24**, 304 (1974).

[QRL 249] Froggatt, P. 'Short-term absence from industry, Parts I, II, III.' *British Journal of Industrial Medicine*, **27**, 199; 211; 297 (1970).

[QRL 250] Fry, J. 'A year of general practice: a study in morbidity.' *British Medical Journal*, **2**, 249 (1952).

[QRL 251] Fry, J. 'Five years of general practice.' *British Medical Journal*, **2**, 1453 (1957).

[QRL 252] Fry, J. *Casualty Services and their Setting—a Study in Medical Care*. London, Oxford University Press for Nuffield Provincial Hospitals Trust, 1960.

[QRL 253] Fry, J. 'Twenty-one years of general practice—changing patterns.' *Journal of the Royal College of General Practitioners*, **22**, 521 (1972).

[QRL 254] Fry, J. *Common Diseases: their Nature, Incidence and Care*. London, Medical and Technical Publications, 1974.

[QRL 255] Fry, J. 'Natural history of hypertension.' *Lancet*, **2**, 431 (1974).

[QRL 256] Fry, J. *et al.* 'Chronic bronchitis in Great Britain.' *British Medical Journal*, **2**, 973 (1961).

[QRL 257] Fulton, M., Julian, D. G. and Oliver, M. F. 'Sudden death and myocardial infarction.' *Circulation*, **39** and **40**, Supplement 4, 182 (1969).

[QRL 258] Garrad, J. and Bennett, A. E. 'A validated interview schedule for use in Population Surveys of Chronic Disease and Disability.' *British Journal of Preventive and Social Medicine*, **25**, 97 (1971).

[QRL 259] Gatley, M. S. 'To be taken as directed.' *Journal of the Royal College of General Practitioners*, **16**, 39 (1968).

[QRL 260] Gedling, P. and Newell, D. J. 'Hospital beds for the elderly.' In *Problems and Progress in Medical Care*, 7th Series, ed. McLachlan, G., pp. 131–145. London, Oxford University Press for Nuffield Provincial Hospitals Trust, 1972.

[QRL 261] Gelson, A. D. N. *et al.* 'Course of patients discharged early after myocardial infarction.' *British Medical Journal*, **1**, 1555 (1976).

[QRL 262] General Register Office. *Analysis of Records for April 1952–March 1954. Studies on Medical and Population Subjects*, No. 9. London, HMSO, 1956.

[QRL 263] Gilhome, K. R. and Newell, D. J. 'Community services for the elderly.' In *Problems and Progress in Medical Care*, 7th Series, ed. McLachlan, G., pp. 147–161. London, Oxford University Press for Nuffield Provincial Hospitals Trust, 1972.

[QRL 264] Gilkes, M. J. and Handa, V. K. 'The duration of pre- and post-operative in-patient stay in ophthalmology.' *Health Trends*, **6**, 76 (1974).

[QRL 265] Gilmore, M., Bruce, N. and Hunt, M. *The Work of the Nursing Team in General Practice*. London, 1974, Council for the Education and Training of Health Visitors.

[QRL 266] Girdwood, R. H. 'Death after taking medicaments.' *British Medical Journal*, **1**, 500 (1974).

[QRL 267] Gish, O. *Doctor Migration and World Health. The Impact of the International Demand for Doctors on Health Services in Developing Countries. Occasional Papers on Social Administration*, No. 43. London, Bell, 1971.

[QRL 268] Girt, J. L., Cooper, L. A. and Abel, R. A. *The Multiple Health Screening Clinic, Rotherham*

1966: A Social and Economic Assessment. DHSS, *Reports on Public Health and Medical Subjects*, No. 121. London, HMSO, 1969.

[QRL 269] Gissane, W. and Bull, J. 'A study of motorway (M1) fatalities.' *British Medical Journal*, 1, 75 (1964).

[QRL 270] Gissane, W. and Bull, J. 'Fatal car occupant injuries after car/lorry collisions.' *British Medical Journal*, 1, 67 (1973).

[QRL 271] Gleisner, J., Hewett, S. and Mann, S. 'Reasons for admission to hospital.' In *Evaluating a Community Psychiatric Service*, ed. Wing, J. K. and Hailey, A. M., pp. 199–220. London, Oxford University Press for Nuffield Provincial Hospitals Trust, 1972.

[QRL 272] Glynn, A. A. 'Vascular diseases of the nervous system.' *British Medical Journal*, 1, 1216 (1956).

[QRL 273] Goldberg, E. M. and Morrison, S. L. 'Schizophrenia and social class.' *British Journal of Psychiatry*, 109, 785 (1963).

[QRL 274] Goldberg, E. M., Mortimer, A. and Williams, B. T. *Helping the Aged: a Field Experiment in Social Work*. London, Allen & Unwin, 1970.

[QRL 275] Goligher, J. C. *et al.* 'Five to eight year results of Leeds/York controlled trial of elective surgery for duodenal ulcer.' *British Medical Journal*, 2, 781 (1968).

[QRL 276] Goligher, J. G. *et al.* 'Five to eight year results of truncal vagotomy and pyloroplasty for duodenal ulcer.' *British Medical Journal*, 1, 7 (1972).

[QRL 277] Goodman, N. and Tizard, J. 'Prevalence of imbecility and idiocy among children.' *British Medical Journal*, 1, 216 (1962).

[QRL 278] Gordon, C., Thomson, J. G. and Emerson, A. R. 'Domiciliary services for over sixties.' *Medical Officer*, 91, 19 (1957).

[QRL 279] Graham, W. L. 'The aged sick-admission to hospital or care at home?' *Lancet*, 1, 304 (1954).

[QRL 280] Gray, P. G. and Cartwright, A. *General Practice Under the NHS*. London, Central Office of Information, 1961.

[QRL 281] Gray, P. G. and Todd, J. E. *Mobility and Reading Habits of the Blind*. London, HMSO, 1968.

[QRL 282] Gray, P. G. *et al. Adult Dental Health in England and Wales in 1968*. Government Social Survey Report 411. London, HMSO, 1970.

[QRL 283] Gregory, D. W. *et al.* 'Natural history of patients with X-ray—negative dyspepsia in general practice.' *British Medical Journal*, 4, 519 (1972).

[QRL 284] Grey, A. M. H. and Topping, A. *The Hospital Survey*, London, HMSO, 1945.

[QRL 285] Gruer, R. *Outpatient Services in the Scottish Border Counties*. *Scottish Health Service Studies*, No. 23. Edinburgh, Scottish Home and Health Department, 1972.

[QRL 286] Gruer, R. *Needs of the Elderly in the Scottish Borders*. *Scottish Health Service Studies*, No. 33. Edinburgh, Scottish Home and Health Department, 1975.

[QRL 287] Grundy, F. *Luton*. Luton, Luton Borough Council, 1945.

[QRL 288] Hall, R. *et al.* 'Observer variation in assessment of results of surgery for peptic ulcer.' *British Medical Journal*, 1, 814 (1976).

[QRL 289] Hamilton, M. *et al.* 'The aetiology of essential hypertension: I. Arterial pressure in the general population.' *Clinical Science*, 13, 11 (1954).

[QRL 290] Hamilton, M. *et al.* 'The aetiology of essential hypertension. IV. The role of inheritance.' *Clinical Science*, 13, 273 (1954).

[QRL 291] Hare, E. H. and Shaw, G. K. *Mental Health on a New Housing Estate: a Comparative Study of Health in Two Districts of Croydon. Maudsley Monograph*, No. 12. London, Oxford University Press, 1965.

[QRL 292] Harkness, J. 'Prevalence of glycosuria and diabetes mellitus.' *British Medical Journal*, 1, 1503 (1962).

[QRL 293] Harnett, R. W. F. and Mair, A. 'Dundee.' In *Further Studies in Hospital and Community*, pp. 73–143. London, Oxford University Press for Nuffield Provincial Hospitals Trust, 1962.

[QRL 294] Harpur *et al.* 'Controlled trial of early mobilisation and discharge from hospital in uncomplicated myocardial infarction.' *Lancet*, 2, 1331 (1971).

[QRL 295] Harris, A. and Norris, V. 'Changes in duration of stay of mental hospital patients during the past 20 years.' *Journal of Mental Science*, 100, 21 (1954).

[QRL 296] Harris, A. I. *Social Welfare for the Elderly*. Government Social Survey Report, No. 366, Vols. I and II. London, HMSO, 1968.

[QRL 297] Harris, A. I., Cox, E. and Smith, C. R. W. *Handicapped and Impaired in Great Britain, Part I. Social Survey Report 418*. London, HMSO, 1971.

[QRL 298] Hart, J. T. 'The management of high blood pressure in general practice.' *Journal of the College of General Practitioners*, 25, 160 (1975).

[QRL 299] Harvey-Smith, E. A. and Cooper, B. 'Patterns of neurotic illness in the community.' *Journal of the Royal College of General Practitioners*, 19, 132 (1970).

[QRL 300] Hawthorne, V. M. *et al.* 'Blood pressure in a Scottish island community.' *British Medical Journal*, **4**, 651 (1969).

[QRL 301] Hawthorne, V. M., Greaves, D. A. and Beevers, D. G. 'Blood pressure in a Scottish town.' *British Medical Journal*, **3**, 600 (1974).

[QRL 302] Hayes, M. J., Morris, G. K. and Hampton, J. R. 'Comparison of mobilisation after two and nine days in uncomplicated myocardial infarction.' *British Medical Journal*, **3**, 10 (1974).

[QRL 303] Haynes, S. 'The rate of discontinuation of orthodontic treatment in the general dental services in Scotland.' *Health Bulletin*, **32**, 253 (1974).

[QRL 304] Heady, J. A. and Heasman, M. A. *Social and Biological Factors in Infant Mortality. GRO Studies on Medical and Population Subjects*, No. 15. London, HMSO, 1959.

[QRL 305] Heasman, M. A. *Mass Miniature Radiography. Report on Three Years' Examinations in England and Wales, 1955–57. GRO Studies on Medical and Population Subjects*, No. 17. London, HMSO, 1961.

[QRL 306] Higgins, I. T. T. 'Tobacco smoking, respiratory symptoms, and ventilatory capacity.' *British Medical Journal*, **1**, 325 (1959).

[QRL 307] Higgins, I. T. T. *et al.* 'Population studies of chronic respiratory disease.' *British Journal of Industrial Medicine*, **16**, 255 (1959).

[QRL 308] Higgins, I. T. T., Cochrane, A. L. and Thomas, A. J. 'Epidemiological studies of coronary disease.' *British Journal of Preventive and Social Medicine*, **17**, 153 (1963).

[QRL 309] Higgins, I. T. T. *et al.* 'Chronic respiratory disease in an industrial town.' *American Journal of Public Health*, **58**, 1667 (1968).

[QRL 310] Higgins, I. T. T. *et al.* 'Coronary disease in Staveley, Derbyshire with an international comparison with three towns in Marion County, West Virginia.' *Journal of Chronic Disease*, **25**, 567 (1972).

[QRL 311] Higgins, I. T. T. *et al.* 'Respiratory symptoms and pulmonary disability in an industrial town.' *British Medical Journal*, **2**, 904 (1956).

[QRL 312] Hill, G. B., Howitt, L. F. and Soaper, A. *Cancer Incidence in Great Britain, 1963–66. GRO Studies on Medical and Population Subjects*, No. 24. London, HMSO, 1972.

[QRL 313] Hill, P. A. and Wigmore, H. M. 'Measurement and control of drug-administration incidents.' *Lancet*, **1**, 671 (1967).

[QRL 314] Hinchcliffe, R. 'The threshold of hearing as a function of age.' *Acustica*, **9**, 303 (1959).

[QRL 315] Hinchcliffe, R. 'Prevalence of the common ear, nose and throat conditions in the adult rural population of Great Britain.' *British Journal of Preventive and Social Medicine*, **15**, 128 (1961).

[QRL 316] Hinks, M. D. *The Most Cruel Absence of Care*. London, King's Fund, 1974.

[QRL 317] Hitchens, R. A. N. and Lowe, C. R. 'Laboratory services in general practice.' *Medical Care*, **4**, 142 (1966).

[QRL 318] Hobbs, M. S. T. 'Survey of general-practitioner maternity units in England and Wales.' *British Medical Journal*, **4**, 287 (1967).

[QRL 319] Hobbs, M. S. T. and Acheson, E. D. 'Perinatal mortality and the organisation of obstetric services in the Oxford area in 1962.' *British Medical Journal*, **1**, 499 (1966).

[QRL 320] Hobbs, M. S. T. and Acheson, E. D. 'Obstetric care in the first pregnancy.' *Lancet*, **1**, 761 (1966).

[QRL 321] Hobson, W. and Pemberton, J. *The Health of the Elderly at Home. Medical, Social and Dietary Study of Elderly People Living at Home in Sheffield*. London, Butterworth, 1955.

[QRL 322] Hockey, L. *Feeling the Pulse. A Survey of District Nursing in Six Areas*. London, Queen's Institute of District Nursing, 1966.

[QRL 323] Hockey, L. *Care in the Balance: a Study of Collaboration Between Hospital and Community Services*. London, Queen's Institute of District Nursing, 1968.

[QRL 324] Hockey, L. 'District nurse attached to hospital.' In *Co-operation in Patient Care*, ed. Hockey, L. London, Queen's Institute of District Nursing, 1970.

[QRL 325] Hockey, L. *Use or Abuse? A Study of the State Enrolled in the Local Authority Nursing Services*. London, Queen's Institute of District Nursing, 1972.

[QRL 326] Hoenig, J. and Ragg, N. 'The non-attending psychiatric out-patient: and administrative problem.' *Medical Care*, **4**, 96 (1966).

[QRL 327] Holland, C. and Heaton, K. W. 'Increasing frequency of gall bladder operations in the Bristol clinical area.' *British Medical Journal*, **3**, 672 (1972).

[QRL 328] Holland, W. W. and Elliott, A. 'Smoking habits in a boarding school and the reaction of the pupils to an anti-smoking demonstration.' *Health Education Journal*, **24**, 186 (1968).

[QRL 329] Holland, W. W. and Elliott, A. 'Cigarette smoking, respiratory symptoms, and anti-smoking propaganda.' *Lancet*, **1**, 41 (1968).

[QRL 330] Holland, W. W. and Reid, D. D. 'The urban factor in chronic bronchitis.' *Lancet*, **1**, 445 (1965).

[QRL 331] Holland, W. W. and Spicer, C. C. 'Influence of weather on respiratory disease.' In *Biometeoreology II*, pp. 30–40. London, Pergamon Press, 1963.

[QRL 332] Hollows, F. C. and Graham, P. A. 'Intraocular pressure, glaucoma, and glaucoma suspects in a defined population.' *British Journal of Ophthalmology*, **50**, 570 (1966).

[QRL 333] Horder, J. and Horder, E. 'Illness in general practice.' *Practitioner*, **173**, 177 (1954).

[QRL 334] Hospitals Consultants and Specialists Association. *Hospital Medical Staffing*. Ascot, The Hospitals Consultants and Specialists Association, 1974.

[QRL 335] Houghton, H. 'Problems of hospital communication: an experimental study.' In *Problems and Progress in Medical Care*, 3rd Series, ed. McLachlan, G., pp. 115–143. London, Oxford University Press for Nuffield Provincial Hospitals Trust, 1968.

[QRL 336] House of Commons. *Fourth Report from the Expenditure Committee. Session 1973–74. Accident and Emergency Services*. Volume I: Report, Volume II: Minutes of Evidence, Appendices and Index. HC 115. London, HMSO, 1974.

[QRL 337] Howie, V. *The Evaluation of an X-ray Unit in a Health Centre. Scottish Health Service Studies*, No. 30. Edinburgh, Scottish Home and Health Department, 1974.

[QRL 338] Hughes, W. and Pugmire, S. L. 'A geriatric hospital service.' *Lancet*, **1**, 1249 (1952).

[QRL 339] Hunt, G. *et al*. 'Predictive features in open myelomeningocele with special reference to sensory level.' *British Medical Journal*, **4**, 197 (1973).

[QRL 340] Hurrell, G. D. 'The prescription and side-effects of steroids.' *Journal of the Royal College of General Practitioners*, **22**, 387 (1972).

[QRL 341] Hurwitz, N. and Wade, O. L. 'Intensive monitoring of adverse reactions to drugs.' *British Medical Journal*, **1**, 531 (1959).

[QRL 342] Hyman, C. A. 'Accidents in the home to children under two.' *Health Visitor*, **47**, 139 (1974).

[QRL 343] Illingworth, C. F. W., Scott, L. D. W. and Jamieson, R. A. 'Acute perforated peptic ulcer.' *British Medical Journal*, **2**, 617, 655 (1944).

[QRL 344] Inman, W. H. W. and Mushin, W. W. 'Jaundice after repeated exposure to halothane; an analysis of reports to the Committee on Safety of Medicines.' *British Medical Journal*, **1**, 5 (1974).

[QRL 345] Inman, W. H. W. and Price Evans, D. A. 'Evaluation of spontaneous reports of adverse reactions to drugs.' *British Medical Journal*, **3**, 746 (1972).

[QRL 346] Innes, G., Kidd, C. and Ross, H. S. 'Mental subnormality in north-east Scotland.' *British Journal of Psychiatry*, **114**, 35 (1968).

[QRL 347] Institute of Municipal Treasurers and Accountants and the Society of County Treasurers. *Education Statistics*. London and Reading, Institute of Municipal Treasurers and Accountants and the Society of County Treasurers (Annual to 1974).

[QRL 348] Institute of Municipal Treasurers and Accountants and the Society of County Treasurers. *Local Health and Social Services Statistics*. London and Reading, Institute of Municipal Treasurers and Accountants and the Society of County Treasurers (Annual to 1974).

[QRL 349] Irvine, D. and Jefferys, M. 'B.M.A. Planning Unit, survey of general practice, 1969.' *British Medical Journal*, **4**, 535 (1971).

[QRL 350] Isaacs, V. 'Studies of illness and death in the elderly in Glasgow.' *Scottish Health Service Studies*, No. 17. Edinburgh, Scottish Home and Health Department, 1971.

[QRL 351] Israel, S. and Draper, P. 'General-practitioner hospital beds: a review.' *British Medical Journal*, **1**, 452 (1971).

[QRL 352] James, U., Brimblecombe, F. S. W. and Wells, J. W. 'The natural history of pulmonary collapse in childhood.' *Quarterly Journal of Medicine*, **25**, 121 (1956).

[QRL 353] Jefferys, M. and Elliott, P. M. *Women in Medicine. The results of an inquiry conducted by the Medical Practitioners' Union in 1962–63*. London, Office of Health Economics, 1966.

[QRL 354] Jefferys, M., Norman-Taylor, W. and Griffiths, G. 'Long-term results of an anti-smoking educational campaign.' *Medical Officer*, **117**, 93 (1967).

[QRL 355] Johnson, H. D. 'Peptic ulcer in hospital.' *Gut*, **3**, 106 (1962).

[QRL 356] Johnston, A. and Goldberg, D. 'Psychiatric screening in general practice.' *Lancet*, **1**, 605 (1976).

[QRL 357] Johnston, R. N. *et al*. 'Chronic bronchitis—measurements and observations over 10 years.' *Thorax*, **31**, 25 (1976).

[QRL 358] Johnston, S. J. *et al*. 'Epidemiology and cause of gastro-intestinal haemorrhage in NE Scotland.' *British Medical Journal*, **3**, 655 (1973).

[QRL 359] Jones, A. and Miles, H. L. 'The Anglesey Mental Health Survey.' In *Problems and Progress in Medical Care*, 1st Series, ed. McLachlan, G., London, Oxford University Press for Nuffield Provincial Hospitals Trust, 1964.

[QRL 360] Jones, D. C. *Food for Thought. The Study of Nursing Care Series 2, Report 4*. London, Royal College of Nursing, 1975.

[QRL 361] Jones, F. A. 'Clinical and social problems of peptic ulcer.' *British Medical Journal*, **1**, 719 and 786 (1957).

[QRL 362] Joyce, C. R. B. *et al.* 'Qualitative study of doctor–patient communication.' *Quarterly Journal of Medicine*, **38**, 183 (1969).

[QRL 363] Joyce, C. R. B., Last, J. M. and Weatherall, M. 'Personal factors as a cause of differences in prescribing by general practitioners.' *British Journal of Preventive and Social Medicine*, **21**, 170 (1967).

[QRL 364] Kaim-Caudle, P. R. and Marsh, G. N. 'Patient-satisfaction survey in general practice.' *British Medical Journal*, **1**, 262 (1975).

[QRL 365] Kay, C. R. *Oral Contraceptives and Health: an Interim Report from the Oral Contraception Study of the Royal College of General Practitioners.* London, Pitman Medical, 1974.

[QRL 366] Kay, O. W. K., Beamish, P. and Roth, M. 'Old age mental disorders in Newcastle upon Tyne.' *British Journal of Psychiatry*, **110**, 146 (1964).

[QRL 367] Keen, H. *et al.* 'The effect of treatment of moderate hyperglycaemia on the incidence of arterial disease.' *Postgraduate Medical Journal*, **46**, supplement, 960 (1968).

[QRL 368] Kellgren, J. H. and Lawrence, J. S. 'Rheumatoid arthritis in a population sample.' *Annals of Rheumatoid Diseases*, **15**, 1 (1956).

[QRL 369] Kessel, W. I. N. 'Psychiatric morbidity in a London general practice.' *British Journal of Preventive and Social Medicine*, **14**, 16 (1960).

[QRL 370] Kessel, W. I. N. and Shepherd, M. 'The health and attitudes of people who seldom consult a doctor.' *Medical Care*, **3**, 6 (1965).

[QRL 371] Khosla, T. and Lowe, C. R. 'Height and weight of British men.' *Lancet*, **1**, 742 (1968).

[QRL 372] Khosla, T. and Lowe, C. R. 'Obesity and smoking habits by social class.' *British Journal of Preventive and Social Medicine*, **26**, 249 (1972).

[QRL 373] Kidd, C. B. 'Misplacement of the elderly in hospital.' *British Medical Journal*, **2**, 1491 (1962).

[QRL 374] Kilpatrick, G. S. 'Prevalence of anaemia in the general population.' *British Medical Journal*, **2**, 1736 (1961).

[QRL 375] Kilpatrick, G. S. and Hardisty, R. M. 'The prevalence of anaemia in the community.' *British Medical Journal*, **1**, 778 (1961).

[QRL 376] Kingsbury, K. J. 'Relation of ABO blood-groups to athero-sclerosis.' *Lancet*, **1**, 199 (1971).

[QRL 377] Kinlen, L. J. *A Community Study of Acute Myocardial Infarction and Sudden Death.* Oxford, Thesis accepted for D.Phil., 1969.

[QRL 378] Kinlen, L. J. 'Incidence and presentation of myocardial infarction in an English community.' *British Heart Journal*, **35**, 616 (1973).

[QRL 379] Knowelden, J., Buhr, A. J. and Dunbar, O. 'Incidence of fractures in persons over 35 years of age.' *British Journal of Preventive and Social Medicine*, **18**, 130 (1964).

[QRL 380] Kosviner, A. *et al.* 'Heroin use in a provincial town.' *Lancet*, **1**, 1189 (1968).

[QRL 381] Kushlick, A. and Cox, G. R. 'The epidemiology of mental handicap.' *Developmental Medicine and Child Neurology*, **15**, 748 (1973).

[QRL 382] Kyle, J. 'An epidemiological study of Crohn's disease in north-east Scotland.' *Gastroenterology*, **61**, 826 (1971).

[QRL 383] Lambert, P. M. and Reid, D. D. 'Smoking, air pollution, and bronchitis in Britain.' *Lancet*, **1**, 853 (1970).

[QRL 384] Lance, H. 'Transport services in general practice.' *Journal of the Royal College of General Practitioners*, **21**, Supplement No. 3 (1971).

[QRL 385] Lane, J. *Vol. II. Statistical Volume, Report of the Committee on the Working of the Abortion Act.* London, HMSO, 1974.

[QRL 386] Last, J. M. 'Regional distribution of general practitioners and consultants in the National Health Service.' *British Medical Journal*, **2**, 796 (1967).

[QRL 387] Last, J. M. and Broadie, E. 'Further careers of young British doctors.' *British Medical Journal*, **4**, 735 (1970).

[QRL 388] Last, J. M., Martin, F. M. and Stanley, G. R. 'Academic record and subsequent career.' *Proceedings of the Royal Society of Medicine*, **60**, 813 (1967).

[QRL 389] Last, J. M. and Stanley, G. R. 'Career preferences of young British doctors.' *British Journal of Medical Education*, **2**, 137 (1968).

[QRL 390] Lawrence, J. S. 'Prevalence of rheumatoid arthritis.' *Annals of Rheumatic Diseases*, **20**, 11 (1961).

[QRL 391] Lawrence, J. S. 'Disc degeneration.' *Annals of Rheumatic Diseases*, **28**, 121 (1969).

[QRL 392] Lawrence, J. S., Laine, V. A. I. and de Graaff, R. 'The epidemiology of rheumatoid arthritis in northern Europe.' *Proceedings of the Royal Society of Medicine*, **54**, 454 (1961).

[QRL 393] Lawther, P. J., Waller, R. E. and Henderson, M. 'Air pollution and exacerbations of bronchitis.' *Thorax*, **25**, 525 (1970).

[QRL 394] Leck, I. *et al.* 'The incidence of malformations in Birmingham, 1950–59.' *Teratology,* **1**, 263 (1969).

[QRL 395] Lee, J. A. H. 'Prescribing and other aspects of general practice in three towns.' *Proceedings of the Royal Society of Medicine,* **57**, 1041 (1964).

[QRL 396] Lee, J. A. H., Draper, P. A. and Weatherall, M. 'Prescribing in three English towns.' *Milbank Memorial Fund Quarterly,* **43**, 285 (1965).

[QRL 397] Lee, J. A. H., Morrison, S. L. and Morris, J. N. 'Fatality from 3 common surgical conditions in teaching and non-teaching hospitals.' *Lancet,* **2**, 785 (1957).

[QRL 398] Lee, T. *et al.* 'Observations on drug prescribing in rheumatoid arthritis.' *British Medical Journal,* **1**, 424 (1974).

[QRL 399] Lewis, B. *et al.* 'Serum lipoprotein abnormalities in patients with ischaemic heart disease.' *British Medical Journal,* **3**, 489 (1974).

[QRL 400] Lightwood, R. *et al.* 'A London trial of home care for sick children.' *Lancet,* **2**, 313 (1957).

[QRL 401] Lister, R. D. and Milson, B. M. 'Car seat-belts.' *Practitioner,* **191**, 332 (1953).

[QRL 402] Litton, A. and Murdoch, W. E. 'Peptic ulcer in south-west Scotland.' *Gut,* **4**, 360 (1963).

[QRL 403] Logan, R. F. L. *et al. Dynamics of Medical Care. The Liverpool Study into Use of Hospital Resources. Memoir No. 14.* London, London School of Hygiene and Tropical Medicine, 1972.

[QRL 404] Logan, W. P. D. *General Practitioners' Records. GRO Studies on Medical and Population Subjects,* No. 7. London, HMSO, 1953.

[QRL 405] Logan, W. P. D. *Morbidity Statistics from General Practice—Vol. II (Occupation). GRO Studies on Medical and Population Subjects,* No. 14. London, HMSO, 1960.

[QRL 406] Logan, W. P. D. and Benjamin, B. *Tuberculosis Statistics for England and Wales 1938–55: an Analysis of Trends and Geographical Distribution. GRO Studies on Medical and Population Subjects,* No. 10. London, HMSO, 1957.

[QRL 407] Logan, W. P. D. and Brooke, E. M. *The Survey of Sickness—1943–1952. GRO Studies on Medical and Population Subjects,* No. 12. London, HMSO, 1957.

[QRL 408] Logan, W. P. D. and Cushion, A. A. *Morbidity Statistics from General Practice—Vol. I (General). GRO Studies on Medical and Population Subjects,* No. 14. London, HMSO, 1958.

[QRL 409] Logie, A. W. *et al.* 'Longitudinal study of untreated chemical diabetes.' *British Medical Journal,* **4**, 630 (1974).

[QRL 410] Long, A. and Atkins, J. B. 'Communications between general practitioners and consultants.' *British Medical Journal,* **4**, 456 (1974).

[QRL 411] Lorber, J. 'Spina bifida cystica: results of treatment of 270 consecutive cases with criteria for selection for the future.' *Archives of Diseases of Childhood,* **47**, 854 (1972).

[QRL 412] Loudon, I. S. L. *The Demand for Hospital Care.* Oxford, United Oxford Hospitals, 1970.

[QRL 413] Loung, K. C., Buckle, A. E. R. and Anderson, M. A. 'Results in 1,000 cases of therapeutic abortion managed by vacuum aspiration.' *British Medical Journal,* **4**, 477 (1971).

[QRL 414] Lowe, C. R., Campbell, H. and Khosla, T. 'Bronchitis in two integrated steel works. III. Respiratory symptoms and ventilatory capacity related to atmospheric pollution.' *British Journal of Industrial Medicine,* **27**, 121 (1970).

[QRL 415] Lowe, C. R. and McKeown, T. 'Arterial pressure in an industrial population.' *Lancet,* **1**, 1086 (1962).

[QRL 416] Lowe, C. R. and MacMahon, B. 'Breast cancer and reproductive history of women in South Wales.' *Lancet,* **1**, 153 (1970).

[QRL 417] Lowe, C. R. *et al.* 'Bronchitis in two integrated steel works.' *British Journal of Preventive and Social Medicine,* **22**, 1 (1968).

[QRL 418] Lunn, J. E. 'School health service work in the ordinary day schools. I. Selective medical inspections (England and Wales 1967).' *Medical Officer,* **118**, 303 (1967).

[QRL 419] Lunn, J. E., Knowelden, J. and Handyside, A. J. 'Patterns of respiratory illness in Sheffield infant schoolchildren.' *British Journal of Preventive and Social Medicine,* **21**, 7 (1967).

[QRL 420] Lunn, J. E., Knowelden, J. and Roe, J. W. 'Patterns of respiratory illness in Sheffield junior schoolchildren.' *British Journal of Preventive and Social Medicine,* **24**, 223 (1970).

[QRL 421] McCance, C. and Hall, D. J. 'Sexual behaviour and contraceptive practice of unmarried female undergraduates at Aberdeen University.' *British Medical Journal,* **2**, 694 (1972).

[QRL 422] McDonald, A. D. 'Maternal health in early pregnancy and congenital defect.' *British Journal of Preventive and Social Medicine,* **15**, 154 (1961).

[QRL 423] McEwan, E. D. 'Effects of early discharge after hospital confinement.' *Lancet,* **2**, 744 (1964).

[QRL 424] McGeown, M. G. 'Chronic renal failure in Northern Ireland, 1968–70.' *Lancet,* **1**, 307 (1972).

[QRL 425] MacGregor, J. E. 'Cervical carcinoma: the beginning of the end?' *Lancet,* **2**, 1296 (1967).

[QRL 426] MacGregor, J. E., Fraser, M. E. and Mann, E. M. F. 'Improved prognosis of cervical cancer due to comprehensive screening.' *Lancet,* **1**, 74 (1971).

[QRL 427] MacGregor, S. W., Heasman, M. A. and Kuenssberg, E. V. *The Evaluation of a Direct Nursing Attachment in a North Edinburgh Practice. Scottish Health Service Studies,* No. 18. Edinburgh, Scottish Home and Health Department, 1971.

[QRL 428] McIntyre, A. D. and Parry, K. M. 'Career attainment—chance or choice. Survey of career experience of doctors graduating in Scottish medical schools in 1962.' *British Journal of Medical Education,* **9**, 70 (1975).

[QRL 429] McKay, A. J., Hawthorne, V. M. and McCartney, H. N. 'Drug taking among medical students at Glasgow.' *British Medical Journal,* **3**, 540 (1973).

[QRL 430] MacKay, C. 'Perforated peptic ulcer in the west of Scotland.' *British Medical Journal,* **1**, 701 (1966).

[QRL 431] Mackay, G. M. 'Some features of traffic accidents.' *British Medical Journal,* **4**, 799 (1969).

[QRL 432] McKennell, A. D. and Thomas, R. K. *Adults' and Adolescents' Smoking Habits and Attitudes.* London, HMSO, Government Social Survey Report 353b. 1967.

[QRL 433] McKenzie, A. *Cancer Statistics for England and Wales 1901–1955. A summary of data relating to mortality and morbidity. GRO Studies on Medical and Population Subjects,* No. 13. London, HMSO, 1957.

[QRL 434] McKeown, T., Mackintosh, J. M. and Lowe, C. R. 'Influence of age upon type of hospital to which patients are admitted.' *Lancet,* **1**, 818 (1961).

[QRL 435] Mackintosh, J. M., McKeown, T. and Garratt, F. N. 'An examination of the need for hospital admission.' *Lancet,* **1**, 815 (1961).

[QRL 436] McKissock, W., Richardson, A. and Taylor, J. 'Primary intracerebral haemorrhage: a controlled trial of surgical and conservative treatment.' *Lancet,* **2**, 221 (1961).

[QRL 437] MacLennan, W. J. 'The young chronic sick at home and in hospital.' *Health Bulletin,* **30**, 1 (1972).

[QRL 438] McLennan, W. J. *et al.* 'Anaemia in the elderly.' *Quarterly Journal of Medicine,* **42**, 1 (1973).

[QRL 439] McMullan, J. J. and Barr, A. 'Out-patient letters: a study of communication.' *Journal of the College of General Practitioners,* **7**, 66 (1964).

[QRL 440] McNeilly, R. H. and Pemberton, J. 'Duration of last attack in 998 fatal cases of coronary artery disease and its relation to possible resuscitation.' *British Medical Journal,* **3**, 139 (1968).

[QRL 441] MacPhail, A. N. and Bradshaw, D. B. 'Delayed in hospital.' *Lancet,* **2**, 89 (1967).

[QRL 442] MacQueen, I. A. G. *A Study of Home Accidents in Aberdeen.* London, Livingstone, 1960.

[QRL 443] Mair, A., Weir, I. B. L. and Wilson, W. A. 'The needs of old people in a Scottish city.' *Public Health,* **70**, 97, 112 (1957).

[QRL 444] Mair, W. J. *et al.* 'Use of radiological facilities by general practitioners.' *British Medical Journal,* **3**, 732 (1974).

[QRL 445] Mann, S. and Sproule, J. 'Reasons for a six-month stay.' In *Evaluating a Community Psychiatric Service,* ed. Wing, J. K. and Hailey, A. M., pp. 233–245. London, Oxford University Press for Nuffield Provincial Hospitals Trust, 1972.

[QRL 446] Marris, T. 'The work of health visitors in London. A survey, 1969.' *Greater London Research Department of Planning and Transportation, Research Report,* No. 12. London, Greater London Council, 1969.

[QRL 447] Marsh, G. and Kaim-Caudle, P. *Team Care in General Practice.* London, Croom Helm, 1976.

[QRL 448] Marsh, G. N., McNay, R. A. and Whewell, J. 'Survey of home visiting by general practitioners in north-east England.' *British Medical Journal,* **1**, 487 (1972).

[QRL 449] Marshall, J. and Kaeser, A. 'Survival after non-haemorrhagic cerebrovascular accidents.' *British Medical Journal,* **2**, 73 (1961).

[QRL 450] Martin, J. and Morgan, M. *Prolonged Sickness and the Return to Work.* London, HMSO, 1975.

[QRL 451] Martin, M. *Colleagues or Competitors? A study of the role of five of the professions supplementary to medicine. Occasional Papers on Social Administration,* No. 31. London, Bell, 1969.

[QRL 452] Mason, A. S. *et al.* 'Epidemiology and clinical picture of Addison's disease.' *Lancet,* **2**, 744 (1968).

[QRL 453] Mather, H. G. *et al.* 'Acute myocardial infarction: home and hospital treatment.' *British Medical Journal,* **3**, 334 (1971).

[QRL 454] Mather, H. G. *et al.* 'Myocardial infarction; a comparison between home and hospital care for patients.' *British Medical Journal,* **1**, 925 (1976).

[QRL 455] Meade, T. W. 'Prescribing of chloramphenicol in general practice.' *British Medical Journal,* **1**, 671 (1967).

[QRL 456] Meade, T. W. *et al.* 'Recent history of ischaemic heart disease and duodenal ulcer in doctors.' *British Medical Journal,* **3**, 701 (1968).

[QRL 457] Meadows, S. H. 'Social class migration and chronic bronchitis.' *British Journal of Preventive and Social Medicine,* **15**, 171 (1961).

[QRL 458] Medical Sociology Research Centre, University College of Swansea, Wales. 'Prescribing in general practice.' *Journal of the Royal College of General Practitioners,* **26**, Supplement No. 1 (1976).

[QRL 459] Meredith, J. S. *et al. 'Hostels' in Hospitals? The Analysis of Beds in Hospitals by Patient Dependency.* London, Oxford University Press for Nuffield Provincial Hospitals Trust, 1968.

[QRL 460] Merrett, J. D. and Adams, G. F. 'Comparison of mortality rates in the elderly hypertensive and normotensive hemiplegic patients.' *British Medical Journal,* **2**, 802 (1966).

[QRL 461] Metters, J. S. and Milton, P. J. D. 'How safe is abortion?' *Lancet,* **1**, 1972 (1972).

[QRL 462] Miall, W. E., Ball, J. and Kellgren, J. H. 'Prevalence of rheumatoid arthritis in urban and rural populations in South Wales.' *Annals of Rheumatic Diseases,* **17**, 263 (1958).

[QRL 463] Miall, W. E. and Chinn, S. 'Screening for hypertension: some epidemiological observations.' *British Medical Journal,* **3**, 595 (1974).

[QRL 464] Miall, W. E. and Oldham, P. D. 'A study of arterial blood pressure and its inheritance in a sample of the general population.' *Clinical Science,* **14**, 459 (1955).

[QRL 465] Miller, D. S., Keighley, A. C. and Langman, M. J. S. 'Changing patterns in epidemiology of Crohn's disease.' *Lancet,* **1**, 691 (1974).

[QRL 466] Miller, F. J. W., Billewicz, W. Z. and Thomson, A. M. 'Growth from birth to adult life of 442 Newcastle upon Tyne children.' *British Journal of Preventive and Social Medicine,* **26**, 224 (1972).

[QRL 467] Miller, F. J. W. *et al. The School Years in Newcastle upon Tyne 1952–1962.* London, Oxford University Press, 1974.

[QRL 468] Miller, F. J. W. *et al. Growing up in Newcastle upon Tyne.* London, Oxford University Press for Nuffield Foundation, 1960.

[QRL 469] Ministry of Health. *Hospital survey of England and Wales in 10 volumes.* London, HMSO, 1945.

[QRL 470] Ministry of Health. *The Development of Consultant Services.* London, HMSO, 1950.

[QRL 471] Ministry of Health. *Recent NHS Prescribing Trends. Reports on Public Health and Medical Subjects,* No. 110. London, HMSO, 1964.

[QRL 472] Ministry of Health. *Enquiry into Sudden Death in Infancy. Reports on Public Health and Medical Subjects,* No. 113. London, HMSO, 1965.

[QRL 473] Ministry of Health. *National Health Service Prescribing 1963. Statistical Report Series,* No. 1. London, HMSO, 1965.

[QRL 474] Ministry of Health. *Report on the Census of Children and Adolescents in Non-Psychiatric Wards of National Health Service Hospitals. June, 1964 and March, 1965. Statistical Report Series,* No. 2. London, HMSO, 1967.

[QRL 475] Ministry of Health. *Care of Younger Chronic Sick Patients in Hospital.* London, Ministry of Health, 1968.

[QRL 476] Ministry of Health. *A Pilot Survey of the Nutrition of Young Children in 1963. Reports on Public Health and Medical Subjects,* No. 118. London, HMSO, 1968.

[QRL 477] Ministry of Health. *Psychiatric Nursing: Today and Tomorrow. Report of the Joint Sub-committee of the Standing Mental Health and the Standing Nursing Advisory Committees.* London, HMSO, 1968.

[QRL 478] Ministry of Health. *Dental Technicians. Report of a Sub-committee of the Central Health Services Council Standing Dental Advisory Committee.* London, HMSO, 1968.

[QRL 479] Ministry of Health, Department of Health for Scotland. *Report of the Joint Working Party on the Medical Staffing Structure in the Hospital Service.* London, HMSO, 1961.

[QRL 480] Ministry of Health, Scottish Home and Health Department. *Report of the Committee on Senior Nursing Staff Structure* (Chairman: Lord Salmon). London, HMSO, 1966.

[QRL 481] Ministry of Health, Scottish Office, Ministry of Housing and Local Government. *The Conduct of the Fluoridation Studies in the United Kingdom and Results Achieved after Five Years. Reports on Public Health and Medical Subjects,* No. 105. London, HMSO, 1962.

[QRL 482] Ministry of Health and Social Services for Northern Ireland. *A Survey of General Practice in Northern Ireland in 1970.* Belfast, HMSO, 1972.

[QRL 483] Model, A. 'A family doctor's work with adolescent patients.' *Proceedings of the Royal Society of Medicine,* **61**, 507 (1968).

[QRL 484] Moir, D. C. *et al.* 'Cardiotoxicity of amitriptyline.' *Lancet,* **2**, 561 (1972).

[QRL 485] Montegriffo, V. M. E. 'Height and weight of a United Kingdom adult population.' *Annals of Human Genetics,* **31**, 389 (1968).

[QRL 486] Morgan, W. *et al.* 'Casual attenders: a socio-medical study of patients attending accident and emergency departments in the Newcastle upon Tyne area.' *Hospital and Health Services Review,* **70**, 189 (1974).

[QRL 487] Morrell, D. C. 'Expressions of morbidity in general practice.' *British Medical Journal,* **2**, 454 (1971).

[QRL 488] Morris, D., Hall, G. A. and Handyside, A. J. 'Admissions from surgical waiting lists.' *British Journal of Preventive and Social Medicine*, **23**, 233 (1969).

[QRL 489] Morris, D., Ward, A. W. M. and Handyside, A. J. 'Early discharge after hernia repair.' *Lancet*, **1**, 681 (1968).

[QRL 490] Morris, J. N. 'A medical examination of 1592 workers.' *Lancet*, **1**, 51 (1941).

[QRL 491] Morris, J. N. *et al.* 'Vigorous exercise in leisure-time and the incidence of coronary heart-disease.' *Lancet*, **1**, 333 (1973).

[QRL 492] Morris, J. N., Heady, J. A. and Barley, R. G. 'Prognosis of coronary heart disease in medical practitioners.' *British Heart Journal*, **19**, 227 (1957).

[QRL 493] Morris, J. N. *et al.* 'Coronary heart disease and physical activity at work.' *Lancet*, **2**, 1053 and 1111 (1953).

[QRL 494] Morris, J. N. *et al.* 'Incidence and prediction of ischaemic heart disease in London busmen.' *Lancet*, **2**, 553 (1966).

[QRL 495] Moss, M. C. and Davies, E. B. *A Survey of Alcoholism in an English County*. Cambridge, Geigy Pharmaceuticals, 1967.

[QRL 496] Murdock, R. and Eva, J. 'Home accidents to children under 15 years: survey of 910 cases.' *British Medical Journal*, **3**, 103 (1974).

[QRL 497] Murray, R. M. 'Alcoholism amongst male doctors in Scotland.' *Lancet*, **2**, 729 (1976).

[QRL 498] National Coal Board. *Medical Service Annual Report 1975–76*. London, National Coal Board, 1976.

[QRL 499] National Dock Labour Board. *Annual Report and Accounts*. London, National Dock Labour Board, 1976.

[QRL 500] Neligan, G., Prudham, D. and Steiner, H. *The Formative Years: Birth, Family and Development in Newcastle upon Tyne*. London, Oxford University Press for Nuffield Provincial Hospitals Trust, 1974.

[QRL 501] Norris, V. *Mental Illness in London. Maudsley Monographs*, No. 6. London, Chapman & Hall for Institute of Psychiatry, 1959.

[QRL 502] Northern Ireland Health and Social Services, Central Services Agency. *Annual Report*. Belfast, Central Services Agency, 1975.

[QRL 503] Northern Ireland Hospitals Authority. *Twenty-fifth Annual Report, year ended 31st December 1972*. Belfast, Northern Ireland Hospitals Authority, 1973.

[QRL 504] Nuffield Provincial Hospitals Trust. *Hospital and Community: I. Hospital Treated Sickness amongst the People of Stirlingshire*. London, Nuffield Provincial Hospitals Trust, 1948.

[QRL 505] Nuffield Provincial Hospitals Trust. *Hospital and Community: II. Hospital Treated Sickness amongst the people of Ayrshire*. London, Nuffield Provincial Hospitals Trust, 1950.

[QRL 506] Nuffield Provincial Hospitals Trust. *Studies in the Function and Design of Hospitals*. London, University of Bristol and Oxford University Press for Nuffield Provincial Hospitals Trust, 1955.

[QRL 507] Nuffield Provincial Hospitals Trust. *Casualty Services and their Setting—a Study in Medical Care*. London, Oxford University Press for Nuffield Provincial Hospitals Trust, 1960.

[QRL 508] Nuffield Provincial Hospitals Trust. *Waiting in Outpatient Departments. A Survey of Outpatient Appointment Systems*. London, Oxford University Press for Nuffield Provincial Hospitals Trust, 1965.

[QRL 509] Office of Population Censuses and Surveys. *Morbidity Statistics from General Practice. Preliminary Report—Method*. London, HMSO, 1973.

[QRL 510] Office of Population Censuses and Surveys. *The General Household Survey Introductory Report*. London, HMSO, 1973.

[QRL 511] Office of Population Censuses and Surveys. *Morbidity Statistics from General Practice. Second National Study. Studies on Medical and Population Subjects*, No. 26. London, HMSO, 1974.

[QRL 512] Office of Population Censuses and Surveys. *The General Household Survey, 1972*. London, HMSO, 1975.

[QRL 513] Office of Population Censuses and Surveys. *The General Household Survey, 1973*. London, HMSO, 1976.

[QRL 514] Oliver, J. E. *et al. Severely Ill-treated Young Children in North-east Wiltshire. Oxford Unit of Clinical Epidemiology—Research Report*, No. 4. Oxford, Oxford Unit of Clinical Epidemiology, 1974.

[QRL 515] Oliver, M. F. 'Ischaemic heart disease in young women.' *British Medical Journal*, **4**, 253 (1974).

[QRL 516] Opit, L. J. and Crawford, J. S. 'Obstetric anaesthesia: a regional audit.' In *Probes for Health*, ed. McLachlan, G., pp. 45–68. London, Oxford University Press for Nuffield Provincial Hospitals Trust, 1975.

[QRL 517] Opit, L. J. and Day, P. R. 'Regional hospital ophthalmic services.' In *Probes for Health*, ed.

McLachlan, G., pp. 85–105. London, Oxford University Press for Nuffield Provincial Hospitals Trust, 1975.

[QRL 518] Osborn, G. R. and Leyshon, V. N. 'Domiciliary testing of cervical smears by home nursing.' *Lancet*, **1**, 256 (1966).

[QRL 519] Oswald, N. C. *et al.* 'Survey of the sputum cytology service in England and Wales.' *Thorax*, **30**, 489 (1975).

[QRL 520] Oswald, N. C., Medvei, V. C. and Waller, R. E. 'Chronic bronchitis: a ten year follow-up.' *Thorax*, **22**, 279 (1967).

[QRL 521] Palmer, J. W. *et al.* 'The use of hospitals by a defined population. A community and hospital study in North Lambeth.' *British Journal of Preventive and Social Medicine*, **23**, 91 (1969).

[QRL 522] Parish, P. A. 'The prescribing of psychotropic drugs in general practice.' *Journal of the Royal College of General Practitioners*, **21**, Supplement No. 4 (1971).

[QRL 523] Parkes, H. G. *Health in the Rubber Industry*. Birmingham, Rubber Manufacturing Employers' Association, 1966.

[QRL 524] Parkhouse, J. and McLaughlin, C. 'Career preferences of doctors graduating in 1974.' *British Medical Journal*, **2**, 630 (1976).

[QRL 525] Parr, D. 'Alcoholism in general practice.' *British Journal of Addiction*, **54**, 25 (1957).

[QRL 526] Parry, W. H. and Wilson, L. A. 'Cervical cytology in Nottingham 1966–1970.' *Medical Officer*, **124**, 85 (1971).

[QRL 527] Parry Jones, A. and Grimoldy, M. R. 'Abortion Act in Somerset.' *British Medical Journal*, **3**, 90 (1973).

[QRL 528] Parsons, P. L. 'Mental health of Swansea's old folk.' *British Journal of Preventive and Social Medicine*, **19**, 43 (1965).

[QRL 529] Pasker, P. and Ashley, J. S. A. 'Interrelationship of different sectors of the total health and social services system.' *Community Medicine*, **126**, 272 (1971).

[QRL 530] Patterson, D. and Slack, J. 'Lipid abnormalities in male and female survivors of myocardial infarction and their first-degree relatives.' *Lancet*, **1**, 393 (1972).

[QRL 531] Patterson, H. R., Fraser, R. C. and Peacock, E. 'Diagnostic procedures and the general practitioner.' *Journal of the Royal College of General Practitioners*, **24**, 237 (1974).

[QRL 532] Pearson, R. C. M. and Peckham, C. 'Preliminary findings at the age of 11 years on children in the national child development study (1958 cohort).' *Community Medicine*, **127**, 113 (1972).

[QRL 533] Pedoe, H. T. *et al.* 'Coronary heart-attacks in East London.' *Lancet*, **2**, 833 (1975).

[QRL 534] Pendreigh, D. M. *et al.* 'Survey of chronic renal failure in Scotland.' *Lancet*, **1**, 304 (1972).

[QRL 535] Perkins, E. S. 'Glaucoma screening from a public health clinic.' *British Medical Journal*, **1**, 417 (1965).

[QRL 536] Petrie, J. C., Howie, J. G. R. and Durno, D. 'Awareness and experience of general practitioners of selected drug interactions.' *British Medical Journal*, **2**, 262 (1974).

[QRL 537] Petrie, J. C., Needham, C. D. and Gillanders, L. A. 'Survey of alimentary radiology findings in the north-east of Scotland region (1967–70).' *British Medical Journal*, **2**, 78 (1972).

[QRL 538] Piachaud, D. and Weddell, J. M. 'Cost of treating varicose veins.' *Lancet*, **2**, 1191 (1972).

[QRL 539] Pike, L. A. 'Screening middle-aged men in a general practice.' *Practitioner*, **209**, 690 (1972).

[QRL 540] Pinker, G. D. and Fraser, A. C. 'Early discharge of maternity patients.' *British Medical Journal*, **2**, 99 (1964).

[QRL 541] Plant, J. C. D. *et al.* 'Incidence of gall bladder disease in Canada, England and France.' *Lancet*, **2**, 249 (1973).

[QRL 542] Platt, Lord, *et al.* 'Dietary sugar intake in men with myocardial infarction.' *Lancet*, **2**, 1265 (1970).

[QRL 543] Pletka, P. *et al.* 'Cadaveric renal transplantation.' *Lancet*, **1**, 1 (1969).

[QRL 544] Pole, J. D. 'Mass radiography: a cost/benefit approach.' In *Problems and Progress in Medical Care*, 5th series, ed. McLachlan, G., pp. 45–55. London, Oxford University Press for Nuffield Provincial Hospitals Trust, 1971.

[QRL 545] Pond, D. A., Bidwell, B. H. and Stein, L. 'A survey of epilepsy in fourteen general practices.' *Psychiatria, Neurologia, Neurochiourgia*, **63**, 217 (1960).

[QRL 546] Porter, A. M. W. 'Drug defaulting in a general practice.' *British Medical Journal*, **1**, 218 (1969).

[QRL 547] Porter, I. A. and Brodie, J. 'General practitioners and a laboratory service.' *Health Bulletin*, **31**, 244 (1972).

[QRL 548] Post Office (1971–5). *Annual Reports on Health and Sick Absence 1969/70–1974/75*. London, Post Office, 1971–75.

[QRL 549] Prior, P. *et al.* 'Mortality in Crohn's disease.' *Lancet*, **1**, 1135 (1970).

[QRL 550] Pulvertaft, C. N. 'Peptic ulcer in town and country.' *British Journal of Preventive and Social Medicine*, **13**, 131 (1959).

[QRL 551] Raffle, P. A. B. and Ager, J. E. *Patterns in Sickness Absence: Experience of London Transport Staff over Two Decades*. London, London Transport, 1973.

[QRL 552] Rang, E. H., Acheson, E. D. and O'Connor, B. T. 'Clinical significance of deaths after discharge from hospital unrecorded in the hospital notes.' *Lancet*, **2**, 908 (1968).

[QRL 553] Raphael, W. *Patients and Their Hospitals*. London, King's Fund, 1973.

[QRL 554] Raphael, W. and Peers, V. *Psychiatric Hospitals Viewed by their Patients*. London, King's Fund, 1972.

[QRL 555] Rawlings, E. E., Smith, E. A. and Wiseberg, E. 'A general practitioner unit, Hope Hospital, Salford.' In *In the Beginning*, ed. McLachlan, G. and Shegog, R., pp. 163–77. London, Oxford University Press for Nuffield Provincial Hospitals Trust, 1970.

[QRL 556] Rea, J. N., Newhouse, M. L. and Halil, T. 'Skin disease in Lambeth.' *British Journal of Preventive and Social Medicine*, **30**, 107 (1976).

[QRL 557] Reedy, B. L. E. C., Philips, P. R. and Newell, D. J. 'Nurses and nursing in primary medical care in England.' *British Medical Journal*, **2**, 1304 (1976).

[QRL 558] Redhead, I. H. 'Incidence of glycosuria and diabetes mellitus in a general practice.' *British Medical Journal*, **1**, 695 (1960).

[QRL 559] Rees, W. D. 'The distress of dying.' *British Medical Journal*, **3**, 105 (1972).

[QRL 560] Reid, D. D. *et al.* 'Cardiorespiratory disease and diabetes among middle-aged male civil servants.' *Lancet*, **1**, 469 (1974).

[QRL 561] Reid, D. D. and Fairbairn, A. S. 'The natural history of chronic bronchitis.' *Lancet*, **1**, 1147 (1958).

[QRL 562] Reid, D. D. *et al.* 'A cardiovascular survey of British postal workers.' *Lancet*, **1**, 614 (1966).

[QRL 563] Reid, D. D. *et al.* 'Smoking and other risk factors for coronary heart-disease in British civil servants.' *Lancet*, **2**, 979 (1976).

[QRL 564] Research Committee of the Council of the College of General Practitioners. *Morbidity Statistics from General Practice*—Vol. III (*Disease in General Practice*). GRO Studies on Medical and Population Subjects, No. 14. London, HMSO, 1962.

[QRL 565] Reynolds, E. *et al.* 'Psychological and clinical investigation of the treatment of anxious out-patients with 3 barbiturates and placebo.' *British Journal of Psychiatry*, **III**, 84 (1965).

[QRL 566] Richards, I. D. G., Donald, E. M. and Hamilton, F. M. W. 'Use of maternity care in Glasgow.' In *In the Beginning*, ed. McLachlan, G. and Shegog, R., pp. 105–31. London, Oxford University Press for Nuffield Provincial Hospitals Trust, 1970.

[QRL 567] Richards, I. D. G. and Lowe, C. R. 'Incidence of congenital defects in South Wales, 1964–6.' *British Journal of Preventive and Social Medicine*, **25**, 59 (1971).

[QRL 568] Richards, N. D. 'Public response to a "Do-it-yourself" cervical cancer test.' In *Cancer Priorities*, ed. Bennette, G., pp. 97–100. London, British Cancer Council, 1972.

[QRL 569] Richardson, I. M. *Age and Need: a Study of Older People in North-east Scotland*. Edinburgh, Livingstone, 1964.

[QRL 570] Richardson, I. M. and Berkeley, J. S. 'General practitioner opinions on medical record content.' *British Medical Journal*, **2**, 788 (1975).

[QRL 571] Richardson, I. M., Brodie, A. S. and Wilson, S. 'Social and medical needs of old people in Orkney.' *Health Bulletin*, **17**, 75, 1959.

[QRL 572] Richardson, I. M. *et al.* 'A study of general practitioner consultations in North-east Scotland.' *Journal of the Royal College of General Practitioners*, **23**, 132 (1973).

[QRL 573] Richardson, J. A. and Dixon, G. 'Effects of legal termination on subsequent pregnancy.' *British Medical Journal*, **1**, 1303 (1976).

[QRL 574] Rimington, J. 'Chronic bronchitis, smoking, and social class.' *British Journal of the Diseases of the Chest*, **63**, 193 (1969).

[QRL 575] Robertson, J. S. and Carr, G. 'Late bookers for ante-natal care.' In *In the Beginning*, ed. McLachlan, G. and Shegog, R., pp. 79–104. London, Oxford University Press for Nuffield Provincial Hospitals Trust, 1970.

[QRL 576] Rocha, J. *Organisers of Voluntary Services in Hospitals*. London, Kings Fund, 1968.

[QRL 577] Rose, H. and Abel-Smith, B., with Deacon, R. A. *Doctors, Patients and Pathology. A Case Study of the Demand for Laboratory Investigations in One Hospital Group. Occasional Papers on Social Administration*, No. 49. London, Bell, 1972.

[QRL 578] Rosin, A. J. 'Why were they in hospital so long?' *Gerontologica clinica*, **12**, 40 (1970).

[QRL 579] Roth, M. 'Natural history of mental disorder in old age.' *Journal of Mental Science*, **101**, 281 (1955).

[QRL 580] Rowe-Jones, D. C. and Aylett, S. O. 'Delay in treatment in carcinoma of colon and rectum.' *Lancet*, **2**, 973 (1965).

[QRL 581] Royal Commission on Medical Education 1965–68 *Report* (Chairman: Lord Todd), Cmnd. 3569. London, HMSO, 1968, reprinted 1969.

[QRL 582] Ruckley, C. V. *et al.* 'Team approach to early discharge and outpatient surgery.' *Lancet,* **1**, 177 (1971).
[QRL 583] Ruckley, C. V. *et al.* 'Major outpatient surgery.' *Lancet,* **2**, 1193 (1973).
[QRL 584] Russell, E. M. *Patient Costing Study. Scottish Health Service Studies*, No. 31. Edinburgh, Scottish Home and Health Department, 1974.
[QRL 585] Russell, J. K. *et al.* 'Maternity in Newcastle upon Tyne.' *Lancet,* **1**, 711 (1963).
[QRL 586] Russell, J. K. and Miller, M. R. 'Care of women with terminal pelvis cancer.' *British Medical Journal,* **1**, 1214 (1964).
[QRL 587] Russell, J. K. and Miller, M. R. 'Family responses to early discharge.' In *In the Beginning*, ed. McLachlan, G. and Shegog, R., pp. 179–86. London, Oxford University Press for Nuffield Provincial Hospitals Trust, 1970.
[QRL 588] Rutter, M., Tizard, J. and Whitmore, K. *Education, Health and Behaviour.* London, Longman, 1970.
[QRL 589] Sadler, J. and Whitworth, T. *Reserves of Nurses. An Enquiry Carried out on Behalf of the Department of Health and Social Security.* London, HMSO, 1975.
[QRL 590] Sansom, D. *et al.* 'Recall of women in a cervical cytology screening programme.' *British Journal of Preventive and Social Medicine,* **29**, 131 (1975).
[QRL 591] Saunders, J. 'Results and costs of a computer-assisted immunization scheme.' *British Journal of Preventive and Social Medicine,* **24**, 187 (1970).
[QRL 592] Saunders, J. and Snaith, A. H. 'Cervical cytology consent rate.' *Lancet,* **2**, 207 (1969).
[QRL 593] Scally, B. G. and MacKay, D. N. 'The special care service in Northern Ireland: origins and structure.' *Irish Journal of Medical Science,* **6**, 267 (1964).
[QRL 594] Scott, C. *The Wearing of Crash Helmets by Motor-cyclists. Social Survey Report*, 227a. London, Central Office of Information, 1960.
[QRL 595] Scott, C., and Jackson, S. *Accidents to Young Motor-cyclists—Statistical Investigation. Report* 227b *from Social Survey.* London, Central Office of Information, 1960.
[QRL 596] Scott, E. 'Prevalence of pernicious anaemia in Great Britain.' *Journal of College of General Practitioners,* **3**, 79 (1960).
[QRL 597] Scott, J. A. *Report on the Heights and Weights of School Pupils in the County of London, 1959.* London, London County Council, 1961.
[QRL 598] Scott, P. J., Durbin, F. C. and Morgan, D. C. 'Accident and emergency services in England and Wales in 1969.' In *Casualty Departments. The Accident Commitment. Report by the British Orthopaedic Association.* London, British Orthopaedic Association, 1973.
[QRL 599] Scott, R. and Gilmore, M. 'Studies of hospital outpatient services—the Edinburgh hospitals.' In *Problems and Progress in Medical Care*, 2nd Series, ed. McLachlan, G., pp. 3–42. London, Oxford University Press for Nuffield Provincial Hospitals Trust, 1966.
[QRL 600] Scott, R. and Robertson, P. D. 'Multiple screening in general practice.' *British Medical Journal,* **2**, 643 (1968).
[QRL 601] Scottish Home and Health Department. *The Future of the Artificial Limb Service in Scotland. Report of a Working Party set up by Secretary of State for Scotland.* Edinburgh, HMSO, 1970.
[QRL 602] Scottish Home and Health Department. *The Future of the Chest Services in Scotland. Report by a Sub-committee of the Scottish Standing Medical Advisory Committee.* Edinburgh, HMSO, 1973.
[QRL 603] Semmence, A. 'Time off work after herniorrhaphy.' *Journal of the Society of Occupational Medicine,* **23**, 36 (1973).
[QRL 604] Shanas, E. *et al. Old People in Three Industrial Societies.* London, Routledge & Kegan Paul, 1968.
[QRL 605] Sharland, D. E. 'Ability of men to return to work after cardiac infarction.' *British Medical Journal,* **2**, 718 (1964).
[QRL 606] Sharp, C. L. 'Diabetes survey in Bedford, 1962.' *Proceedings of the Royal Society of Medicine,* **57**, 193 (1964).
[QRL 607] Sheiham, A. *et al.* 'Orthodontic treatment in the general dental service in England and Wales.' *British Dental Journal,* **131**, 535 (1971).
[QRL 608] Sheldon, J. H. *The Social Medicine of Old Age.* London, Oxford University Press, 1948.
[QRL 609] Sheldon, J. H. 'On the natural history of falls in old age.' *British Medical Journal,* **2**, 1685 (1960).
[QRL 610] Shepherd, M. *et al. Psychiatric Illness in General Practice.* London, Oxford University Press, 1966.
[QRL 611] Sidel, V. W., Jefferys, M. and Mansfield, P. J. 'General practice in the London Borough of Camden.' *Journal of the Royal College of General Practitioners,* **22**, Supplement No. 3 (1972).
[QRL 612] Silversin, J. B. *et al.* 'Patterns of dental practice of British general dental practitioners.' *British Dental Journal,* **137**, 433 (1974).

[QRL 613] Silversin, J. B. *et al.* 'The pattern of use of the dental surgery assistant by British dentists.' *Community Dentistry and Oral Epidemiology,* **2**, 282 (1974).

[QRL 614] Skinner, F. W. *Physical Disability and Community Care.* London, Bedford Square Press, 1969.

[QRL 615] Slack, J. and Evans, K. A. 'The increased risk of death from ischaemic heart disease in first degree relatives of 121 men and 96 women with ischaemic heart disease.' *Journal of Medical Genetics,* **3**, 239 (1966).

[QRL 616] Sleet, R. A. 'The prevalence of cortico-steroid administration in the general population.' *Journal of the Royal College of General Practitioners,* **17**, 261 (1969).

[QRL 617] Smith, S. M., Hanson, R. and Noble, S. 'Parents of battered babies: a controlled study.' *British Medical Journal,* **4**, 388 (1973).

[QRL 618] Smithells, R. W. 'Incidence of congenital abnormalities in Liverpool, 1960–64.' *British Journal of Preventive and Social Medicine,* **22**, 36 (1968).

[QRL 619] Sorsby, A. *Causes of Blindness in England and Wales—MRC Memorandum 24.* London, HMSO, 1950.

[QRL 620] Sorsby, A. *The Causes of Blindness in England, 1948–50.* London, HMSO, 1953.

[QRL 621] Sorsby, A. *Blindness in England, 1951–54.* London, HMSO, 1956.

[QRL 622] Sorsby, A. *The Incidence and Causes of Blindness in England and Wales 1948–1962. Reports on Public Health and Medical Subjects,* No. 114. London, HMSO, 1966.

[QRL 623] Spence, J. *et al. A Thousand Families in Newcastle upon Tyne: an Approach to the Study of Health and Illness in Children.* London, Oxford University Press, 1954.

[QRL 624] Spicer, C. C. and Lipworth, L. *Regional and Social Factors in Infant Mortality. GRO Studies on Medical and Population Subjects,* No. 19. London, HMSO, 1966.

[QRL 625] Stallworthy, J. A., Moolgaoker, A. S. and Walsh, J. J. 'Legal abortion: a critical assessment of its risks.' *Lancet,* **2**, 1245 (1971).

[QRL 626] Stanley, G. R. and Last, J. M. 'The careers of young medical women.' *British Journal of Medical Education,* **2**, 204 (1968).

[QRL 627] Stanton, B. R. and Exton-Smith, A. N. *Longitudinal Study of the Dietary of Elderly Women.* London, King's Fund, 1970.

[QRL 628] Stephens, F. O. and Dudley, H. A. F. 'An organisation for outpatient surgery.' *Lancet,* **1**, 1042 (1961).

[QRL 629] Stevenson, A. C. and Cheeseman, E. A. 'Hereditary deaf mutism with particular reference to Northern Ireland.' *Annals of Human Genetics,* **20**, 177 (1955–6).

[QRL 630] Stewart, I. McD. G. 'Long-term observations on high blood-pressure presenting in fit young men.' *Lancet,* **1**, 355 (1971).

[QRL 631] Stitt, F. *et al.* 'Clinical and biochemical indicators of cardio-vascular disease among men living in hard and soft water areas.' *Lancet,* **1**, 122 (1973).

[QRL 632] Stockwell, F. *The Unpopular Patient. The Study of Nursing Care,* Series 1, No. 2. London, Royal College of Nursing, 1972.

[QRL 633] Sutherland, A. *A Study of Long-stay Admissions to the Acute Medical Wards in the Aberdeen Hospitals. Scottish Health Service Studies,* No. 22. Edinburgh, Scottish Home and Health Department, 1972.

[QRL 634] Talbot, S. *et al.* 'ABO blood-groups and venous thromboembolic disease.' *Lancet,* **1**, 1257 (1970).

[QRL 635] Taylor, Lord, and Chave, S. *Mental Health and Environment.* London, Longmans, 1964.

[QRL 636] Taylor, P. J. 'Individual variations in sickness absence.' *British Journal of Industrial Medicine,* **24**, 169 (1967).

[QRL 637] Taylor, P. J. 'Occupational and regional associations of death, disablement, and sickness absence among Post Office Staff, 1972–75.' *British Journal of Industrial Medicine,* **33**, 230 (1976).

[QRL 638] Taylor, P. J. and Pocock, S. J. 'Mortality of shift and day workers 1956–68.' *British Journal of Industrial Medicine,* **29**, 210 (1972).

[QRL 639] Taylor, P. J. and Pocock, S. J. 'Commuter travel and sickness absence of London office workers.' *British Journal of Preventive and Social Medicine,* **26**, 165 (1972).

[QRL 640] Taylor, P. J., Pocock, S. J. and Sergean, R. 'Absenteeism of shift and day workers: a study of six types of shift systems in 29 organisations.' *British Journal of Industrial Medicine,* **29**, 208 (1972).

[QRL 641] Theobald, G. W. 'Home on the second day; the Bradford experiment.' *British Medical Journal,* **2**, 1364 (1959).

[QRL 642] Thomas, A. J., Cotes, J. E. and Higgins, I. T. T. 'Prevalence of coronary heart disease in elderly coal-workers.' *Lancet,* **1**, 414 (1956).

[QRL 643] Thomas, K. B. 'Temporarily dependent patient in general practice.' *British Medical Journal,* **1**, 625 (1974).

[QRL 644] Thomas, M. and Morton-Williams, J. *Overseas Nurses in Britain. A PEP Survey for the United Kingdom Council for Overseas Student Affairs*, Broadsheet, 539. London, Political and Economic Planning, 1972.

[QRL 645] Thomson, A. A., Billewicz, W. Z. and Holliday, R. M. 'Secular changes in the physique of Aberdeen mothers, 1950–64.' *British Journal of Preventive and Social Medicine*, **21**, 137 (1967).

[QRL 646] Thomson, D. 'Sickness absence in the civil service.' *Proceedings of the Royal Society of Medicine*, **65**, 572 (1972).

[QRL 647] Thorn, J. B. *et al.* 'Costs of detecting and treating cancer of the uterine cervix in North-east Scotland in 1971.' *Lancet*, **1**, 674 (1975).

[QRL 648] Timms, N. W. 'Child guidance service.' In *Problems and Progress in Medical Care*, 3rd Series, ed. McLachlan, G., pp. 91–114. London, Oxford University Press for Nuffield Provincial Hospitals Trust, 1968.

[QRL 649] Todd, G. F. *Statistics of Smoking in the United Kingdom. Research Paper* No. 1, 6th edition. London, Tobacco Research Council, 1972.

[QRL 650] Todd, J. E. *Children's Dental Health in England and Wales 1973. OPCS Social Survey Division Report*, 1011. London, HMSO, 1975.

[QRL 651] Todd, J. E. and Gray, P. G. 'Information for the prescriber.' Appendix 2 to the *Report of the Committee of Enquiry into the Relationship of the Pharmaceutical Industry with the National Health Service 1965–67*, Cmnd. 3410. London, HMSO, 1967.

[QRL 652] Todd, J. E. and Whitworth, A. *Adult Dental Health in Scotland, 1972. OPCS Social Survey Division Report*, 1009. London, HMSO, 1974.

[QRL 653] Tooth, G. C. and Brooke, E. M. 'Trends in the mental hospital population and their effect on future planning.' *Lancet*, **1**, 710 (1961).

[QRL 654] Topliss, E. P. 'Selection procedure for hospital and domiciliary confinements.' In *In the Beginning*, ed. McLachlan, G. and Shegog, R., pp. 59–78. London, Oxford University Press for Nuffield Provincial Hospitals Trust, 1970.

[QRL 655] Torrance, N. *et al.* 'Acute admissions to medical beds.' *Journal of the Royal College of General Practitioners*, **22**, 211 (1972).

[QRL 656] Townsend, P. *The Family Life of Old People: an Enquiry in East London*. London, Routledge & Kegan Paul, 1957.

[QRL 657] Townsend, P. *The Last Refuge*. London, Routledge & Kegan Paul, 1962.

[QRL 658] Townsend, P. and Wedderburn, D. *The Aged in the Welfare State. Occasional Papers on Social Administration*, No. 14. London, Bell, 1965.

[QRL 659] Trapnell, J. E. and Duncan, E. H. L. 'Patterns of incidence in acute pancreatitis.' *British Medical Journal*, **2**, 179 (1975).

[QRL 660] Trotter, W. R. *et al.* 'A goitre survey in the Vale of Glamorgan.' *British Journal of Preventive and Social Medicine*, **16**, 16 (1962).

[QRL 661] Tunbridge, R. E. 'Sociomedical aspects of diabetes mellitus.' *Lancet*, **2**, 893 (1953).

[QRL 662] Tunbridge, R. E. *The Rehabilitation and Resettlement of Disabled Persons. Memorandum of evidence from Council of BMA*. London, British Medical Association, 1954.

[QRL 663] Tunstall, J. *Old and Alone: a Sociological Study of Old People*. London, Routledge & Kegan Paul, 1966.

[QRL 664] Turnbull, A. C. *et al.* 'Perinatal mortality in a mining area and its implications for the obstetric service.' In *In the Beginning*, ed. McLachlan, G. and Shegog, R., pp. 151–162. London, Oxford University Press for Nuffield Provincial Hospitals Trust, 1970.

[QRL 665] UK Atomic Energy Authority. *Annual Report on Radiological Protection and Occupational Health*. Harwell, UK AEA, 1971.

[QRL 666] Vere, D. W. 'Errors in complex prescribing.' *Lancet*, **1**, 370 (1965).

[QRL 667] Wade, O. L., Hadden, D. R. and Hood, H. 'The prescribing of drugs in the treatment of diabetes.' *British Journal of Preventive and Social Medicine*, **27**, 44 (1973).

[QRL 668] Wade, O. L. and Hood, H. 'The prescribing of drugs reported to cause adverse reactions.' *British Journal of Preventive and Social Medicine*, **26**, 205 (1972).

[QRL 669] Wadsworth, M. E. J., Butterfield, W. J. H. and Blaney, R. *Health and Sickness: The Choice of Treatment*, London, Tavistock, 1971.

[QRL 670] Wadsworth, M. E. J. and Jarrett, R. J. 'Incidence of diabetes in the first 26 years of life.' *Lancet*, **2**, 1172 (1974).

[QRL 671] Wager, R. *Care of the Elderly—an Exercise in Cost Benefit Analysis*. London, Institute of Municipal Treasurers and Accountants, 1972.

[QRL 672] Waite, M. 'Health visitors and birth control advice 1970/71, parts 1 and 2.' *Nursing Times*, **68**, 157, 161 (1972).

[QRL 673] Waite, M. 'Domiciliary midwives and birth control advice 1970–71, parts 1 and 2.' *Nursing Times*, **68**, 193, 197 (1972).

[QRL 674] Waite, M. 'Consultant surgeons and vasectomy.' *British Medical Journal*, **2**, 629 (1973).

[QRL 675] Wakefield, J. *et al*. 'Relation of abnormal cytological smears and carcinoma of cervix uter to husband's occupation.' *British Medical Journal*, **2**, 142 (1973).

[QRL 676] Walker, A. L. *et al*. *Report on Confidential Enquiries into Maternal Deaths in England and Wales, 1952–54. Reports on Public Health and Medical Subjects*, No. 97. London, HMSO, 1957.

[QRL 677] Walker, A. L. *et al*. *Report on Confidential Enquiries into Maternal Deaths in England and Wales, 1955–1957. Reports on Public Health and Medical Subjects*, No. 103. London, HMSO, 1960.

[QRL 678] Walker, A. L. *et al*. *Report on Confidential Enquiries into Maternal Deaths in England and Wales, 1958–1960. Reports on Public Health and Medical Subjects*, No. 108. London, HMSO, 1963.

[QRL 679] Walker, A. L. *et al*. *Report on Confidential Enquiries into Maternal Deaths in England and Wales, 1961–1963. Reports on Public Health and Medical Subjects*, No. 115. London, HMSO, 1966.

[QRL 680] Wallace, J. *et al*. 'An epidemiological study of lens opacities among steel workers.' *British Journal of Industrial Medicine*, **28**, 265 (1971).

[QRL 681] Waller, R. E. and Brooks, A. G. F. 'Heights and weights of men visiting a public exhibition.' *British Journal of Preventive and Social Medicine*, **26**, 180 (1972).

[QRL 682] Waller, R. E. and Commins, B. J. 'Studies of the smoke and polycyclic aromatic hydrocarbon content of the air in large urban areas.' *Environmental Research*, **1**, 295 (1967).

[QRL 683] Waller, R. E., Commins, B. J. and Lawther, P. J. 'Air pollution in a city street.' *British Journal of Industrial Medicine*, **22**, 128 (1965).

[QRL 684] Walls, A. D. F. and Ruckley, C. V. 'A five year follow-up of Lord's dilation for haemorrhoids.' *Lancet*, **1**, 1212 (1976).

[QRL 685] Wansbrough, N. and Miles, A. *Industrial Therapy in Psychiatric Hospitals. The report of a fact-finding survey of industrial units in psychiatric hospitals in England and Wales which establishes the scope of such units and the variations in their management*. London, King Edward's Hospital Fund for London, 1968.

[QRL 686] Ward, A. W. M. 'Terminal care in malignant disease.' *Social Science and Medicine*, **8**, 413 (1974).

[QRL 687] Ward, I. V. and Irvine, E. D. 'The incidence of congenital abnormality in infants born to Exeter mothers 1954–60.' *Medical Officer*, **106**, 381 (1961).

[QRL 688] Warin, J. F. 'An evaluation of whooping cough vaccination in Oxford.' *Royal Society of Health Journal*, **88**, 21 (1968).

[QRL 689] Warren, M. D. and Cooper, J. 'Medical officer of health. The job, the man and the career.' *Medical Officer*, **117**, 41 (1966).

[QRL 690] Warren, M. D. and Cooper, J. 'Local government medical staff.' *Medical Officer*, **118**, 185 (1967).

[QRL 691] Warren, M. D., Cooper, J. and Warren, J. L. 'Problems of emergency admissions to London hospitals.' *British Journal of Preventive and Social Medicine*, **21**, 141 (1967).

[QRL 692] Waterhouse, J. A. H. *Cancer Handbook of Epidemiology and Prognosis*. Edinburgh, Churchill Livingstone, 1974.

[QRL 693] Waters, W. E. 'Headache and the eye.' *The Lancet*, **2**, 1 (1970).

[QRL 694] Waters, W. E. 'Smoking and neuroticism.' *British Journal of Preventive and Social Medicine*, **25**, 162 (1971).

[QRL 695] Waters, W. E., Elwood, P. C. and Asscher, A. W. 'Community survey of analgesic consumption and kidney function in women.' *Lancet*, **1**, 341 (1973).

[QRL 696] Waters, W. E. *et al*. 'Clinical significance of dysuria in women.' *British Medical Journal*, **2**, 754 (1970).

[QRL 697] Waters, W. E. *et al*. 'Ten-year haematological follow-up mortality and haematological changes.' *British Medical Journal*, **4**, 761 (1969).

[QRL 698] Watkinson, G. 'The incidence of chronic peptic ulcer found at necropsy.' *Gut*, **1**, 14 (1960).

[QRL 699] Watson, L. M. 'Cigarette smoking in school children.' *Health Bulletin*, **24**, 5 (1966).

[QRL 700] Weatherall, J. A. C. 'A follow-up study of children notified with spina bifida.' In *Child Health: a collection of studies. Studies on Medical and Population Subjects*, No. 31, pp. 15–24. London, HMSO, 1976.

[QRL 701] Weatherall, J. A. C. and White, G. C. 'A study of survival of children with spina bifida.' In *Child Health: a collection of studies. Studies on Medical and Population Subjects*, No. 31, pp. 1–14. London, HMSO, 1976.

[QRL 702] Weatherall, M. 'Pharmacological aspects of prescribing and classification of drugs.' *Proceedings of the Royal Society of Medicine*, **57**, 1043 (1964).

[QRL 703] Webb, B. and Williams, W. M. 'Mobility of general practitioners during the first few years in general practice.' *Sociological Review*, **20**, 591 (1972).

[QRL 704] Weddell, J. M. 'Varicose veins pilot survey, 1966.' *British Journal of Preventive and Social Medicine*, **23**, 179 (1969).
[QRL 705] Weir, R. D. 'Perforated peptic ulcer in North-east Scotland.' *Scottish Medical Journal*, **5**, 257 (1960).
[QRL 706] Weir, R. D., McKenzie, M. and Richardson, I. M. 'Aberdeen.' In *Further Studies in Hospital and Community*, pp. 143–204. London, Oxford University Press for Nuffield Provincial Hospitals Trust, 1962.
[QRL 707] Welsh Hospital Board. *Children in Hospital in Wales. Final report of the Working Party on Children in Hospital in Wales*, Cardiff, Welsh Hospital Board, 1972.
[QRL 708] Wilkes, E. 'Terminal cancer at home.' *Lancet*, **1**, 799 (1965).
[QRL 709] Wilkes, E., Dixon, R. A. and Knowelden, J. 'Modern obstetrics and the general practitioner.' *British Medical Journal*, **4**, 687 (1975).
[QRL 710] Willcox, D. R. C., Gillan, R. and Hare, E. H. 'Do psychiatric out-patients take their drugs?' *British Medical Journal*, **2**, 790 (1965).
[QRL 711] Willcox, R. R. 'Immigration and venereal diseases in England and Wales.' *British Journal of Venereal Diseases*, **46**, 412 (1970).
[QRL 712] Williams, B. T. and Knowelden, J. 'General-practitioner deputizing services—their spread and control.' *British Medical Journal*, **1**, 9 (1974).
[QRL 713] Williams, W. O. *A study of general practitioners' workload in South Wales 1965–1966. Reports from General Practice*, No. 12. London, The Royal College of General Practitioners, 1970.
[QRL 714] Williamson, I. *et al*. 'Old people at home: their unreported needs.' *Lancet*, **1**, 1117 (1964).
[QRL 715] Wilson, L. A., Lawson, I. R. and Brass, W. 'Multiple disorders in the elderly.' *Lancet*, **2**, 841 (1962).
[QRL 716] Wilson, T. S. 'Scottish local health authorities—medical staffing as at January, 1966.' *Health Bulletin*, **24**, 81 (1966).
[QRL 717] Wing, J. K. 'Pilot experiment in the rehabilitation of long hospitalised male schizophrenic patients.' *British Journal of Preventive and Social Medicine*, **14**, 173 (1960).
[QRL 718] Wing, J. K. *et al*. 'Residential services for the mentally ill: developments, 1964–71.' In *Evaluating a Community Psychiatric Service*, ed. Wing, J. K. and Hailey, A. M., pp. 115–40. London, Oxford University Press for Nuffield Provincial Hospitals Trust, 1972.
[QRL 719] Wing, J. K. and Hailey, A. M. 'Statistical projections of service utilization.' In *Evaluating a Community Psychiatric Service*, ed. Wing, J. K. and Hailey, A. M., pp. 165–72. London, Oxford University Press for Nuffield Provincial Hospitals Trust, 1972.
[QRL 720] Wing, L. 'Severely retarded children in a London area: prevalence and provision of services.' *Psychological Medicine*, **1**, 405 (1971).
[QRL 721] Wing, L. *et al*. 'An epidemiological and experimental evaluation of industrial rehabilitation of chronic psychiatric patients in the community.' In *Evaluating a Community Psychiatric Service*, ed. Wing, J. K. and Hailey, A. M., pp. 283–308. London, Oxford University Press for Nuffield Provincial Hospitals Trust, 1972.
[QRL 722] Wood, A. J. J. *et al*. 'Medicines evaluation and monitoring group: central nervous system effects of pentazocine.' *British Medical Journal*, **1**, 305 (1974).
[QRL 723] Wood, M. M. and Elwood, P. C. 'Symptoms of iron deficiency anaemia.' *British Journal of Preventive and Social Medicine*, **20**, 117 (1966).
[QRL 724] Woodford-Williams, E. *et al*. 'The day hospital in the community care of the elderly.' *Gerontologica clinica*, **4**, 241 (1962).
[QRL 725] Woodruff, M. F. A. *et al*. 'Renal transplantation in man.' *Lancet*, **1**, 6 (1969).
[QRL 726] Wright, H. J. *General Practice in South-west England. Reports from General Practice*, No. 8. London, Royal College of General Practitioners, 1968.
[QRL 727] Younie, D. 'Mental subnormality and the general practitioner.' *Journal of the Royal College of General Practitioners*, **25**, 293 (1975).
[QRL 728] Department of Health and Social Security, Department of Education and Science, Welsh Office. *Fit for the Future. Report of the Committee on Child Health Services*, Vol. II (Chairman: S. D. M. Court), Cmnd 6684-1. London, HMSO, 1976.

BIBLIOGRAPHY

[B 1] Abel-Smith, B. *The Hospitals 1800–1948. A Study in Social Administration in England and Wales*. London, Heinemann, 1964.

[B 2] Abramson, J. H. *Survey Methods in Community Medicine*. Edinburgh, Churchill Livingstone, 1974.

[B 3] Accident Services Review Committee of Great Britain and Ireland. *Report of a Pilot Study conducted by a Working Party on Progress in the Provision of Accident Services*. London, British Medical Association, 1970.

[B 4] Acheson, E. D. *Medical Record Linkage*. London, Oxford University Press for Nuffield Provincial Hospitals Trust, 1967.

[B 5] Acheson, E. D. and Forbes, J. A. 'Experiment in the retrieval of information in general practice.' *British Journal of Social and Preventive Medicine*, **22**, 105 (1968).

[B 6] Acheson, R. M. and Hall, D. J. 'Epilogue.' In *Seminars in Community Medicine*, Vol. 2: *Health Information, Planning and Monitoring*, ed. Acheson, R. M., Hall, D. J. and Aird, L. London, Oxford University Press, 1976.

[B 7] Adler, M. W., Dunnell, K. and Weddell, J. M. 'Experiments in medical care.' *British Medical Bulletin*, **30**, 242 (1974).

[B 8] Aird, L. A. and Silver, P. H. S. 'Women doctors from The Middlesex Hospital Medical School (University of London) 1947–67.' *British Journal of Medical Education*, **5**, 232 (1971).

[B 9] Akhtar, A. J. 'Refusal to participate in a survey of the elderly.' *Gerontologica clinica*, **14**, 205 (1971).

[B 10] Alderson, M. R. 'Referral to hospital amongst a representative sample of adults who died.' *Proceedings of the Royal Society of Medicine*, **59**, 719 (1966).

[B 11] Alderson, M. R. 'Data on sickness absence in some recent publications of the Ministry of Pensions and National Insurance.' *British Journal of Preventive and Social Medicine*, **21**, 1 (1967).

[B 12] Alderson, M. R. 'Social class and the health service.' *Medical Officer*, **124**, 50 (1970).

[B 13] Alderson, M. R. 'Information systems in the unified health service.' In *The Future and Present Indicatives*, ed. McLachlan, G. London, Oxford University Press for Nuffield Provincial Hospitals Trust, 1973.

[B 14] Alderson, M. R. 'Central government routine health statistics.' In *Reviews of United Kingdom Statistical Sources*, Vol. II, ed. Maunder, W. F. London, Heinemann, 1974.

[B 15] Alderson, M. R. 'Towards a health information system.' *WHO Chronicle*, **28**, 52 (1974).

[B 16] Alderson, M. R. 'Statistics as a basis for health management and planning.' In *The Theory and Practice of Public Health*, 4th edition, ed. Hobson, W., p. 29. London, Oxford University Press (1974).

[B 17] Alderson, M. R. 'Evaluation of health information systems.' *British Medical Bulletin*, **30**, 203 (1974).

[B 18] Alderson, M. R. *An Introduction to Epidemiology*. London, Macmillan (1976).

[B 19] Alderson, M. R. 'A review of the national health service's computing policy in the 1970's.' *British Journal of Preventive and Social Medicine*, **30**, 11 (1976).

[B 20] Alderson, M. R. 'Progress towards health information systems.' In *Scientific Aids in Hospital Diagnosis*, ed. Nicholson, J. P., p. 207. New York, Plenum Press, 1976.

[B 21] Anderson, J. A. D. and Draper, P. A. 'The attachment of local authority staff to general practices.' *Medical Officer*, **117**, 111 (1967).

[B 22] Anderson, J. A. D. and Warren, E. A. 'Communications with general practitioners.' *Medical Officer*, **116**, 333 (1966).

[B 23] Arie, T. 'A new deal for half our doctors.' *Lancet*, **2**, 1073 (1976).

[B 24] Armitage, P. *Statistical Methods in Medical Research*. Oxford, Blackwell (1971).

[B 25] Armitage, P. *et al.* 'The variability of measurements of casual blood pressure—II. Survey experience.' *Clinical Science*, **30**, 337 (1966).

[B 26] Arthur, L. J. H. *et al.* 'Non-accidental injury in children: what we do in Derby.' *British Medical Journal*, **1**, 1363 (1976).

[B 27]   Ash, R. and Mitchell, H. D. 'Doctor migration 1962–4. With an addendum for 1964–5 from the Ministry of Health.' *British Medical Journal*, **1**, 569 (1968).

[B 28]   Asher, P. 'One thousand school children.' *Medical Officer*, **117**, 327 (1967).

[B 29]   Ashford, J. 'How can quantitative methods help the health services manager?' In *Measuring for Management*, ed. McLachlan, G., p. 1. London, Oxford University Press for Nuffield Provincial Hospitals Trust, 1975.

[B 30]   Babson, J. H. 'Hospital costing in Great Britain.' *Hospital*, **67**, 106 (1971).

[B 31]   Backett, E. M., Heady, J. A. and Evans, J. C. G. 'Studies of a general practice. The doctor's job in an urban area.' *British Medical Journal*, **1**, 109 (1954).

[B 32]   Bailey, N. T. J. 'Statistics in hospital planning and design.' *Applied Statistics*, **5**, 146 (1956).

[B 33]   Bain, D. J. G. 'Prescribing psychotropic drugs for children.' *Journal of the Royal College of General Practitioners*, **25**, 49 (1975).

[B 34]   Bain, D. J. G. and Haines, A. J. 'A treatment room survey in a health centre in a New Town.' *Health Bulletin*, **32**, 111 (1974).

[B 35]   Bain, D. J. G. and Haines, A. J. 'A year's study of drug prescribing in general practice using computer-assisted records.' *Journal of the Royal College of General Practitioners*, **25**, 41 (1975).

[B 36]   Baker, G. and Bevan, J. M. *A Bibliography on Health Centres in the United Kingdom*. London, Update Publications Ltd., 1974.

[B 37]   Baldwin, J. A. (ed.). *Aspects of the Epidemiology of Mental Illness: Studies in Record Linkage*. Boston, Little, Brown & Co., 1971.

[B 38]   Baldwin, J. A. *The Mental Hospital in the Psychiatric Service. A Case-Register Study*. London, Oxford University Press for Nuffield Provincial Hospitals Trust, 1971.

[B 39]   Barber, J. H. *et al*. 'Health centre X-ray unit.' *British Medical Journal*, **2**, 423 (1974).

[B 40]   Barr, A. 'Measuring nursing care.' In *Problems and Progress in Medical Care*, ed. McLachlan, G. London, Oxford University Press for Nuffield Provincial Hospitals Trust, 1964.

[B 41]   Barrett, R. E. 'Health supervision of school children by selective and routine examination.' *Medical Officer*, **118**, 316 (1967).

[B 42]   Bedson, S. P. and Camps, F. E. 'Need for and suggested scheme of investigation into sudden death in infancy. Memorandum to Ministry of Health.' *Reports on Public Health and Medical Subjects*, Appendix I, No. 113, London, HMSO, 1951.

[B 43]   Belson, W. A. and Thompson, B. A. *Bibliography of Methods of Social and Business Research*. London, London School of Economics and Political Science, and Crosby Lockwood Staples, 1973.

[B 44]   Benjamin, B. 'Assessment of medical care.' *Proceedings of the Royal Society of Medicine*, **60**, 17 (1967).

[B 45]   Benjamin, B. and Ash, R. 'Prescribing information and management of the N.H.S. pharmaceutical services.' *Journal of The Royal Statistical Society*, Series A, *General*, **127**, 165 (1964).

[B 46]   Bennett, A. E. 'Evaluating the role of the community hospital.' *British Medical Bulletin*, **30**, 223 (1974).

[B 47]   Bennett, A. E. and Ritchie, K. *Questionnaires in Medicine: a Guide to their Design and Use*. London, Oxford University Press for Nuffield Provincial Hospitals Trust, 1975.

[B 48]   Bevan, J. M., Dowie, R. and Kay, P. G. 'Transport for patients in general practice.' *Update*, **11**, 1033 (1975).

[B 49]   Bewley, B. R. and Bewley, T. H. 'Hospital doctors' career structure and misuse of medical womanpower.' *Lancet*, **2**, 270 (1975).

[B 50]   Bewley, B. R., Day, I. and Ide, L. *Smoking by Children in Great Britain—a review of the literature*. London, SSRC and MRC, 1973.

[B 51]   Bewley, B. R., Halil, T. and Snaith, A. H. 'Smoking by primary school children—prevalence and associated respiratory symptoms.' *British Journal of Preventive and Social Medicine*, **27**, 150 (1973).

[B 52]   Bewley, T. H. 'Heroin and cocaine addiction.' *Lancet*, **1**, 808 (1965).

[B 53]   Bispham, K., Thorne, S. and Holland, W. W. 'Information for area health planning.' In *Challenges for Change*, ed. McLachlan, G., p. 235. London, Oxford University Press for Nuffield Provincial Hospitals Trust, 1972.

[B 54]   Blackburn, H. *et al*. 'The electrocardiogram in population studies: a classification system.' *Circulation*, **21**, 1160 (1960).

[B 55]   Bone, M. 'Measures of contraceptive effectiveness and their use.' *Studies on Medical and Population Subjects*, No. 28. London, HMSO, 1975.

[B 56]   Bone, M., Spain, B. and Martin, F. M. *Plans and Provisions for the Mentally Handicapped*. London, George Allen & Unwin, 1972.

[B 57]   Bradford, S. C. *Documentation*. London, Crosby Lockwood, 1948.

[B 58] Bradford, T. C. 'Community electrocardiography.' *Journal of the Royal College of General Practitioners*, **25**, 445 (1975).

[B 59] Bradshaw, J. 'A toxonomy of social need.' In *Problems and Progress in Medical Care*, 7th Series, ed. McLachlan, G., p. 69. London, Oxford University Press for Nuffield Provincial Hospitals Trust, 1972.

[B 60] Brennan, M. E. and Knox, E. G. 'An investigation into the purposes, accuracy, and effective use of the blind register in Scotland.' *British Journal of Preventive and Social Medicine*, **27**, 154 (1973).

[B 61] Brennan, M. E. and Opit, L. J. 'Extension of family planning service in general practice.' *British Medical Journal*, **3**, 30 (1974).

[B 62] Breslow, L. 'A quantitive approach to the WHO definition of health: physical, mental and social well-being.' *International Journal of Epidemiology*, **1**, 347 (1972).

[B 63] British Medical Journal. 'Two for the price of one. New hospitals at Bury St. Edmunds and at lFrimley.' *British Medical Journal*, **2**, 113 (1968).

[B 64] British Medical Journal. 'Costing the NHS.' *British Medical Journal*, **4**, 122 (1973).

[B 65] British Medical Journal. 'Quality of life.' *British Medical Journal*, **1**, 1168 (1976).

[B 66] British Medical Journal. 'Patients' days.' *British Medical Journal*, **2**, 491 (1976).

[B 67] Brodman, K., Erdman, A. J. and Wolff, H. G. *Cornell Medical Index—Health Questionnaire—Manual*. New York, Cornell University Medical College, 1956.

[B 68] Bronte-Stewart, B. and Pickering, G. W. 'Cardiovascular diseases.' *Medical Surveys and Clinical Trials*, ed. Witts, L. J. London, Oxford University Press, 1959.

[B 69] Brotherston, J. H. F. 'The use of the hospital: review of research in the United Kingdom.' *Medical Care*, **1**, 142 and 225 (1963).

[B 70] Brotherston, J. H. F. 'Change and the National Health Service.' In *Management and the Health Services*, ed. Gatherer, A. and Warren, M. D., p. 1. London, Pergamon Press, 1971.

[B 71] Brown, C. G. 'Prescribing Mandrax.' *British Medical Journal*, **2**, 54 (1973).

[B 72] Brown, G. W. 'The mental hospital as an institution.' *Social Science and Medicine*, **7**, 407 (1973).

[B 73] Brown, R. G. S. 'The supply of general practitioners to East Yorkshire.' *Yorkshire Bulletin of Economic and Social Research*, **22**, 164 (1970).

[B 74] Brown, R. G. S. and Walker, C. 'The distribution of medical manpower.' In *Problems and Progress in Medical Care*, 5th Series, ed. McLachlan, G. London, Oxford University Press for Nuffield Provincial Hospitals Trust, 1971.

[B 75] Brown, R. G. S. and Walker, C. 'Motivation and morale in general practice.' *Journal of the Royal College of General Practitioners*, **23**, 194 (1973).

[B 76] Buck, C., Fry, J. and Irvine, D. H. 'A framework for good primary medical care—the measurement and achievement of quality.' *Journal of the Royal College of General Practitioners*, **24**, 599 (1974).

[B 77] Burdon, J. F. 'Display by spectrum.' *Journal of the Royal College of General Practitioners*, **4**, 106 (1961).

[B 78] Butler, J. R. and Knight, R. 'General practice, manpower and health service reorganisation.' *Journal of Social Policy*, **3**, 235 (1974).

[B 79] Butler, J. R. and Knight, R. 'The choice of practice location.' *Journal of the Royal College of General Practitioners*, **25**, 496 (1975).

[B 80] Butler, J. R. and Knight, R. 'Designated areas: a review of problems and policies.' *British Medical Journal*, **2**, 571 (1975).

[B 81] Buxton, M. J. and Klein, R. E. 'Distribution of hospital provision: policy themes and resource variations.' *British Medical Journal*, **1**, 345 (1975).

[B 82] du Cann, E. 'Public accounts.' *Hansard*, **655**, 9/12/76.

[B 83] Canvin, R. W. 'Improving general practice facilities for rural patients—an experimental mobile surgery.' A paper presented to the Royal Society for Health at a meeting at Civic Centre, Exeter, 24/11/71.

[B 84] Capstick, I. 'Medical audit: need for pilot studies in general practice.' *British Medical Journal*, **1**, 278 (1974).

[B 85] Cardew, B. 'An appointment system service for general practitioners: its growth and present usage.' *British Medical Journal*, **4**, 542 (1967).

[B 86] Carne, S. 'Sickness absence certification. Analysis of one group practice in 1967.' *British Medical Journal*, **1**, 147 (1969).

[B 87] Carstairs, V. and Skrimshire, A. 'The provision of out-patient care at health centres: a review of data available for planning.' *Health Bulletin*, **26**, 12 (1968).

[B 88] Cartwright, A. 'General practitioners and family planning.' *Medical Officer*, **120**, 43 (1968).

[B 89] Cartwright, A. 'Studies of patients.' *British Medical Bulletin*, **30**, 218 (1974).

[B 90] Cartwright, A. and Marshall, R. 'General practice in 1963: its conditions, contents and satisfactions.' *Medical Care*, **3**, 69 (1965).

[B 91] Cartwright, A. and O'Brien, M. 'Social class variations in health care and in the nature of general practitioner consultations.' *Sociological Review Monograph*, **22**, 77 (1976).

[B 92] Cartwright, K. *et al.* 'Design and implementation of a developmental paediatric programme.' In *Bridging in Health*, ed. McLachlan, G., p. 161. London, Oxford University Press for Nuffield Provincial Hospitals Trust, 1975.

[B 93] Case, R. A. M. and Pearson, J. T. 'Tables for comparative composite cohort analysis in cancer.' In *Studies on Medical and Population Subjects*, No. 13, pp. 30–99. London, HMSO, 1967.

[B 94] Central Health Services Council. *The Organisation of the Inpatients' Day*, London, HMSO, 1976.

[B 95] Central Statistical Office. *Guide to Official Statistics*. London, HMSO, 1976.

[B 96] Chaplin, N. W. (ed.). *The Hospitals and Health Services Year Book*. London, The Institute of Health Service Administrators (Annual).

[B 97] Chapman, J. M. and Coulson, A. 'Community diagnosis: an analysis of indicators of health and disease in a metropolitan area.' *International Journal of Epidemiology*, **1**, 75 (1972).

[B 98] Chave, S. and Taylor, S. (1961). Personal communication to Hare and Shaw (1966), q.v.

[B 99] Cheeseman, E. A. 'Medical record linkage in Northern Ireland.' In *Record Linkage in Medicine*, ed. Acheson, E. D., p. 70. Edinburgh, Livingstone, 1968.

[B 100] Chen, M. K. and Bryant, B. E. 'The measurement of health—a critical and selective overview.' *International Journal of Epidemiology*, **4**, 257 (1975).

[B 101] Cherns, A. B., Sinclair, R. and Jenkins, W. I. (eds.). *Social Science and Government: Policies and Problems*. London, Tavistock, 1972.

[B 102] Chiang, C. L. and Cohen, R. B. 'How to measure health: a stochastic model for an index of health.' *International Journal of Epidemiology*, **2**, 7 (1973).

[B 103] Christopher, L. J. *et al.* 'Spontaneous reporting of adverse drug reactions.' *Health Trends*, **8**, 74 (1976).

[B 104] Churchill Livingstone. *The Medical Directory*, 2 volumes. Edinburgh, Churchill Livingstone (Annual).

[B 105] Clark, E. M. 'Disease coding in a problem-orientated general practice.' *Journal of the Royal College of General Practitioners*, **24**, 469 (1974).

[B 106] Clarke, M. and Bennett, A. E. 'Problems in the measurement of hospital utilization.' *Proceedings of the Royal Society of Medicine*, **64**, 795 (1971).

[B 107] Cochrane, A. L. 'Detection of pulmonary tuberculosis in a community.' *British Medical Bulletin*, **10**, 91 (1954).

[B 108] Cochrane, A. L. *Effectiveness and Efficiency*. London, Nuffield Provincial Hospitals Trust, 1972.

[B 109] Cochrane, A. L., Chapman, P. J. and Oldham, P. D. 'Observers' errors in taking medical history.' *Lancet*, **1**, 1007 (1951).

[B 110] Cocking, J. 'In-patient waiting lists.' *Health and Social Services Journal*, **84**, 1102 (1974).

[B 111] College of General Practitioners Research Committee. 'Classification of morbidity.' *Journal of the College of General Practitioners*, **2**, 140 (1959).

[B 112] College of General Practitioners. 'Chronic bronchitis in Great Britain—a national survey carried out by the respiratory disease study group of the College.' *British Medical Journal*, **2**, 973 (1961).

[B 113] College of General Practitioners Research Committee. 'Classification of morbidity.' *Journal of the College of General Practitioners*, **6**, 207 (1963).

[B 114] College of General Practitioners. 'Present state and future needs of general practice.' *Reports from General Practice*. II. *Council of the College of General Practitioners*. London, 1965.

[B 115] Colombotis, J., Elinson, J. and Lowenstein, R. 'Effect of interviewers on interview responses.' *Public Health Reports*, **83**, 685 (1968).

[B 116] Cooper, C. 'The doctor's dilemma—a paediatrician's view.' In *Concerning Child Abuse*, ed. Franklin, A. W., p. 21. Edinburgh, Churchill Livingstone, 1975.

[B 117] Cooper, J. E. *et al.* 'Psychiatric diagnosis in New York and London—a comparative study of mental hospital admissions.' *Maudsley Monograph* No. 20. London, Oxford University Press, 1972.

[B 118] Cooper, M. H. and Culyer, A. J. *Health Economics*. Harmondsworth, Penguin, 1973.

[B 119] Court, S. M. D. *Fit for the Future. Report of the Committee on Child Health Services*, Vols. 1 and 2, Cmnd. 6684. London, HMSO, 1976.

[B 120] Crawford, M. D. and Morris, J. N. 'Ruptured ventricle: incidence in population of London, 1957–58.' *British Medical Journal*, **2**, 1624 (1960).

[B 121] Crichton, A. and Crawford, M. P. *Disappointed Expectations. Report on a Survey of Professional and Technical Staff in the Hospital Service in Wales 1963*. Cardiff, Welsh Staff Advisory Committee, Welsh Hospital Board (no date).

[B 122] Crombie, D. L. 'A casualty survey.' *Journal of the College of General Practitioners*, **2**, 346 (1959).

[B 123] Crombie, D. L. 'A model of the medical care system: a general systems approach.' In *The Economics of Medical Care*, ed. Hauser, M. M., p. 61. London, Allen & Unwin, 1972.

[B 124] Crombie, D. L. Personal communication, 1975.

[B 125] Crombie, D. L. and Pinsent, R. J. F. H. 'Medical records in general practice.' *Health Trends*, **1**, 1 (1969).

[B 126] Crombie, D. L. *et al*. 'Comparison of the first and second national morbidity surveys.' *Journal of the Royal College of General Practitioners*, **25**, 874 (1975).

[B 127] Crooks, J. *et al*. 'Prescribing and administration of drugs in hospital.' *Lancet*, **1**, 373 (1965).

[B 128] Crooks, J. *et al*. 'Evaluation of a method of prescribing drugs in hospital, and a new method of recording their administration.' *Lancet*, **1**, 668 (1967).

[B 129] Cross, K. W., Hassall, C. and Gath, D. 'Psychiatric day-care. The new chronic population?' *British Journal of Preventive and Social Medicine*, **26**, 199 (1972).

[B 130] Culyer, A. J., Lavers, R. J. and Williams, A. 'Health indicators.' In *Social Indicators and Social Policy*, ed. Schonfield, A. and Shaw, S., p. 94. London, Heinemann, 1972.

[B 131] Curtis, P. 'Medical audit in general practice.' *Journal of the Royal College of General Practitioners*, **24**, 607 (1974).

[B 132] Davies, B. P. *Social Needs and Resources in Local Services*. London, Michael Joseph, 1968.

[B 133] Davies, B. P. and Murray, G. J. *Personal Social Services and Voluntary Organizations in the Personal Social Service Field. Reviews of United Kingdom Statistical Sources*, Vol. 1, ed. Maunder, W. F. London, Heinemann, 1974.

[B 134] Davis, R. H. and Williams, J. E. 'X-ray unit for general practitioners.' *British Medical Journal*, **1**, 502 (1968).

[B 135] Dawes, K. S. 'Survey of general practice records.' *British Medical Journal*, **3**, 219 (1972).

[B 136] Department of Education and Science. *The Health of the School Child. Report of the Chief Medical Officer of the Department of Education and Science for the Years 1971–1972*. London, HMSO, 1974.

[B 137] Department of Education and Science. *The School Health Service 1908–1974*. London, HMSO, 1975.

[B 138] Department of Employment. *Family Expenditure Survey, 1975*. London, HMSO, 1976.

[B 139] Department of the Environment. *The Monitoring of the Environment in the UK—first report of the Central Unit on Environmental Pollution*. London, HMSO, 1974.

[B 140] Department of Health and Social Security. *A Pilot Survey of Patients attending Day Hospitals. Statistical Report Series*, No. 7, London, HMSO, 1969.

[B 141] Department of Health and Social Security. *Organisation of the Work of Junior Hospital Doctors. A Management Services (NHS) Study commissioned by the Joint Working Party on the Organisation of Medical Work in Hospitals*. London, HMSO, 1971.

[B 142] Department of Health and Social Security. Hospital Services for the Mentally Ill. Circular, December 1971.

[B 143] Department of Health and Social Security. *Report of the Working Party on Medical Administrators* (Chairman: Dr. R. B. Hunter). London, HMSO, 1972.

[B 144] Department of Health and Social Security. *Management Arrangements for the Reorganised National Health Service*. London, HMSO, 1972.

[B 145] Department of Health and Social Security. *National Health Service Reorganisation: England*. London, HMSO, 1972.

[B 146] Department of Health and Social Security. Services for Mental Illness Related to Old Age. Circular, October 1972.

[B 147] Department of Health and Social Security. *First report by the Sub-committee on Nutritional Surveillance. Reports on Health and Social Subjects*, No. 6. London, HMSO, 1973.

[B 148] Department of Health and Social Security. *Mentally Handicapped Children in Residential Care*. London, HMSO, 1974.

[B 149] Department of Health and Social Security. *Health and Personal Social Services Statistics for England (with summary tables for Great Britain)*. London, HMSO (Annual).

[B 150] Department of Health and Social Security. *Diet and Coronary Heart Disease. Reports on Health and Social Subjects*, No. 9. London, HMSO, 1974.

[B 151] Department of Health and Social Security. *Better Services for the Mentally Ill*, Cmnd. 6233. London, HMSO, 1975.

[B 152] Department of Health and Social Security. *On the State of the Public Health—The Annual Report of the Chief Medical Officer of the Department of Health and Social Security*. London, HMSO (Annual).

[B 153] Department of Health and Social Security. *Priorities for Health and Personal Social Services in England. A Consultative Document*. London, HMSO, 1976.

[B 154] Department of Health and Social Security. *Sharing Resources for Health in England. Report of the Resource Allocation Working Party*. London, HMSO, 1976.

[B 155] Department of Health and Social Security, Welsh Office. *Better Services for the Mentally Handicapped*, Cmnd. 4683. London, HMSO, 1971.

[B 156] Department of Health and Social Security, Welsh Office. *Community Hospitals. Their Role and Development in the National Health Service*. London, Department of Health and Social Security, 1974.

[B 157] Department of Health and Social Security, Welsh Office. *The Facilities and Services of Mental Illness and Mental Handicap Hospitals in England and Wales 1972. Statistical and Research Report Series*, No. 8. London, HMSO, 1974.

[B 158] Diggle, G. and Jackson, G. 'Child injury intensive monitoring systems.' *British Medical Journal*, 3, 334 (1973).

[B 159] Dixon, P. N. 'Work of a nurse in a health centre treatment room.' *British Medical Journal*, 4, 292 (1969).

[B 160] Dixon, P. N. and Morris, A. S. 'Casual attendances at an accident department and a health centre.' *British Medical Journal*, 4, 214 (1971).

[B 161] Doll, R. 'Monitoring the National Health Service.' *Proceedings of the Royal Society of Medicine*, 66, 729 (1973).

[B 162] Doll, R. and Hill, A. B. 'Smoking and carcinoma of the lung.' *British Medical Journal*, 2, 729 (1950).

[B 163] Doll, R. and Hill, A. B. 'Mortality in relation to smoking. Ten years' observation of British doctors.' *British Medical Journal*, 1, 1399 (1964).

[B 164] Dollery, C. T. 'The quality of health care.' In *Challenges for Change*, ed. McLachlan, G., p. 3. London, Oxford University Press for Nuffield Provincial Hospitals Trust, 1971.

[B 165] Dollinger, J. *Statistique des Personnes Atteintes de Cancer*. Budapest, Pub. Statist. Hong. Nouv. Ser. 19, 1907.

[B 166] Douglas, J. W. B. and Blomfield, J. N. 'The reliability of longitudinal surveys.' *Millbank Memorial Fund Quarterly*, 34, 227 (1956).

[B 167] Downie, B. N. 'The elderly in Scottish hospitals 1961–1966.' *Scottish Health Service Studies*, 21. Edinburgh, Scottish Home and Health Department, 1972.

[B 168] Dudley, H. A. F. 'Necessity for medical audit.' *British Medical Journal*, 1, 275 (1974).

[B 169] Dunlop, B. D. 'Need for and utilization of long-term care among elderly Americans.' *Journal of Chronic Diseases*, 29, 75 (1976).

[B 170] Dunlop, D. *Medicines in Our Time*. London, Nuffield Provincial Hospitals Trust, 1973.

[B 171] Durnin, J. V. G. A. *et al*. 'Food intake and energy expenditure of elderly females with varying family size.' *Journal of Nutrition*, 75, 73 (1961).

[B 172] Durnin, J. V. G. A. *et al*. 'The food intake and energy expenditure of elderly females living alone.' *British Journal of Nutrition*, 15, 499 (1961).

[B 173] Earthrowl, B. and Stacey, M. Personal communication, 1976.

[B 174] Eastern Health and Social Services Board, Northern Ireland. *First Annual Report. Year Ended 31st December 1974 (incorporating period 1st October, 1973–31st December, 1973)*. Belfast, Eastern Health and Social Services Board, 1975.

[B 175] Eccles, J. D. and Powell, M. 'The health of dentists. A survey in South Wales, 1965/1966.' *British Dental Journal*, 123, 379 (1967).

[B 176] Edmonds, D. 'Need—do we need it?' *Burisa*, 17, 21 (1975).

[B 177] Edwards, B. *Sources of Social Statistics*. London, Heinemann, 1974.

[B 178] Edwards, D. A. W. *et al*. 'Design and accuracy of calipers for measuring subcutaneous tissue thickness.' *British Journal of Nutrition*, 9, 133 (1955).

[B 179] Eimerl, T. S. 'Organised curiosity.' *Journal of the Royal College of General Practitioners*, 3, 246 (1960).

[B 180] Eimerl, T. S. and Laidlaw, A. J. *A Handbook for Research in General Practice*, 2nd ed. London, Livingstone, 1969.

[B 181] Elwood, J. H. and Nevin, N. C. 'Factors associated with anencephalus and spina bifida in Belfast.' *British Journal of Social and Preventive Medicine*, 27, 73 (1973).

[B 182] Eysenck, H. J. *Smoking, Health and Personality*, p. 119. London, Weidenfeld & Nicolson, 1965.

[B 183] Fairbairn, A. S., Wood, C. A. and Fletcher, C. M. 'Variability in answers to a questionnaire on respiratory systems.' *British Journal of Preventive and Social Medicine*, 19, 175 (1959).

[B 184] Fairley, J. and Hewett, W. C. 'Survey of casualty departments in Greater London.' *British Medical Journal*, 2, 375 (1969).

[B 185] Fanshel, S. 'A meaningful measure of health for epidemiology.' *International Journal of Epidemiology*, 1, 319 (1972).

[B 186] Farmer, R. D. T. and Cross, K. W. 'An automated records system for general practice.' *British Journal of Preventive and Social Medicine*, 26, 148 (1972).

[B 187] Farmer, R. D. T. *et al*. 'Executive council lists and general practitioner files.' *British Journal of Preventive and Social Medicine*, 28, 49 (1974).

[B 188] Farndale, J. *The Day Hospital Movement in Great Britain*. London, Pergamon Press, 1961.

[B 189] Farr, W. *Second Annual Report of the Registrar-General for Births, Marriages, Deaths in England*. London, HMSO, 1841.

[B 190] Fein, R. 'On measuring economic benefits of health programmes.' In *Medical History and Medical Care*, ed. McLachlan, G. and McKeown, T., p. 179. London, Oxford University Press for Nuffield Provincial Hospitals Trust, 1971.

[B 191] Feldstein, M. S. 'Effects of differences in hospital bed scarcity on type of use.' *British Medical Journal*, **2**, 562 (1964).

[B 192] Ferster, G. 'The role of economic analysis in health services management.' In *Measuring for Management*, ed. McLachlan, G., p. 25. London, Oxford University Press for Nuffield Provincial Hospitals Trust, 1975.

[B 193] Fletcher, C. M. *Communication in Medicine*. London, Nuffield Provincial Hospitals Trust, 1973.

[B 194] Fletcher, C. M. and Tinker, C. M. 'Chronic bronchitis—a further study of simple diagnostic methods in the working population.' *British Medical Journal*, **1**, 1491 (1961).

[B 195] Flood Page, C. M. and Slack, G. L. 'A contented profession? A survey of Old Londoner dentists: 1968.' *British Dental Journal*, **127**, 220 (1969).

[B 196] Floyd, C. B. 'Car service in general practice: a two-year survey.' *British Medical Journal*, **2**, 614 (1968).

[B 197] Floyd, C. B. and Livesey, A. 'Self-observation in general practice—the bleep method.' *Journal of the Royal College of General Practitioners*, **25**, 425 (1975).

[B 198] Flynn, C. A. and Gardner, F. 'The careers of women graduates from the Royal Free Hospital School of Medicine, London.' *British Journal of Medical Education*, **3**, 28 (1969).

[B 199] Fottrell, E., Peermohamed, R. and Kothari, R. 'Identification and definition of long-stay mental hospital population.' *British Medical Journal*, **4**, 675 (1975).

[B 200] Franklin, A. W. (ed.). *Concerning Child Abuse: Papers Presented to the Tunbridge Wells Study Group on Non-accidental Injury to Children*. Edinburgh, Churchill Livingstone, 1975.

[B 201] Fry, J. *Profiles of Disease: A Study in the Natural History of Common Diseases*. Edinburgh and London, Livingstone, 1966.

[B 202] Fry, J. 'Hospital referrals: must they go up? Changing patterns over 20 years.' *Lancet*, **2**, 148 (1971).

[B 203] Fry, J. 'Present state and future needs of general practice.' *Report from General Practice*, No. 16. London, The Royal College of General Practitioners, 1973.

[B 204] Fry, J. and Blake, P. 'Keeping of records in general practice.' *British Medical Journal*, **1**, 339 (1956).

[B 205] Fyfe, T. and Maclean, N. M. 'A health centre E.C.G. service: its use and abuse.' *British Medical Journal*, **1**, 563 (1975).

[B 206] Gardiner, A. Q., Petersen, J. and Hall, D. J. 'A survey of general practitioners' referrals to a psychiatric out-patient service.' *British Journal of Psychiatry*, **124**, 536 (1974).

[B 207] Gardner, M. J. and Heady, J. A. 'Some effects of within-person variability in epidemiological studies.' *Journal of Chronic Diseases*, **26**, 781 (1973).

[B 208] Garfield, S. R. 'A new ambulatory health care delivery system model.' In *Medinfo 1974*, Vol. 1, ed. Anderson, J. and Forsythe, J. M., pp. 481–6. Amsterdam, North-Holland, 1975.

[B 209] Gath, D. H., Hassall, C. and Cross, K. W. 'Whither psychiatric day care? A study of day patients in Birmingham.' *British Medical Journal*, **1**, 94 (1973).

[B 210] Gauvain, S. *Occupational Health—a Guide to Sources of Information*. London, Heinemann Medical Books, 1974.

[B 211] General Medical Council. *The Medical Register*, 2 vols. London, General Medical Council (Annual).

[B 212] General Register Office. 'Area of Residence of Mental Hospital Patients. Admissions to Mental Hospitals in England and Wales in 1957, according to Area of Residence, Diagnosis, Sex and Age.' *Studies on Medical and Population Subjects*, No. 16. London, HMSO, 1960.

[B 213] General Register Office. *Census, 1961–Great Britain, General Report*. London, HMSO, 1968.

[B 214] Gillum, R. F. *et al.* 'Community surveillance for cardiovascular disease: the Framingham cardiovascular disease survey.' *Journal of Chronic Diseases*, **29**, 289 (1976).

[B 215] Gish, O. 'British doctor migration 1962–67.' *British Journal of Medical Education*, **4**, 279 (1970).

[B 216] Glennerster, H. 'The Plowden research.' *Journal of the Royal Statistical Society*, Series A, **132**, 194 (1969).

[B 217] Godfrey, S. *et al.* 'Repeatability of physical signs in airways obstruction.' *Thorax*, **24**, 4 (1969).

[B 218] Goodman, M. 'The diagnostic index and the family record card.' *Journal of the Royal College of General Practitioners*, **21**, 590 (1971).

[B 219] Graham, N. G., de Dombal, F. T. and Goligher, J. G. 'Reliability of physical signs in patients with severe attacks of ulcerative colitis.' *British Medical Journal*, **2**, 746 (1971).

[B 220] Graham, R. C. 'The Tayside master patient index—how and why.' *Hospital and Health Services Review*, **70**, 385 (1974).

[B 221] Gray, P. G. and Parr, E. A. *The Medresco Hearing-aid Service in 1955: an inquiry made for the Ministry of Health*. London, Central Office of Information, 1956.

[B 222] Gray, S. *The Electoral Register: Practical Information for Use when Drawing Samples*, both for *Interview and Postal Surveys*. London, OPCS Social Survey Division, 1971.

[B 223] Green, R. H. 'General practitioners and open-access pathology services.' *Journal of the Royal College of General Practitioners*, **23**, 316 (1973).

[B 224] Greenfield, C. C. 'Revised procedure for dual round surveys in estimating vital events.' *Journal of the Royal Statistical Society*, **139**, 389 (1976).

[B 225] Greenwood, M. 'Discussion on paper by Cotton, H.' *Journal of the Royal Statistical Society*, **111**, 32 (1948).

[B 226] Grogono, A. W. and Woodgate, D. J. 'Index for measuring health.' *Lancet*, **2**, 1024 (1971).

[B 227] Hailey, A. M. 'The chronic mental hospital population: a six-year follow-up study.' *British Journal of Preventive and Social Medicine*, **27**, 255 (1973).

[B 228] Hall, J. 'Subjective measures of quality of life in Britain: 1971–75.' In *Social Trends*, ed. Thompson, E. J., p. 47. London, HMSO, 1976.

[B 229] Hall, M. 'A view from the emergency and accident department.' In *Concerning Child Abuse*, ed. Franklin, A. W., p. 7. Edinburgh, Churchill Livingstone, 1975.

[B 230] Hannay, D. R. 'Accuracy of health centre records.' *Lancet*, **2**, 371 (1972).

[B 231] Hannay, D. R. and Maddox, E. J. 'Incongruous referrals.' *Lancet*, **2**, 1195 (1975).

[B 232] Harris, A. I. and Head, E. *Sample Surveys in Local Authority Areas, with Particular Reference to the Handicapped and Elderly*. London, OPCS Social Survey Division, 1971.

[B 233] Hart, J. T. 'The health of coal mining communities.' *Journal of the Royal College of General Practitioners*, **21**, 517 (1971).

[B 234] Hart, J. T. 'The inverse care law.' *Lancet*, **1**, 405 (1971).

[B 235] Hassall, C., Gath, D. and Cross, K. W. 'Psychiatric day-care in Birmingham.' *British Journal of Preventive and Social Medicine*, **26**, 112 (1972).

[B 236] Hauser, M. M. *The Economics of Medical Care*. London, Allen & Unwin, 1972.

[B 237] Haward, R. A. 'Scale of under notification of infectious diseases by general practitioners.' *Lancet*, **1**, 873 (1973).

[B 238] Hawthorn, P. J. *The Nurse Working with the General Practitioner—an evaluation of research and a review of the literature*. London, Department of Health and Social Security, 1971.

[B 239] Hayward, J. *Information—a prescription against pain. RCN Study of Nursing Care*, Series 2, No. 5. London, Royal College of Nursing, 1975.

[B 240] Health Bulletin. 'The Woodside story.' *Health Bulletin*, **31**, 105 (1973).

[B 241] Heasman, M. A. 'The use of computers in a central organization and record linkage.' In *Principles and Practice of Medical Computing*, ed. Whitby, I. G. and Lutz, W., p. 75. Edinburgh, Churchill Livingstone, 1971.

[B 242] Heasman, M. A. and Carstairs, V. 'Inpatient management: variations in some aspects of practice in Scotland.' *British Medical Journal*, **1**, 495 (1971).

[B 243] Heasman, M. A. and Lipworth, L. *Accuracy of Certification of Cause of Death. General Register Office Studies on Medical and Population Subjects*, No. 20. London, HMSO, 1966.

[B 244] Hewitt, D. and Milner, J. 'Components of the demand for hospital care.' *International Journal of Epidemiology*, **1**, 61 (1972).

[B 245] Hobbs, P. *Aptitude or Environment. A study of the group teaching activities of health visitors*. London, Royal College of Nursing and National Council of Nurses of the United Kingdom, 1973.

[B 246] Hodgkin, G. K. *Towards Earlier Diagnosis: A family doctor's approach. First, Second and Third edition*. Edinburgh, Churchill Livingstone, 1963, 1966, 1973.

[B 247] Hodgkin, G. K. 'Evaluating the doctor's work.' *Journal of the Royal College of General Practitioners*, **23**, 759 (1973).

[B 248] Holland, W. W. and Waller, J. 'Population studies in the London Borough of Lambeth.' *Community Medicine*, **126**, 153 (1971).

[B 249] Holland, W. W., and Whitehead, T. P. 'Value of new laboratory tests in diagnosis and treatment.' *Lancet*, **2**, 391 (1974).

[B 250] Holohan, A. M. 'Accident and emergency departments: illness and accident behaviour.' *Sociological Review Monograph*, **22**, 111 (1976).

[B 251] Holohan, A. M., Newell, D. J. and Walker, J. H. 'Practitioners, patients and the accident department.' *Hospital and Health Services Review*, **71**, 80 (1975).

[B 252] Horowitz, O. and Wilbek, E. 'Effect of tuberculosis infection on mortality risk.' *American Review of Respiratory Disease*, **104**, 643 (1971).

[B 253] Hospital Advisory Service. *Annual Report, 1969–70*. London, HMSO, 1971.

[B 254] Hospital Advisory Service. *Annual Report, 1971*. London, HMSO, 1972.

[B 255] Hospital Advisory Service. *Annual Report, 1972*. London, HMSO, 1973.

[B 256] Hospital Advisory Service. *Annual Report, 1973*. London, HMSO, 1974.

[B 257] Hull, F. M. 'Disease coding.' *Journal of the Royal College of General Practitioners*, **21**, 581 (1971).

[B 258] Huskisson, E. C. 'Measurement of pain.' *Lancet*, **2**, 1127 (1974).

[B 259] Ingram, R. M. 'Role of the school eye clinic in modern ophthalmology.' *British Medical Journal*, **1**, 278 (1973).

[B 260] Inman, W. H. W. 'Role of drug-reaction monitoring in the investigation of thrombosis and "the pill".' *British Medical Bulletin*, **26**, 248 (1970).

[B 261] Isaacs, B. and Neville, Y. 'The needs of old people.' *British Journal of Preventive and Social Medicine*, **30**, 79 (1976).

[B 262] Jefferys, M. *An Anatomy of Social Welfare Services. A Survey of Social Welfare Staff and their Clients in the County of Buckinghamshire*. London, Michael Joseph, 1965.

[B 263] Jefferys, M. *et al.* 'A set of tests for measuring motor impairment in prevalence studies.' *Journal of Chronic Diseases*, **22**, 303 (1969).

[B 264] Johnson, D. A. W. 'A further study of psychiatric out-patient services in Manchester. An operational study of general practitioner and patient expectation.' *British Journal of Psychiatry*, **123**, 185 (1973).

[B 265] Jones, D. and Bourne, A. 'Monitoring the distribution of resources in the national health service.' *Social and Economic Administration*, **10**, 92 (1976).

[B 266] Jones, D. and Masterman, S. 'NHS resources: scales of variation.' *British Journal of Social and Preventive Medicine*, **30**, 244 (1976).

[B 267] Jones, K. *A History of the Mental Health Services*. London, Routledge & Kegan Paul, 1972.

[B 268] Jones, K. *et al. Opening the Door. A study of new policies for the mentally handicapped*. London, Routledge & Kegan Paul, 1975.

[B 269] Kaeser, A. C. and Cooper, B. 'The psychiatric patient, the general practitioner, and the outpatient clinic: an operational study and a review.' *Psychological Medicine*, **1**, 312 (1971).

[B 270] Kalimo, E. and Rubin, D. L. 'Relationship among indicators of morbidity: cross national comparisons.' *Journal of Chronic Diseases*, **29**, 1 (1976).

[B 271] Kannell, C. F., Marquis, A. H. and Laurent, A. *An Experimental Study on the Effect of Reinforcement, Question Length, and Re-interviewing in Reporting Selected Chronic Conditions in Household Interviews*. Michigan, Survey Research Centre University of Michigan, 1969.

[B 272] Kay, C. R. 'A comparison of two methods of determining social status.' *Journal of the Royal College of General Practitioners*, **16**, 162 (1968).

[B 273] Kent, H. M. 'Cervical cytology in Herefordshire.' *Public Health, London*, **88**, 275 (1974).

[B 274] Kessel, W. I. N. and Walton, H. *Alcoholism*. Harmondsworth, Penguin, 1969.

[B 275] King's Fund. *Accounting for Health*. London, King Edward's Fund for London, 1973.

[B 276] Knox, E. G. 'Research and health services.' In *Probes for Health*, ed. McLachlan, G., p. 1. London, Oxford University Press for Nuffield Provincial Hospitals Trust, 1975.

[B 277] Kohn, R. and White, K. L. (eds.). *Health Care. An International Study. Report of the World Health Organization/International Collaborative Study of Medical Care Utilization*. London, Oxford University Press, 1976.

[B 278] Kuenssberg, E. V. 'Recording of morbidity of families "F" book.' *Journal of the Royal College of General Practitioners*, **7**, 410 (1964).

[B 279] Lambert, P. M. Personal communication, 1972.

[B 280] *Lancet*. 'Another go at measuring outcome.' *Lancet*, **2**, 613 (1976).

[B 281] Last, J. M. 'The iceberg: "completing the clinical picture" in general practice.' *Lancet*, **2**, 28 (1963).

[B 282] Last, J. M. 'Overseas movement of British doctors.' *Social and Economic Administration*, **1**, 20 (1967).

[B 283] Last, J. M. and Stanley, G. R. 'Performance in medical school examinations.' *British Journal of Medical Education*, **3**, 43 (1969).

[B 284] Lawrie, J. E., Newhouse, M. L. and Elliott, P. M. 'Working capacity of women doctors.' *British Medical Journal*, **1**, 409 (1966).

[B 285] Lee, J. A. H. 'The effectiveness of routine examination of schoolchildren.' *British Medical Journal*, **1**, 573 (1958).

[B 286] Lee, R. H. *et al.* 'Rehabilitation policy. A study of a regional rehabilitation hospital.' *Hospital and Health Services Review*, **70**, 346 (1974).

[B 287] Lees, D. S. and Cooper, M. H. 'The work of the general practitioner.' *Journal of the College of General Practitioners*, **6**, 408 (1963).

[B 288] Levitt, H. N. 'Diagnostic facilities for general practitioners in England and Wales.' *Journal of the College of General Practitioners*, **8**, 312 (1964).

[B 289] Lilienfeld, A. M. and Pasamanick, B. 'The association of maternal and fetal factors with the development of cerebral palsy and epilepsy.' *American Journal of Obstetrics and Gynecology*, **70**, 93 (1955).

[B 290] Logan, R. F. L. 'Studies in the spectrum of medical care.' In *Problems and Progress in Medical Care*, ed. McLachlan, G. London, Oxford University Press for Nuffield Provincial Hospitals Trust, 1964.

[B 291] Luckman, J. and Murray, F. 'Management policies for a gynaecological department: a case study.' *Health Trends*, **4**, 33 (1972).

[B 292] Lunn, J. E. 'School health service work in the ordinary day schools. II. A modified selective inspection procedure derived from a study of the periodic entrance inspection.' *Medical Officer*, **118**, 313 (1967).

[B 293] McColl, I. and Fernow, L. C. 'Audit of audit.' *Lancet*, **2**, 738 (1976).

[B 294] McColl, I., Mackie, L. C. and Rendall, M. 'Communication as a method of medical audit.' *Lancet*, **1**, 1341 (1976).

[B 295] McCowen, P., and Wilder, J. *Lifestyle of 100 Psychiatric Patients: some costs and policy implications for rehabilitation*. London, Psychiatric Rehabilitation Association, 1975.

[B 296] MacGregor, J. E., Fraser, M. E. and Mann, E. M. F. 'The cytopipette in the diagnosis of early cervical carcinoma.' *Lancet*, **1**, 252 (1966).

[B 297] McGregor, R. M. 'The review of a family practice.' *Health Bulletin*, **11**, 14 and **12**, 41 (1953).

[B 298] McKeown, T. *et al. Screening in Medical Care: Reviewing the Evidence*. London, Oxford University Press for Nuffield Provincial Hospitals Trust, 1968.

[B 299] McLachlan, G. (ed.). *Problems and Progress in Medical Care. Essays on Current Research, Second Series*. London, Oxford University Press for Nuffield Provincial Hospitals Trust, 1966.

[B 300] McLachlan, G. *Portfolio for Health. 2. The developing programme of the DHSS in health services research*. London, Oxford University Press for Nuffield Provincial Hospitals Trust, 1973.

[B 301] McSherry, C. K. 'Quality assurance: the cost of utilization review and the educational value of medical audit in a university hospital.' *Surgery*, **80**, 122 (1976).

[B 302] Malleson, A. *Need Your Doctor be so Useless?* London, Allen & Unwin, 1973.

[B 303] Mansfield, P. 'The study and evaluation of general practice.' *Journal of the Royal College of General Practitioners*, **23**, 887 (1973).

[B 304] Marr, J. W. 'Individual weighed dietary surveys.' *Nutrition*, **19**, 18 (1965).

[B 305] Marsh, G. N. and McNay, R. A. 'Team workload in an English general practice. I.' *British Medical Journal*, **1**, 315 (1974) (I).

[B 306] Marsh, G. N. and McNay, R. A. 'Factors affecting workload in general practice. II.' *British Medical Journal*, **1**, 319 (1974) (II).

[B 307] Marshall, T., Farmer, R. D. T. and Cross, K. W. 'A new method of comparing consulting patterns in general practice.' In *Probes for Health*, ed. McLachlan, G., p. 125. London, Oxford University Press for Nuffield Provincial Hospitals Trust, 1975.

[B 308] Marson, W. S. *et al.* 'Measuring the quality of general practice.' *Journal of the Royal College of General Practitioners*, **23**, 23 (1973).

[B 309] Martin, A. and Millard, P. H. 'The new patient index—a method of measuring the activity of day hospitals.' *Age and Ageing*, **4**, 119 (1975).

[B 310] Martin, J. P. *Social Aspects of Prescribing*. London, Heinemann, 1957.

[B 311] Matthew, G. K. 'Measuring need and evaluating services.' In *Portfolio for Health—Problems and Progress in Medical Care*, 6, ed. McLachlan, G., p. 27. London, Oxford University Press for Nuffield Provincial Hospitals Trust, 1971.

[B 312] Maynard, A. 'Inequalities in psychiatric care in England and Wales.' *Social Science and Medicine*, **6**, 221 (1972).

[B 313] Maynard, A. and Tingle, R. 'The mental health services: a review of the statistical sources and a critical assessment of their usefulness.' *British Journal of Psychiatry*, **124**, 317 (1974).

[B 314] Meade, T. W. *et al.* 'Observer variation in recording the peripheral pulses.' *British Heart Journal*, **40**, 661 (1968).

[B 315] Mechanic, D. *Medical Sociology*. New York, Free Press, 1968.

[B 316] Mechanic, D. 'General practice in England and Wales: results from a survey of a national sample of general practitioners.' *Medical Care*, **6**, 245 (1968).

[B 317] Mechanic, D. 'Practice orientations among general medical practitioners in England and Wales.' *Medical Care*, **8**, 15 (1970).

[B 318] Mechanic, D. 'General medical practice: some comparisons between the work of primary care physicians in the United States and England and Wales.' *Medical Care*, **10**, 402 (1972).

[B 319] Medical Research Council: Committee on research into chronic bronchitis. *Questionnaire on Respiratory Symptoms*. London, Medical Research Council, 1966.

[B 320] Mencher, S. *British Private Medical Practice and the National Health Service*. Pittsburgh, University of Pittsburgh, 1968.

[B 321] Miller, D. M. 'Cervical cytology consent rate.' *Lancet*, **2**, 491 (1969).

[B 322] Milne, J. S., Maule, M. M. and Williamson, J. 'Methods of sampling in the study of older people, with comparison of respondents and non-respondents.' *British Journal of Preventive and Social Medicine,* **25**, 37 (1971).

[B 323] Milne, J. S. and Williamson, J. 'Comparison of a teaching machine with an observer in the detection of angina pectoris by questionnaire.' *British Journal of Preventive and Social Medicine,* **25**, 105 (1971).

[B 324] Ministry of Health. *A Hospital Plan for England and Wales,* Cmnd. 1604. London, HMSO, 1962.

[B 325] Ministry of Health. *Accident and Emergency Services. Report of the Sub-committee of the Standing Medical Advisory Committee* (Chairman: Sir Harry Platt). London, HMSO, 1962.

[B 326] Ministry of Health. *The Hospital Building Programme. A Revision of the Hospital Plan for England and Wales,* Cmnd. 3000. London, HMSO, 1966.

[B 327] Ministry of Health, Department of Health for Scotland, Ministry of Education. *An Inquiry into Health Visiting. Report of a Working Party on the Field of Work, Training and Recruitment of Health Visitors* (Chairman: Sir Wilson Jameson). London, HMSO, 1956, reprinted 1974.

[B 328] Ministry of Housing and Local Government. *Report of the Committee on Local Authority and Allied Personal Social Services* (Chairman: F. Seebohm), Cmnd. 3703. London, HMSO, 1968.

[B 329] Mitton, R. 'Some area variations in birth control services.' *Community Medicine,* **129**, 183 (1972).

[B 330] Mitton, R. 'Family planning clinics in 1970.' *Family Planning,* **22**, 30 (1973).

[B 331] Moir, D. C. and Hedley, E. A. 'Re-evaluation of a method of prescribing drugs in hospital.' *Health Bulletin,* **29**, 131 (1971).

[B 332] Montacute, C. *Costing and Efficiency in Hospitals.* London, Oxford University Press for Nuffield Provincial Hospitals Trust, 1962.

[B 333] Montgomery, K. 'Out-patients of a London teaching hospital.' *British Journal of Preventive and Social Medicine,* **22**, 50 (1968).

[B 334] Morgan, M. *The Census of Residential Accommodation: 1970. II. Residential Accommodation for the Mentally Ill and for the Mentally Handicapped.* London, Department of Health and Social Security, Welsh Office, 1975.

[B 335] Morrell, D. C. 'Symptom interpretation in general practice.' *Journal of the Royal College of General Practitioners,* **22**, 297 (1972).

[B 336] Morrell, D. C., Gage, H. G. and Robinson, N. A. 'Patterns of demand in general practice.' *Journal of the Royal College of General Practitioners,* **19**, 331 (1970).

[B 337] Morrell, D. C., Gage, H. G. and Robinson, N. A. 'Referral to hospital by general practitioners.' *Journal of the Royal College of General Practitioners,* **21**, 77 (1971).

[B 338] Morrell, D. C. and Kasap, H. S. 'The effect of an appointment system on demand for medical care.' *International Journal of Epidemiology,* **2**, 143 (1972).

[B 339] Morrell, D. C. and Nicholson, S. 'Measuring the results of changes in the method of delivering primary medical care—a cautionary tale.' *Journal of the Royal College of General Practitioners,* **24**, 111 (1974).

[B 340] Morris, J. N. 'Recent history of coronary disease.' *Lancet,* **1**, 1 and 69 (1951).

[B 341] Morton-Williams, J. and Berthoud, R. *Nurses Attitude Survey.* London, Social and Community Planning Research, 1971.

[B 342] Moser, C. A. and Kalton, G. *Survey methods in social investigation.* London, Heinemann, 1971.

[B 343] Munday, A. 'Physiological measures of anxiety in hospital patients.' *RCN Study of Nursing Care,* Series 2, No. 3. London, Royal College of Nursing, 1973.

[B 344] Munro, J. E. and Ratoff, L. 'The accuracy of general practice records.' *Journal of the Royal College of General Practitioners,* **23**, 821 (1973).

[B 345] Murray, R. M. 'Survey of analgesic consumption.' *Lancet,* **1**, 554 (1973).

[B 346] National Centre of Health Statistics. *Reporting of Hospitalization in the Health Interview Survey.* Washington, U.S. Department of Health, Education, and Welfare, 1965.

[B 347] *National Health Service Reorganization Act 1973,* Chapter 32. London, HMSO, 1973.

[B 348] Newson, J. and Newson, E. *Infant Care in an Urban Community.* London, Allen & Unwin, 1963.

[B 349] Newson, J. and Newson, E. *Four Year Olds in an Urban Community.* London, Allen & Unwin, 1968.

[B 350] Newson, J. and Newson, E. *Seven Year Olds in an Urban Environment.* London, Allen & Unwin, 1976.

[B 351] Nightingale, F. *Notes on Hospitals.* London, Longmans Green, 1863.

[B 352] Northern Ireland General Health Services Board, *Twenty-fifth Annual Report Year 1972–73.* Belfast, Northern Ireland General Health Services Board, 1973.

[B 353] Northern Ireland Health and Personal Social Services. *Directory.* Belfast, Northern Ireland Health and Personal Social Services, 1976.

[B 354] Northern Ireland Hospitals Authority. *Hospital Directory for period ending 31st March 1973.* Belfast, Northern Ireland Hospitals Authority, 1972.

[B 355] Nuffield Provincial Hospitals Trust. *Studies in the Functions and Design of Hospitals.* Chapter 2:

'The Outpatient Service'. London, Oxford University Press for Nuffield Provincial Hospitals Trust, 1955.

[B 356] Nuffield Provincial Hospitals Trust. *Studies in the Function and Design of Hospitals*. Chapter 7: 'Planning to meet demand.' London, Oxford University Press for Nuffield Provincial Hospitals Trust, 1955.

[B 357] Nuffield Provincial Hospitals Trust. *Towards a Clearer View. The Organization of Diagnostic X-ray Departments*. London, Oxford University Press for Nuffield Provincial Hospitals Trust, 1962.

[B 358] Nuffield Provincial Hospitals Trust. *Portfolio of Health, 2. Problems and Progress in Medical Care*, 8th series, ed. McLachlan, G. London, Oxford University Press for Nuffield Provincial Hospitals Trust, 1973.

[B 359] Oddie, J. A. *et al.* 'The community hospital. A pilot trial.' *Lancet,* **2**, 308 (1971).

[B 360] Office of Health Economics. *The NHS Reorganisation*. London, Office of Health Economics, 1974.

[B 361] Opit, L. J. and Farmer, R. D. T. 'Cost of dispensing in the pharmaceutical services.' *Lancet,* **1**, 160 (1974).

[B 362] Oppenheim, A. N. *Questionnaire Design and Attitude Measurement*. London, Heinemann, 1966.

[B 363] Parkhouse, J. 'Where do graduates do their jobs?' *British Journal of Medical Education,* **10**, 408 (1976).

[B 364] Parkhouse, J. 'A follow-up of career preferences.' *British Journal of Medical Education,* **10**, 480 (1976).

[B 365] Parry, W. H. and Seymour, M. W. 'Epidemiology of battered babies in Nottingham.' *Community Medicine,* **126**, 121 (1971).

[B 366] Parsons, T. *The Social Systems*. Glencoe, The Free Press, 1951.

[B 367] Pemberton, J. 'Illness in general practice.' *British Medical Journal,* **1**, 306 (1949).

[B 368] Piachaud, D. and Weddell, J. M. 'The economics of treating varicose veins.' *International Journal of Epidemiology,* **1**, 287 (1972).

[B 369] Pickett, K. G. *Sources of Official Data*. London, Longman, 1974.

[B 370] Pickles, W. N. *Epidemiology in Country Practice*. Bristol, Wright 1939; Devonshire Press, reissued 1972.

[B 371] Pike, L. A. 'A screening programme for the elderly in general practice.' *Practitioner,* **203**, 805 (1969).

[B 372] Pinker, R. *English Hospital Statistics 1861–1938*. London, Heinemann, 1966.

[B 373] Pinnock, R. Personal communication, 1976.

[B 374] Raftery, E. B. and Holland, W. W. 'Examination of the heart: an investigation into variation.' *American Journal of Epidemiology,* **85**, 438 (1967).

[B 375] Rankine, R. and Weir, R. M. L. 'Enquiry into the incidence of chronic illness and disability in the young and middle-aged.' Quoted in Scottish Home and Health Department Report (B 406).

[B 376] Rawnsley, K. and Loudon, J. B. 'Factors influencing the referral of patients to psychiatrists by general practitioners.' *British Journal of Preventive and Social Medicine,* **16**, 174 (1962).

[B 377] Rawson, A. 'Deafness: report of a departmental inquiry into the promotion of research.' *DHSS Reports on Health and Social Subjects*, No. 4. London, HMSO, 1973.

[B 378] Records and Statistics Unit of the College of General Practitioners. 'The analysis of routine medical records.' *Journal of the College of General Practitioners,* **11**, 34 (1966).

[B 379] Redman, N. R., Toby, J. P. and Peniket, J. B. 'Hospital junior doctors: survey at Northampton General Hospital.' *British Medical Journal,* **3**, 522 (1969).

[B 380] Reedy, B. L. E. C. 'Usefulness of a gazetteer of general practice.' *British Medical Journal,* **4**, 419 (1975).

[B 381] Rein, M. 'Social class and the health service.' *New Society,* **14**, 807 (1969).

[B 382] Research Unit, Royal College of General Practitioners. 'The analysis of summarized data using "S" cards.' *Journal of the Royal College of General Practitioners,* **22**, 377 (1972).

[B 383] Research Unit, Royal College of General Practitioners. 'A general practice glossary.' *Journal of the Royal College of General Practitioners,* **23**, Supplement No. 3 (1973).

[B 384] Richardson, I. M. 'General practitioners and district nurses.' *British Journal of Preventive and Social Medicine,* **28**, 187 (1974).

[B 385] Rickard, J. H. 'The costs of domiciliary nursing care.' *Journal of the Royal College of General Practitioners,* **24**, 839 (1974).

[B 386] Rickard, J. H. 'Per capita expenditure of the English area health authorities.' *British Medical Journal,* **1**, 299 (1976).

[B 387] Rickard, J. H. *A Cost Effectiveness Analysis of the Oxford Community Hospital Programme*. Oxford, Department of the Regius Professor of Medicine and the Oxford Regional Health Authority, 1976.

[B 388] Riddell, J. 'Scottish local health authorities—medical staffing.' *Health Bulletin,* **20**, 72 (1962).

[B 389] Roberts, J. A. 'Economics evaluation of health care: a survey.' *British Journal of Social and Preventive Medicine*, **28**, 210 (1974).

[B 390] Robertson, N. C. 'The incidence of referrals to the psychiatric services by individual general practitioners.' In *Proceedings of the Conference on Psychiatric Case Registers at the University of Aberdeen March 1973*, ed. Hall, D. J., Robertson, N. C. and Eason, R. J. *Statistical and Research Report Series*, No. 7. London, HMSO, 1974.

[B 391] Robinson, R. B. *General Practitioner Hospital Beds—a regional census and survey of patients and facilities*. Croydon, South-East Metropolitan Regional Hospital Board, 1973.

[B 392] Rose, G. A. 'The diagnosis of heart pain and intermittent claudication in field surveys.' *Bulletin of the World Health Organization*, **27**, 645 (1962).

[B 393] Rose, G. A. and Blackburn, H. 'Cardiovascular survey methods.' *WHO Monograph Series*, No. 56. Geneva, World Health Organization, 1968.

[B 394] Rose, G. A., Holland, W. W. and Crowley, E. A. 'A sphygmomanometer for epidemiologists.' *Lancet*, **1**, 296 (1964).

[B 395] Ross, A. 'Acute bed requirements.' *British Medical Journal*, **2**, 430 (1972).

[B 396] Rosser, R. M. and Watts, V. C. 'The measurement of hospital output.' *International Journal of Epidemiology*, **1**, 361 (1972).

[B 397] Rowntree, B. S. *Old People*. London, Oxford University Press, 1947.

[B 398] Royal College of General Practitioners. *The Practice Nurse. Further development of her role in general practice and its effect on the doctor's work*. Reports from General Practice No. 10. London, Royal College of General Practitioners, 1968.

[B 399] Ruiz, L., Colley, J. R. P. and Hamilton, P. J. S. 'Measurement of triceps skinfold thickness: an investigation of sources of variation.' *British Journal of Preventive and Social Medicine*, **25**, 165 (1971).

[B 400] Rutstein, D. D. *et al.* 'Measuring the quality of medical care: a clinical method.' *New England Journal of Medicine*, **294**, 582 (1976).

[B 401] Sainsbury, P. 'A comparative evaluation of a comprehensive community psychiatric service.' In *Policy for Action*, ed. Cawley, R. and McLachlan, G., p. 129. London, Oxford University Press for Nuffield Provincial Hospitals Trust, 1973.

[B 402] Sanazaro, P. J. 'Medical audit: experience in the U.S.A.' *British Medical Journal*, **1**, 271 (1974).

[B 403] Sansom, C. D., Wakefield, J. and Yule, R. 'Cervical cytology in the Manchester region: changing patterns of response.' *Medical Officer*, **123**, 357 (1970).

[B 404] Saunders, J. and Snaith, A. H. 'Cervical cytology. A computer-assisted population screening programme.' *Medical Officer*, **117**, 299 (1967).

[B 405] Scottish Home and Health Department. *Experimental Nurse Training at Glasgow Royal Infirmary*. Edinburgh, HMSO, 1963.

[B 406] Scottish Home and Health Department. *The Young Chronic Sick. Report of a sub-committee of the Scottish Health Services Council*. Edinburgh, HMSO, 1964.

[B 407] Scottish Home and Health Department. *Doctors in an Integrated Health Service—report of a joint working party appointed by the Secretary of State for Scotland*. Edinburgh, HMSO, 1971.

[B 408] Scottish Home and Health Department. *Scottish Health Statistics*. Edinburgh, HMSO (Annual).

[B 409] Scottish Hospital Advisory Service. *Quinquennial report, 1970–74*. Edinburgh, Scottish Home and Health Department, 1975.

[B 410] Seglow, J., Kellmer-Pringle, M. and Wedge, P. *Growing Up Adopted*. London, National Foundation for Educational Research in England and Wales, 1972.

[B 411] Seymour, J., Conway, N. and Bridger, E. 'Electrocardiograph service for general practitioners: an appraisal.' *British Medical Journal*, **1**, 305 (1968).

[B 412] Sharpe, J. E. *et al.* 'Prevalence of chronic bronchitis in an American male urban and industrial population.' *American Review of Respiratory Disease*, **91**, 510 (1965).

[B 413] Sheffield Regional Hospital Board. *Hospital Statistics Year 1972*. Sheffield, Statistics Section, Sheffield Regional Hospital Board [1973].

[B 414] Silversin, J. B., Shafer, S. M. and Sheiham, A. 'Dental education in Great Britain and the United States.' *Journal of Dental Education*, **38**, 497 (1974).

[B 415] Smith, F. and Seddon, T. M. 'Transport of patients in general practice.' *Journal of the Royal College of General Practitioners*, **15**, 52 (1968).

[B 416] Smith, J. W. *et al.* 'Comparative study of district and community hospitals.' *British Medical Journal*, **2**, 471 (1973).

[B 417] Smithells, R. W. 'The Liverpool congenital abnormalities registry.' *Developmental Medicine and Child Neurology*, **4**, 320 (1962).

[B 418] South East Metropolitan Regional Hospital Board Management Services Division. *Hospital Statistics 1972*, 2 volumes. Croydon, Statistics and O.R. Department, South East Metropolitan Regional Hospital Board, 1973.

[B 419] South East Thames Regional Health Authority. *Directory*. Croydon, South East Thames Regional Health Authority, 1974.

[B 420] South Western Regional Hospital Board. *In-patient and Out-patient Statistics for the Year 1972*. Bristol, South Western Regional Hospital Board [1973].

[B 421] Sowerby, P. R. 'The use of transport in a rural practice.' *Journal of the Royal College of General Practitioners*, **17**, 131 (1969).

[B 422] Specialist Group on Management Services and Statistics. 'Report from the sub-group on statistical services..Appendix C.' In *A Report from the Working Party on Collaboration between the NHS and Local Government on its activities from January to July 1973*. London, HMSO, 1973.

[B 423] Spencer, J. T. 'A diagnostic work study index.' *Journal of the Royal College of General Practitioners*, **13**, 39 (1967).

[B 424] Starey, C. J. H. 'A hospital outpatient referral survey.' *Journal of the College of General Practitioners*, **4**, 214 (1961).

[B 425] Stewart, R. and Sleeman, J. *Continuously under Review. A study of the management of out-patient departments. Occasional Papers on Social Administration*, No. 20. London, Bell, 1967.

[B 426] Stocks, P. 'The measurement of morbidity.' *Proceedings of the Royal Society of Medicine*, **37**, 593 (1944).

[B 427] Stocks, P. *Sickness in th   ̫pulation of England and Wales, 1944–1947*. London, HMSO, 1949.

[B 428] Stuart, A. *Basic Ideas ̫ ̫cientific Sampling*. London, Griffin, 1968.

[B 429] Sutcliffe, E. M. 'The social accounting of health.' In *The Economics of Medical Care*, ed. Hauser, M. M., p. 238. London, Allen & Unwin, 1972.

[B 430] Taylor, T. 'The quality of health care.' *Scottish Medical Journal*, **20**, 45 (1975).

[B 431] Thompson, A. M. C. (ed.). *A Bibliography of Nursing Literature 1859–1960. With an Historical Introduction*. London, Library Association for The Royal College of Nursing, 1968.

[B 432] Thompson, A. M. C. (ed.). *A Bibliography of Nursing Literature 1961–1970*. London, Library Association for the Royal College of Nursing, 1974.

[B 433] Thompson, P. 'Cervical cytology consent rate.' *Lancet*, **2**, 385 (1969).

[B 434] Thould, A. K. 'Medical audit: necessary, but rigidity greatest danger.' *British Medical Journal*, **1**, 279 (1974).

[B 435] Titmus, R. *Commitment to Welfare*. London, Allen & Unwin, 1968.

[B 436] Todd, G. F. *Reliability of Statements about Smoking Habits: supplementary report*. London, Tobacco Research Council, 1966.

[B 437] Townsend, P. *The Disabled in Society*. London, Royal College of Surgeons, 1967.

[B 438] Trent Regional Health Authority. *Directory and Code List of Premises in the Region according to Area and District Health Authority*. Sheffield, Statistics and Medical Records Section, Sheffield Regional Hospital Board, 1974.

[B 439] Trevelyan, M. H. and Cooke, J. 'Use of acute medical and general-practitioner beds by the practitioners working in one new town.' *Journal of the Royal College of General Practitioners*, **24**, 477 (1974).

[B 440] Trout, K. *An Experiment in Out-patient Information*. Sheffield, Chesterfield Hospital Management Committee, and Sheffield Regional Hospital Board, 1972.

[B 441] Trout, K. and Martindale, A. *An Experiment in Out-patient Information*. Sheffield, Statistics Section, Trent Regional Health Authority, 1974.

[B 442] Twaddle, A. C. 'The concept of health status.' *Social Science and Medicine*, **8**, 29 (1974).

[B 443] Vaananen, I. 'The role of the medical record in hospital planning systems.' In *Information Processing of Medical Records*, ed. Anderson J. and Forsythe, J. M., p. 160. Amsterdam, North-Holland, 1970.

[B 444] Vere, D. 'Primum non nocere, or the pharmacological lucky dip.' *British Medical Journal*, **2**, 816 (1976).

[B 445] Vessey, M. P., Johnston, B. and Donnelly, J. 'Reliability of reporting by women taking part in a prospective contraceptive study.' *British Journal of Preventive and Social Medicine*, **28**, 104 (1974).

[B 446] Wade, O. L. 'Prescribing of chloramphenicol and aplastic anaemia.' *Journal of the College of General Practitioners*, **12**, 277 (1966).

[B 447] Wade, O. L. 'The computer and drug prescribing.' In *Computers in the Service of Medicine*, Vol. I, ed. McLachlan, G. and Shegog, R. A. London, Oxford University Press for Nuffield Provincial Hospitals Trust, 1968.

[B 448] Wade, O. L. and Hood, H. E. 'An analysis of prescribing of an hypnotic in the community.' *British Journal of Preventive and Social Medicine*, **26**, 121 (1972).

[B 449] Wade, O. L. and McDevitt, G. D. 'Prescribing and the British National Formulary.' *British Medical Journal*, **2**, 635 (1966).

[B 450] Waite, M. *Consultant Gynaecologists and Birth Control*. London, Birth Control Trust, 1974.

[B 451] Waite, M. 'Consultant psychiatrists and abortion.' *Journal of Psychological Medicine*, **4**, 74 (1974).

[B 452] Walker, R. G., Miller, W. R. and McLean, I. G. *A Study of the Work of Hospital Junior Medical Staff. Scottish Health Services Studies*, No. 10. Edinburgh, Scottish Home and Health Department, 1969.

[B 453] Wallace, B. B. *et al.* 'Unrestricted access by general practitioners to a department of diagnostic radiology.' *Journal of the Royal College of General Practitioners*, **23**, 337 (1973).

[B 454] Ward, A. W. M. 'Women doctors graduating at Sheffield, 1933–1957.' *Medical Officer*, **122**, 287 (1969).

[B 455] Warren, M. D. 'Interview surveys of handicapped people: the accuracy of statements about the underlying medical conditions.' *Rheumatology and Rehabilitation*, **15**, 295 (1976).

[B 456] Welsh Office. *Health and Personal Social Services Statistics for Wales*. Cardiff, HMSO (Annual).

[B 457] Western Health and Social Services Board, Northern Ireland. *The First Annual Report of the Western Health and Social Services Board for the Year 1974*. Londonderry, Western Health and Social Services Board, 1975.

[B 458] Wheeler, M. 'How many acute beds do we really need?' *British Medical Journal*, **4**, 220 (1972).

[B 459] Whitehead, F. 'Social security statistics.' In *Reviews of United Kingdom Statistical Sources*, Vol. II, ed. Maunder, W. F. London, Heinemann, 1974.

[B 460] Whitehead, T. P. *Progress in Medical Computing*. London, Elliott Medical Automation, 1965.

[B 461] Whitehead, T. P. 'Quality control techniques in laboratory services.' *British Medical Bulletin*, **30**, 237 (1974).

[B 462] Whitfield, A. G. W. 'Higher medical and surgical degrees of the University of Birmingham.' *British Journal of Medical Education*, **1**, 359 (1967).

[B 463] Whitfield, A. G. W. 'Emigration of Birmingham medical graduates 1959–63.' *Lancet*, **1**, 667 (1969).

[B 464] Whitfield, A. G. W. 'Current work of Birmingham medical graduates 1959–63.' *Lancet*, **1**, 882 (1969).

[B 465] Whitfield, M. J. 'The relationship between year of registration and morbidity in general practice.' *Journal of the Royal College of General Practitioners*, **22**, 675 (1972).

[B 466] Whyte, R. 'Psychiatric new-patient clinic non-attenders.' *British Journal of Psychiatry*, **127**, 160 (1975).

[B 467] Wilkerson, H. L. C. and Krall, L. P. 'Diabetes in a New England town.' *Journal of the American Medical Association*, **135**, 209 (1947).

[B 468] Williams, A. 'Measuring the effectiveness of health care systems.' *British Journal of Preventive and Social Medicine*, **28**, 196 (1974).

[B 469] Williams, A. '"Need" as a demand concept (with special reference to health).' In *Economic Policies and Social Goals*, ed. Culyer, A. J., p. 60. London, Robertson, 1974.

[B 470] Williams, B. T., Dixon, R. A. and Knowelden, J. 'Emergency admission to hospital from a deputizing service. A controlled study of duration of stay and outcome.' *British Journal of Preventive and Social Medicine*, **27**, 126 (1973).

[B 471] Williams, B. T., Dixon, R. A. and Knowelden, J. 'B.M.A. deputizing service in Sheffield, 1970.' *British Medical Journal*, **1**, 593 (1973).

[B 472] Williams, B. T., Dixon, R. A. and Knowelden, J. 'The impact of general-practitioner deputising services on accident and emergency departments in the Sheffield hospital region.' *Journal of the Royal College of General Practitioners*, **23**, 638 (1973).

[B 473] Williamson, P. M. 'The adoption of new drugs by doctors practising in group and solo practice.' *Social Science and Medicine*, **9**, 233 (1975).

[B 474] Wilson, C. W. M. *et al.* 'Influence of different sources of therapeutic information on prescribing by general practitioners.' *British Medical Journal*, **2**, 599 (1963).

[B 475] Wilson, C. W. M. *et al.* 'Pattern of prescribing in general practice.' *British Medical Journal*, **2**, 604 (1963).

[B 476] Wing, J. K. 'Principles of evaluation.' In *Evaluating a Community Psychiatric Service. The Camberwell Register 1964–71*, ed. Wing, J. K. and Hailey, A. M., p. 11. London, Oxford University Press for Nuffield Provincial Hospitals Trust, 1972.

[B 477] Wing, J. K. and Hailey, A. M. (eds.). *Evaluating a Community Psychiatric Service. The Camberwell Register 1964–71*. London, Oxford University Press for Nuffield Provincial Hospitals Trust, 1972.

[B 478] Wolff, H. Z. 'The place of psychotherapy in the district psychiatric services.' In *Policy for Action*, ed. Cawley, R. and McLachlan, G., p. 117. London, Oxford University Press for Nuffield Provincial Hospitals Trust, 1973.

[B 479] Wood, P. H. N. 'Epidemiology of rheumatic disorders: problems of classification.' *Proceedings of the Royal Society of Medicine*, **63**, 189 (1970).

[B 480] Wood, P. H. N. '2. Recent trends in sickness absence and mortality.' *Annals of the Rheumatic Diseases,* **29**, 324 (1970).

[B 481] Wood, P. H. N. '4. Morbidity and mortality, and hospital services for rheumatism sufferers.' *Annals of the Rheumatic Diseases,* **31**, 522 (1972).

[B 482] Wood, P. H. N. and Benn, R. T. 'Digest of data on the rheumatic diseases. 1. Digest of morbidity and mortality data on the rheumatic diseases.' *Annals of the Rheumatic Diseases,* **28**, 443 (1969).

[B 483] Wood, P. H. N. and Benn, R. T. '3. Handicap and disability, and international comparisons of morbidity and mortality.' *Annals of the Rheumatic Diseases,* **31**, 72 (1972).

[B 484] Wood, P. H. N. and McLeish, C. L. '5. Morbidity in industry, and rheumatism in general practice.' *Annals of the Rheumatic Diseases,* **33**, 93 (1974).

[B 485] Woodcock, K. 'How useful are our present statistics on sexually transmitted disease?' *British Journal of Venereal Diseases,* **51**, 153 (1975).

[B 486] Woodford-Williams, E. and Alvarez, A. S. 'Four years experience of a day hospital in geriatric practice.' *Gerontologica clinica,* **7**, 96 (1965).

[B 487] World Health Organization. *Report of the International Pilot Study of Schizophrenia.* Geneva, World Health Organization, 1973.

[B 488] World Health Organization. 'Clearing house on health indexes.' *World Health Statistical Reports,* **29**, 140 (1976).

[B 489] Wright, B. M. and McKerrow, C. B. 'Maximum forced expiratory flow rate as a measure of ventilatory capacity, with description of a new portable instrument for measuring.' *British Medical Journal,* **1**, 1041 (1959).

[B 490] Yasin, S. *et al.* 'Assessment of habitual physical activity apart from occupation.' *British Journal of Preventive and Social Medicine,* **21**, 163 (1967).

[B 491] Yates, J. M. 'Information for the management of clinical work in hospitals.' In *The Future and Present Indicatives,* ed. McLachlan, G., p. 137. London, Oxford University Press for Nuffield Provincial Hospitals Trust, 1973.

[B 492] Yerushalmy, J. 'Statistical problems in assessing methods of medical diagnosis, with special reference to X-ray techniques.' *Public Health Reports,* **62**, 1432 (1947).

[B 493] Yule, R. 'The frequency of cytologic testing.' *Acta Cytologica,* **16**, 389 (1972).

[B 494] Scottish Home and Health Department. *The Health Service in Scotland. The Way Ahead.* Edinburgh, HMSO, 1976.

[B 495] Bates, M. M. and Sharratt, M. 'The King's Fund Emergency Bed Service, London.' *Health Trends,* **7**, 73 (1975).

[B 496] Ministry of Health. *Review Body on Doctors' and Dentists' Remuneration. Seventh Report* (Chairman: Lord Kindersley), Cmnd. 2992. London, HMSO, 1966.

SUBJECT INDEX

Abnormality, congenital, 2.1.2; 2.5.10.2
Abortion, 2.1.2; 2.5.1; 3.1; 5.1.2.5
Absence from work, 1.4.5; 2.1.2; 2.4; 5.1.1; 6.2.5.2
Abstracts of published articles, 1.10.1
Acceptability of medical care, 6.2.3
Accessibility of medical care, 6.2.1
Accident and emergency department, 3.2; 5.4.2
Accident and emergency services, use of, 5.4.1
Accidents, 1.4.5; 2.5.2
Accidents, domestic, 2.5.2
Accidents, motor-cycle, 2.5.2
Accidents, road, 2.5.3; 5.4.2
Accuracy of biochemical measures, 1.7.5
Accuracy of data, 1.7.2; 1.7.3; 1.7.4; 1.7.5
Accuracy of haematological measures, 1.7.5
Accuracy of medical records, 2.3.2; 5.1.2
Accuracy of subjects' responses, 1.7.3
Activity limitation, 2.2.1.2
Acute bed provision, 4.1.2; 5.6.2
Acute beds, use of, 5.6.2; 6.2.4.1
Acute stroke, 2.1.2
Addiction, 2.5.3; 5.6.5.2
Addisonian anaemia, 2.2.2.2
Admission, emergency, 3.4
Adolescents in hospital, 5.6.2
Adopted children, 2.5.10.1
Adverse drug reactions, 2.2.1.2; 2.5.4; 6.2.5.2
AHA annual reports, 5.6.6
Aims of the NHS, 6.1
Alcoholism, 2.5.3; 5.6.5.2
Alimentary disease, 2.5.5
Ambulances, 4.1.1; 5.3
Amphetamines, 5.1.2.8
Anaemia, 2.2.2.2; 2.5.7
Anaemia, Addisonian, 2.2.2.2
Anaemia, iron-deficiency, 2.2.2.2
Anaemia, pernicious, 2.5.7
Anaesthetic, death under, 2.5.22
Analgesics, 2.2.1.2; 2.2.2.2
Angina questionnaire, WHO, 2.2.2.4
Annual reports, AHA, 5.6.6
Annual reports, BG, 5.6.6
Annual reports, Northern Ireland, 4; 5.6.6
Annual reports, RHA, 5.6.6
Annual reports, RHB, 5.6.6
Ante-natal records, 2.5.10.1
Anti-depressant drugs, 5.1.2.8
Anti-diabetic drugs, 5.1.2.8
Apnoeic attack, 2.5.10.1
Appointment systems, 2.3.2; 3.1; 5.1.2.3
Appointments, failure to keep, 6.2.3

Appointments, out-patient, 3.3; 5.4.3.2
Archive, SSRC Survey, 1.10.5
Archived statistics, 1.10.5
Area health authority, 1.4.4
Area Medical Officer, 1.4.4; 4.2.1
Arterial blood pressure, inheritance of, 2.2.2.2
Arthritis, 2.2.2.2; 2.5.6
Arthritis, rheumatoid, 2.2.2.2; 6.2.4.1
Artificial limb-fitting centres, 5.8
Asian subjects, 2.2.2.2
Association of Clinical Pathologists, 5.5.1
Association of Psychiatric Social Workers, 5.3.3
Asthma, 2.5.28
Audit, medical, 6.2.4
Audit of health care, 6.2.6
Autopsy data, coroners, 2.1.2
Available beds, 3.6

Barbiturate drugs, 5.1.2.8
Bed norms, 4.1.2
Bed provision, acute, 4.1.2; 5.6.2
Beds, available, 3.6
Beds, critical number of, 4.1.2
Beds, maternity, 4.1.4; 4.3.6
Beds, occupied, 3.6
Beds, use of, 2.3.3
Beds, use of acute, 5.6.2; 6.2.4.1
Bermondsey and Southwark, 2.2.2.3
Best buy hospitals, 4.1.2
BG annual reports, 5.6.6
Bias in data collection, 1.7.2; 1.7.3; 1.7.6; 2.1.1
Bias, memory, 1.7.3; 2.1.1; 2.2.1.1; 5.3.1; 5.4.1
Bibliographies of published works, 1.10.2
Biochemical measures, accuracy of, 1.7.5
Blindness, 2.5.17
Blood disease, 2.5.7
Blood pressure, high, 1.7.4
Blood pressure, inheritance of arterial, 2.2.2.2
Blood pressure, measurement of, 1.7.2; 1.7.4; 2.1.1;
    2.2.2.2
Blood pressure, systolic, 2.2.2.2
Breast cancer, 2.5.8
Breathalizer tests, 2.5.3
British Co-operative Clinic Group, 2.5.30
British Medical Association, 2.5.2; 4.2.6; 5.1.2.1;
    5.1.2.4
British National Formulary, 4.5.1
British Orthopaedic Association, 5.4.2
Bronchodilator aerosols, 5.1.2.8

Cancer, 2.1.2; 2.5.8

Cancer, breast, 2.5.8
Cancer, oral, 2.5.8
Cancer registration, 2.1.2; 2.5.8
CANCERLINE, 1.10.3
Carcinoma of the cervix, 1.7.5; 1.7.6; 2.3.1; 2.5.8; 6.2.3
Cardiac arrest in infants, 2.5.10.1
Cardiorespiratory disease, 1.7.6; 2.2.2.2; 2.2.2.4
Cardiovascular disease, 1.7.2; 1.7.4; 1.7.5; 2.1.2; 2.5.9; 2.5.25
Careers of medical graduates, 4.2.5
Casualty Surgeons Association, 5.4.2
Central Services Agency, Northern Ireland, 4
Centre for Extension Training in Community Medicine, 4.2.1
Cerebral irritations in infants, 2.5.10.1
Cerebral vessels, 2.5.9
Certificates, National Insurance, 5.1.2; 5.1.2.10
Certificates, private sickness, 5.1.2.10
Cervical cytology, 1.7.5; 1.7.6; 5.1.2; 5.3; 6.2.3; 7.2.1.5
Cervix, carcinoma of the, 1.7.5; 1.7.6; 2.3.1; 2.5.8; 6.2.3
Chest services, 5.5.1
Child abuse, 2.5.10.4
Child birth, 2.5.10.1
Child development, Newcastle Survey of, 2.5.10.1
Child development study, national, 2.5.10.1
Child guidance, 2.5.23; 5.3.3
Child health, institute of, 2.5.26
Child psychiatry, 5.3.3
Children, 2.5.10
Children, adopted, 2.5.10.1
Children, dental health of, 5.2.1
Children, educationally subnormal, 2.5.10.5; 2.5.24
Children, handicapped, 2.5.10.5
Children, height of, 2.5.26
Children in hospital, 5.6.2
Children, mentally handicapped, 2.5.24
Children, weight of, 2.5.26
Chiropodists, 2.1; 2.5.19; 4.4
Chiropody, 5.3
Chiropractor, 3
Chloramphenicol drugs, 5.1.2.8
Chronic sick, young, 2.5.21.1
Chronostamps, 4.3.7; 5.1.2.2
Classification of disease, international, 2.3.2.1; 2.3.2.2
Clearing house of health indexes, 2.1
Clinical Pathologists, Association of, 5.5.1
Committee on Medical Aspects of Food Policy, 2.5.25
Committee on Nursing, 4.3.1
Committee on Safety of Medicines, 6.2.5.2
Communication between patient and staff, 6.2.5.3
Community health doctor, 4.2.1
Community Health Services, 5.3
Community Health Services costs, 5.3
Community Health Services, referral to, 5.3.2
Community Health Services, use of, 5.3.1
Community Medicine, Centre for Extension Training in, 4.2.1

Community Medicine, Specialist in, 1.4.4
Community nurse attachment schemes, 4.3.2
Community nurses, 4.3.2; 5.3
Complaints in hospital, 6.2.5.3
Congenital abnormality, 2.1.2; 2.5.10.2
Consultants, 4.2.2
Consultants and Specialists Association, Hospital, 4.2.5
Consultation with general practitioner, 2.2.1.2; 5.1.2
Contraception, 2.5.18; 5.1.2.5; 6.2.3
Contraceptives, effects of oral, 2.3.2.3; 5.1.2.5
Convulsions in infants, 2.5.10.1
Cornell Medical Index, 2.2.2.2; 2.5.23
Coronary artery disease, 1.7.6; 6.2.5.2
Coronary heart disease, 2.1.2; 2.2.2.2; 2.5.9; 2.5.25
Coroner's autopsy data, 2.1.2
Corticosteroid drugs, 5.1.2.8
Cost of hospital drugs, 4.5.1; 5.5.2
Cost of pregnancy, 2.5.10.1
Costs, Community Health Services, 5.3
Costs, dental, 5.2.2
Costs, Northern Ireland prescribing, 4.5.1
Costs, prescribing, 4.5.1; 6.2.4.2
Costs, School Health Service, 5.3
Council for the Education and Training of Health Visitors, 4.3.2; 4.3.3
Court Committee, 2.3.1; 4.1.5; 5.3.3; 7.3.2.3
Critical number of beds, 4.1.2
CSO survey control unit, 1.10.4
Cyanotic attack, 2.5.10.1

Davies kit, 6.2.3
Day centres, 4.1.3
Day hospitals, 4.1.3
Day hospitals, geriatric, 5.7.1
Day hospitals, psychiatric, 5.7.2
Day patients, mental illness, 5.7.2
Deafness, 2.5.11
Death under anaesthetic, 2.5.22
Definition of need, 2.1
Degrees, higher medical and surgical, 4.2.5
Delay in referral to hospital, 3.1; 3.2; 5.4.3.2; 7.2.1.2
Delay in seeking care, 6.2.3
Dental clinic, school, 5.2.1
Dental costs, 5.2.2
Dental Estimates Board, 4.2.3; 5; 5.2.2
Dental health, 2.5.12; 5.2; 6.2.5.2
Dental health of children, 5.2.1
Dental hygienists, 5.2.2
Dental manpower, 4.2
Dental practitioners, 4.2.3; 5.2
Dental services, 5.2
Dental services, use of, 5.2.1
Dental surgery assistants, 5.2.2
Dentists, junior hospital, 4.2.5
Dentists, private, 5.2.2
Dentists' workload, 5.2.2
Denver development screening test, 2.5.10.1
Depression, 2.5.23
Deputizing services, general practitioner, 5.1.2.4
Designated area allowance, 4.2.4
Development screening test, Denver, 2.5.10.1

DHSS, 1.4.3; 2.2.1.2
Diabetes, 2.5.13
Diagnostic departments, hospital, 5.5
Diagnostic Index E-book, 2.3.2.2
Diagnostic procedures, evaluation of, 6.2.4.1
Diary records, 2.1.1
Diary records, general practitioner, 5.1.2.6
Diary records, health visitors', 4.3.3
Dietary intake, 1.7.2; 2.5.25
Dietary surveys, 2.5.25
Dietitians, 4.4
Direct-access investigation, 3.1; 5.1.2.7
Directories, health service, 5.6.6
Directory, the Medical, 4.2; 4.2.1; 4.2.8
Distribution of medical manpower, 4.2.4
Distribution of resources, 4; 6.2.1
District community physician, 1.4.4; 4.2.1
District management team, 1.4.4
District Nursing, Queen's Institute of, 4.3.2; 4.3.4
Doctor index, 4.2; 4.2.4; 4.2.6
Doctors' careers, women, 4.2.5; 4.2.8
Doctors, junior hospital, 4.2.5
Doctors, student, 4.2.7
Domestic accidents, 2.5.2
Drinking habits, 2.5.3; 2.5.8
Drug abuse, 2.5.3
Drug reactions, adverse, 2.2.1.2; 2.5.4; 6.2.5.2
Drug taking, 2.5.3; 5.6.5.2
Drugs, anti-depressant, 5.1.2.8
Drugs, anti-diabetic, 5.1.2.8
Drugs, barbiturate, 5.1.2.8
Drugs, chloramphenicol, 5.1.2.8
Drugs, corticosteroid, 5.1.2.8
Drugs, cost of hospital, 4.5.1; 5.5.2
Drugs, hypnotic, 5.1.2.8
Drugs, psychotropic, 5.1.2.8
Drugs, thyroid, 5.1.2.8
Dual-record systems, 7.3.1.5
Duodenal ulcer, 2.2.2.4
Duty of junior doctors, hours of, 4.2.5

Economic evaluation of care, 6.2.5.4
Economics, Office of Health, 7.4
Education Authority, Local, 1.4.3
Educational Research, National Foundation for, 2.5.10.5; 4.2.7
Educationally subnormal children, 2.5.10.5; 2.5.24
Effects of oral contraceptives, 2.3.2.3; 5.1.2.5
Elderly, 2.5.14
Elderly, Panel on Nutrition of the, 2.5.25
Electrocardiogram, 1.7.2; 1.7.5; 2.2.2.2; 5.1.2.7
Emergency admission, 3.4
Emergency Bed Service, 3.4; 5.6.3
Emergency Obstetric Services, 5.8; 6.2.6
Emigration of doctors, 4.2.5; 4.2.6
Environmental pollution, 2.5.15
Epilepsy, 2.5.16
Errors, measurement, 2.1.1
Errors, random, 1.7.2; 2.1.1
European Economic Community, 1.10.3
Evaluation of care, economic, 6.2.5.4
Evaluation of diagnostic procedures, 6.2.4.1

Evaluation of outcome of care, 6.2.5
Evaluation of psychiatric services, 6.2.6
Evaluation of treatment, 6.2.4.1
Excerpta Medica, 1.10.1
Executive Council, 1.4.3
Expectation of life, 2.1.2
Expenditure on private care, 3.6
Eye clinic, school, 5.3.3
Eye disease, 2.5.17

Facilities for care, 6.2.2
Failure to keep appointments, 6.2.3
Faith healer, 3
Family Expenditure Survey, 2.2.1.2; 3.6
Family planning, 2.5.18; 5.1.2.5; 5.3; 6.2.3
Family Practitioner Committee, 5.1.2
Fear of cancer, 6.2.3
Fees, general practitioner, 5.1.2
Feet, 2.5.19
First national morbidity study, 2.3.2; 2.3.2.1; 7.3.2.1
Fluoridation, 6.2.5.2
Food Policy, Committee on Medical Aspects of, 2.5.25
Food Survey, National, 2.5.25
Formulary, British National, 4.5.1
FPC Index, 5.1.2
Functional disability, 2.2.2.4
Functioning of out-patient services, 2.2.2.3; 5.4.3.1

General Health Services Board, Northern Ireland, 4; 4.2.3
General Household Survey, 1.7.3; 2.2.1.2; 2.5.6; 3.3; 5.1.1; 5.3.1; 5.4.1; 5.6.1; 7.3.2.1
General Medical Council, 4.2; 4.2.6; 4.2.8
General Nursing Council, 4.3.8
General practice, 3.1; 5.1
General practice data, 2.3.2; 2.3.2.1; 2.3.2.2; 2.3.2.3; 5.1.2; 5.1.2.1
General practice in Northern Ireland, 5.1.2.1
General practice nurses, 4.3.7
General practice records, 2.3.2; 2.3.2.1; 2.3.2.2; 5.1.2
General practitioner, 4.2.4
General practitioner attitudes, 5.1.2.1
General practitioner, consultation with, 2.2.1.2; 5.1.2
General practitioner deputizing services, 5.1.2.4
General practitioner diary records, 5.1.2.6
General practitioner fees, 5.1.2
General practitioner hospitals, 4.1.4; 5.6.4
General practitioner investigations, 5.1.2.7
General practitioner list size, 4.2.4
General practitioner mobility, 4.2.4
General practitioner prescribing habits, 4.5.1; 5.1.2.8; 6.2.4.2
General practitioner previous medical experience, 4.2.4
General practitioner receptionists, 5.1.2.3
General practitioner referral, 5.1.2.7; 5.1.2.9; 5.4.3.1
General practitioner services, use of, 5.1.1
General practitioner use of pathology, 5.1.2.7

General practitioner use of radiology, 5.1.2.7
General practitioner working time, 5.1.2.2
General practitioner workload, 5.1.2
General Practitioners, Royal College of, 2.3.2;
    2.3.2.1; 2.3.2.2; 2.5.13; 4.1.4; 4.3.2; 5.1.2
Genito-urinary disease, 2.5.20
Geriatric day hospitals, 5.7.1
Geriatric hospitals, 4.1.3
Glaucoma, 2.2.2.2; 2.5.17
Goitre, 2.2.2.2
Government publications, indexes to, 1.10.3
Graduates, careers of medical, 4.2.5
Greater London Council, 1.4.3
Group interview, 2.1.1
Group practice allowance, 5.1.2.1
Group practices, 5.1.2.1
Guide to official statistics, 1.10.2
Gymnasts, remedial, 4.4
Gynaecology services, 5.1.2.5

Haematological measures, accuracy of, 1.7.5
Halothane anaesthesia, 6.2.5.2
Halsbury Committee, 4.3.5; 4.4
Handicapped, 1.7.2; 2.1.2; 2.5.21
Handicapped children, 2.5.10.5
Handicapped children, mentally, 2.5.24
Handicapped, private consultation by, 3.6
Headaches, 2.2.2.2
Health agencies' records, 5.3.1
Health and Social Services Board, Northern Ireland,
    4; 5.6.6
Health centre treatment room, 5.4.2
Health centre usage, 2.2.1.2
Health centres, 4.1.5; 4.3.7; 5.1.2.1; 5.3; 7.3.2.3
Health Examination Survey, 2.1.1
Health indexes, clearing house of, 2.1
Health information system, 7.1; 7.2; 7.3
Health Interview Survey, 2.1.1
Health Service Directories, 5.6.6
Health Status Index, 2.1
Health Symptoms Index, 6.2.5.3
Health visitors, 4.3.2; 4.3.3; 5.3
Health Visitors, Council for the Education and
    Training of, 4.3.2; 4.3.3
Health visitors' diary records, 4.3.3
Hearing aids, use of, 6.2.3
Hearing test, STYCAR, 2.5.10.1
Heart disease, coronary, 2.1.2; 2.2.2.2; 2.5.9; 2.5.25
Heart disease, ischaemic, 2.2.2.2
Height of children, 2.5.26
Helpers to professions supplementary to medicine,
    4.4
Herbalist, 3
Hernia, 6.2.5.2
High blood pressure, 1.7.4
Higher medical and surgical degrees, 4.2.5
Home nurses, 4.3.4; 5.3
Home visits, 3.1; 5.1.2.1; 5.1.2.6
Hospital activity analysis, 5.4.3.1; 5.6.2
Hospital Advisory Service, 6.2.6
Hospital Consultants and Specialists Association,
    4.2.5

Hospital dentists, junior, 4.2.5
Hospital diagnostic departments, 5.5
Hospital doctors, junior, 4.2.5
Hospital in-patient enquiry, 1.4.3; 2.3.3; 5.6.2
Hospital management committee, 1.4.3
Hospital morbidity data, 2.1.2; 2.3.3
Hospital nurses, 4.3.5
Hospital pharmacies, 5.5.2
Hospital pharmacy staffing, 4.4
Hospitalization rate, 5.6.1
Hours of duty of junior doctors, 4.2.5
Hypertension, 2.2.2.2; 2.5.9
Hypnotic drugs, 5.1.2.8

Illegitimate children, 2.5.10.1
Immunization, 5.1.2; 7.2.1.5
Inappropriate care, 3.5
Income from private practice, 3.6
Index, Cornell Medical, 2.2.2.2; 2.5.23
Index, doctor, 4.2; 4.2.4; 4.2.6
Index, FPC, 5.1.2
Index, Health Status, 2.1
Index, Health Symptoms, 6.2.5.3
Index Medicus, 1.10.3
Index, Science Citation, 1.10.3
Indexes, clearing house of health, 2.1
Indexes to government publications, 1.10.3
Indexes to research in progress, 1.10.4
Indicator of well-being, 6.2.5.2
Industrial therapy in mental illness hospitals, 5.6.5.2
Infancy, 2.5.10.3
Infancy, sudden death in, 2.5.10.3
Infant mortality, 2.1.2; 2.5.10.3
Infant welfare clinic, 2.3.1
Infants, cardiac arrest in, 2.5.10.1
Infants, cerebral irritations in, 2.5.10.1
Infants, convulsions in, 2.5.10.1
Infectious disease, 2.1.2
Infectious disease, reporting of, 5.1.2
Influenza epidemic, 2.2.1.1
Information requirements, planners', 7.2.2
Information System, Health, 7.1; 7.2; 7.3
Information systems, management requirements
    from, 7.2
Inheritance of arterial blood pressure, 2.2.2.2
Initial practices allowance, 4.2.4
In-patient data, non-psychiatric, 5.6.2
In-patient services, 5.6
In-patient services, use of, 5.6.1
In-patients' day, 6.2.5.3
Institute of Child Health, 2.5.26
Institute of Municipal Treasurers and Accountants,
    4.1.1; 4.1.5; 4.3.2; 5.3
Insurance company records, 2.1.2
International Agency for Research on Cancer,
    1.10.3
International classification of disease, 2.3.2.1;
    2.3.2.2
Interpretation of data, 1.7.9
Interpretation of X-rays, 1.7.5
Interview, group, 2.1.1
Interview survey, health, 2.1.1

Interviewers, 1.7.3
Intra-ocular pressure, 2.2.2.2
Investigations, general practitioner, 5.1.2.7
Iron therapy, oral, 2.2.2.2
Iron-deficiency anaemia, 2.2.2.2
Ischaemic heart disease, 2.2.2.2

Junior doctors, hours of duty of, 4.2.5
Junior hospital dentists, 4.2.5
Junior hospital doctors, 4.2.5
Junior hospital doctors' staffing requirements, 4.2.5

Kidney function, 2.2.2.2

Labour, 2.5.10.1
Lambeth, 2.2.2.4
Leisure activity, 1.7.2
Library Services, Royal College of General Practitioners, 1.10.1
List size, general practitioner, 4.2.4
Local Education Authority, 1.4.3
Local government medical staff, 4.2.1
Local Government, Working Party on Collaboration between NHS and, 7.3
Local Health Authority, 1.4.3
Local population studies, 2.1; 2.1.1; 2.2.2
Long-stay patients, 4.1.2; 5.6.2
Long-stay psychiatric patients, 5.6.5.3

Malignant disease, 1.7.6; 2.1.2; 2.5.8
Management requirements from information systems, 7.2
Management services and statistics, specialist group on, 7.3
Mandrax, 6.2.4.1
Manpower, dental, 4.2
Manpower, distribution of medical, 4.2.4
Manpower, medical, 4.2
Manpower, nursing and midwifery, 4.3
Manpower, professional and technical, 4.4
Manpower sources of information, 4.2
Mass miniature radiography, 2.5.33; 5.5.1
Master patient registers, 7.3.3
Maternal mortality, 2.5.22
Maternity, 2.5.10.1; 2.5.22
Maternity and Midwifery Advisory Committee, Standing, 4.3.6
Maternity beds, 4.1.4; 4.3.6
Measurement errors, 2.1.1
Measurement of blood pressure, 1.7.2; 1.7.4; 2.1.1; 2.2.2.2
Measurement of pain, 6.2.5.2
Measurement of respiratory function, 2.2.2.2
Measurement of skinfold thickness, 1.7.4; 2.2.2.2; 2.5.26
Medical audit, 6.2.4
Medical Directory, the, 4.2; 4.2.1; 4.2.8; 5.1.2.7
Medical graduates, careers of, 4.2.5
Medical manpower, 4.2
Medical manpower, distribution of, 4.2.4
Medical Officer of Health, 1.4.3; 1.4.4; 4.2.1
Medical Officers of Health, Society of, 4.2.1; 4.3.3

Medical Practices Committee, 4.2.4
Medical Practitioners Union, 4.2.8
Medical records, 2.3.2; 2.3.2.1; 2.3.2.2; 5.1.2
Medical records, accuracy of, 2.3.2; 5.1.2
Medical Register, the 4.2; 4.2.1
Medical Research Council, 1.10.3
Medical Women's Federation, 4.2.8
Medication, side effects of, 2.5.4; 6.2.5.2
Medicine taking, 2.2.1.2; 2.2.2.2; 2.5.29; 5.1.2.8; 6.2.3
Medicines, Committee on Safety of, 6.2.5.2
MEDLARS, 1.10.3
MEDLINE, 1.10.3
Memory bias, 1.7.3; 2.1.1; 2.2.1.1; 5.3.1; 5.4.1
Mental handicap services, 5.6.5
Mental health enquiry, 2.5.23; 5.6.5
Mental illness, 2.2.2.2; 2.5.23; 5.6.5.2
Mental illness day patients, 5.7.2
Mental illness hospitals, industrial therapy in, 5.6.5.2
Mental illness services, 5.6.5
Mental subnormality, 2.5.23; 2.5.24; 5.6.5
Mentally handicapped children, 2.5.24
Mentally handicapped patients, 5.6.5.1
Midwifery Advisory Committee, Standing Maternity and, 4.3.6
Midwifery Manpower, Nursing and, 4.3
Midwives, 4.3.6; 4.3.7; 5.3
Midwives, pay and related conditions of nurses and, 4.3.5
Migraine, 2.2.2.2
Ministry of Health, 1.4.3
Morbidity data, hospital, 2.1.2; 2.3.3
Morbidity study, first national, 2.3.2; 2.3.2.1; 7.3.2.1
Morbidity study, second national, 2.1.2; 2.2.1.2; 2.3.2.2; 5.1.2.1; 5.1.2.9; 5.3.2; 7.3.2.1
Mortality data, 2.1.2; 6.2.5.1
Mortality, infant, 2.1.2; 2.5.10.3
Mortality, maternal, 2.5.22
Mortality, neonatal, 2.5.10.1; 2.5.10.3
Mortality, perinatal, 2.5.10.1; 6.2.5.1
Mortality, post-neonatal, 2.5.10.3
Motor-cycle accidents, 2.5.2
MRC respiratory questionnaire, 2.2.2.4

National Birthday Trust, 2.5.10.1; 7.3.2.1
National Child Development Study, 2.5.10.1
National Food Survey, 2.5.25
National Foundation for Educational Research, 2.5.10.5; 4.2.7
National Insurance Certificates, 5.1.2; 5.1.2.10
National Morbidity Study, first, 2.3.2; 2.3.2.1; 7.3.2.1
National Morbidity Study, second, 2.1.2; 2.2.1.2; 2.3.2.2; 5.1.2.1; 5.1.2.9; 5.3.2; 7.3.2.1
National population studies, 2.1; 2.1.1; 2.2.1
Need, definition of, 2.1
Neonatal mortality, 2.5.10.1; 2.5.10.3
Neurotic patients, 2.5.23
Newcastle Survey of Child Development, 2.5.10.1
NHS and local government, working party on collaboration between, 7.3
NHS, organization of the, 1.4.1

NHS, reorganization of the, 1.4.1; 2.1; 5.3
NHS resources, 4
Night calls, 3.1; 5.1.2
Noise in hospitals, 6.2.5.3
Non-psychiatric in-patient data, 5.6.2
Non-response, 1.7.6
Northern Ireland annual reports, 4; 5.6.6
Northern Ireland Central Services Agency, 4
Northern Ireland General Health Services Board, 4;
    4.2.3
Northern Ireland, general practice in, 5.1.2.1
Northern Ireland Health and Social Services Board,
    4; 5.6.6
Northern Ireland Hospitals Authority, 4; 5.6.6
Northern Ireland prescribing costs, 4.5.1
Northern Ireland resources, 4
Nuffield Foundation, 5.1.2.3
Nuffield Provincial Hospitals Trust, 1.10.3; 2.3.3;
    3.3; 4.1.2; 4.2.4; 4.2.6; 4.3.4; 4.3.8; 4.4;
    5.1.2.3; 5.4.2; 5.4.3.1
Number of private patients, 3.6
Nurseries, 2.5.10.1
Nurses and midwives, pay and related conditions of,
    4.3.5
Nurses, community, 4.3.2; 5.3
Nurses, general practice, 4.3.7
Nurses, home, 4.3.4; 5.3
Nurses, hospital, 4.3.5
Nurses, overseas, 4.3.1
Nurses, State Enrolled, 4.3.4
Nurses, State Registered, 4.3.4
Nurses, student, 4.3.8
Nursing and midwifery manpower, 4.3
Nursing, Committee on, 4.3.1
Nursing, Royal College of, 4.3.1; 4.3.2
Nursing staff, senior, 4.3.5
Nutrition, 2.5.25
Nutrition of the Elderly, Panel on, 2.5.25

Obstetric care, 2.5.10.1
Obstetric services, emergency, 5.8; 6.2.6
Occupational Health Services, 1.4.5
*Occupational Health—Guide to Sources of Infor-
    mation*, 1.10.2
Occupational morbidity, 2.3.2.1
Occupational prevalence of respiratory disease,
    2.2.2.2
Occupational therapists, 4.4
Occupied beds, 3.6
Office of Health Economics, 7.4
Oral cancer, 2.5.8
Oral contraceptives, effects of, 2.3.2.3; 5.1.2.5
Oral hygiene, 2.5.12
Oral iron therapy, 2.2.2.2
Organization of out-patient departments, 5.4.3.2
Organization of the NHS, 1.4.1
Orthodontics, 5.2.2
Orthoptists, 4.4
Osteopath, 3.6
Outcome of care, evaluation of, 6.2.5
Outcome of radium treatment, 6.2.5.1
Out-patient appointments, 3.3; 5.4.3.2

Out-patient department, waiting time at, 3.3; 5.4.3;
    5.4.3.2
Out-patient departments, organization of, 5.4.3.2
Out-patient services, 5.4.3
Out-patient services, functioning of, 2.2.2.3; 5.4.3.1
Out-patient services, peripheral, 5.4.3.3
Out-patient services, psychiatric, 5.1.2.9; 5.4.3.1
Out-patient services, use of, 5.4.1
Overseas nurses, 4.3.1

Pain, measurement of, 6.2.5.2
Pain relief, 6.2.5.2
Panel on Nutrition of the Elderly, 2.5.25
Pathology, general practitioner, use of, 5.1.2.7
Pathology services, 5.5.1
Patient registers, master, 7.3.3
Patient transportation systems, 5.1.2.6
Patients' views of hospital care, 6.2.5.3
Pay and related conditions of nurses and midwives,
    4.3.5
Perinatal mortality, 2.5.10.1; 6.2.5.1
Peripheral out-patient services, 5.4.3.3
Pernicious anaemia, 2.5.7
Pharmacies, hospital, 5.5.2
Pharmacy staffing, hospital, 4.4
Physiotherapists, 4.4
Physique, 2.5.26
Planners' information requirements, 7.2.2
Play groups, 2.5.10.1
Pneumoconiosis, 1.7.6; 2.2.2.2
Pollution, environmental, 2.5.15
Population studies in South Wales, 2.2.2.2
Population studies, local, 2.1; 2.1.1; 2.2.2
Population studies, national, 2.1; 2.1.1; 2.2.1
Portfolio for health, 2, 1.10.4
Post-neonatal mortality, 2.5.10.3
Pregnancy, 2.5.10.1; 3.1; 5.1.2.1
Pregnancy, cost of, 2.5.10.1
Prescribed disease statistics, 1.4.5
Prescribing costs, 4.5.1; 6.2.4.2
Prescribing costs, Northern Ireland, 4.5.1
Prescribing habits, general practitioner, 4.5.1;
    5.1.2.8; 6.2.4.2
Prescriptions, 5.1.2; 6.2.4.1
Private care, 3; 3.6
Private care, expenditure on, 3.6
Private consultation by handicapped, 3.6
Private dentists, 5.2.2
Private patients, number of, 3.6
Private practice, income from, 3.6
Private sickness certificates, 5.1.2.10
Professional and technical manpower, 4.4
Professional and Technical Whitby Council, 4.4
Professions supplementary to medicine and speech
    therapists, 4.4
Professions supplementary to medicine, helpers to,
    4.4
Prophylactic procedures, 5.1.2.1
Psychiatric case registers, 5.6.5.3
Psychiatric day hospitals, 5.7.2
Psychiatric hospitals, 4.1.3
Psychiatric illness, 2.5.23; 5.1.2.9

Psychiatric out-patient services, 5.1.2.9; 5.4.3.1
Psychiatric referral, 5.1.2.9
Psychiatric screening, 2.5.23
Psychiatric services, 5.6.5
Psychiatric services, evaluation of, 6.2.6
Psychiatric Social Workers, Association of, 5.3.3
Psychiatry, child, 5.3.3
Psychotherapy, 3
Psychotropic drugs, 5.1.2.8
Puberty, 2.5.26
Public Accounts Committee, 6.2.5.4

Queen's Institute of District Nursing, 4.3.2; 4.3.4
Questionnaire, MRC respiratory, 2.2.2.4
Questionnaire, WHO angina, 2.2.2.4
Questionnaires, 1.7.2; 1.7.3
Questionnaires, self-completion, 1.7.3; 2.1.1
Queues for care, 3; 7.2.1.2; 7.3.2.2

Radiographers, 4.4
Radiography, 5.5.1
Radiography, mass miniature, 2.5.33; 5.5.1
Radiology, general practitioner use of, 5.1.2.7
Radiology services, 5.5.1
Radium treatment, outcome of, 6.2.5.1
Random errors, 1.7.2; 2.1.1
Receptionists, general practitioner, 5.1.2.3
Record linkage, 2.1.2; 2.5.10.2; 6.2.5.2; 7.3.3
Record systems, dual, 7.3.1.5
Records, accuracy of medical, 2.3.2
Records, ante-natal, 2.5.10.1
Records, diary, 2.1.1
Records, general practice, 2.3.2; 2.3.2.1; 2.3.2.2;
    5.1.2
Records, health agencies, 5.3.1
Records, medical, 2.3.2; 2.3.2.1; 2.3.2.2; 5.1.2
Referral, general practitioner, 5.1.2.7; 5.1.2.9;
    5.4.3.1
Referral, psychiatric, 5.1.2.9
Referral to community health services, 5.3.2
Referral to hospital, delay in, 3.1; 3.2; 5.4.3.2;
    7.2.1.2
Regional Health Authority, 1.4.4
Regional Hospital Board, 1.4.3
Register, the medical, 4.2; 4.2.1
Registers, master patient, 7.3.3
Registers, psychiatric case, 5.6.5.3
Rehabilitation, 2.5.27; 5.8
Reliability of data, 1.7.2; 1.7.3
Remedial gymnasts, 4.4
Reorganization of the NHS, 1.4.1; 2.1; 5.3
Report of Medical Officer of Health, 5.3
Reporting of age, 1.7.3
Reporting of infectious disease, 5.1.2
Research in progress, indexes to, 1.10.4
Resource allocation working party, 4
Resources, NHS, 4
Resources, Northern Ireland, 4
Respiratory disease, 1.7.6; 2.2.2.2; 2.5.28
Respiratory disease, occupational prevalence of,
    2.2.2.2

Respiratory disease, symptoms of, 1.7.2; 1.7.3;
    2.2.2.2
Respiratory function, measurement of, 2.2.2.2
Respiratory questionnaire, MRC, 2.2.2.4
Response rate, 1.7.6
Review body on doctors' and dentists' remuneration,
    4.2.4; 4.2.5
RHA annual reports, 5.6.6
RHA resources, 4
RHB annual reports, 5.6.6
Rheumatism, 2.2.2.2; 2.5.6
Rheumatoid arthritis, 2.2.2.2; 6.2.4.1
Road accidents, 2.5.3; 5.4.2
Road Research Laboratory, Traffic and, 2.5.2
Royal College of General Practitioners, 2.3.2;
    2.3.2.1; 2.3.2.2; 2.5.13; 4.1.4; 4.3.2; 5.1.2
Royal College of General Practitioners Library Ser-
    vices, 1.10.1
Royal College of Nursing, 4.3.1; 4.3.2

Satisfaction with care, 6.2.5.3
Schizophrenia, 1.7.3
School children, 2.5.10.1; 2.5.10.5; 5.3.3
School dental clinic, 5.2.1
School eye clinic, 5.3.3
School Health Service, 1.4.3; 2.5.10.1; 5.3; 5.3.3;
    7.3.2.3
School Health Service costs, 5.3
Schoolboy smoking, 2.5.31
Science Citation Index, 1.10.3
Screening, 1.7.6; 2.1; 2.1.1; 2.3.1; 2.5.7; 2.5.10.5;
    6.2.3
Screening, psychiatric, 2.5.23
Second National Morbidity Study, 2.1.2; 2.2.1.2;
    2.3.2.2; 5.1.2.1; 5.1.2.9; 5.3.2; 7.3.2.1
Self-care, 2.3.2
Self-completion questionnaires, 1.7.3; 2.1.1
Self-medication, 2.2.1.2; 2.5.29; 3; 5.1.2.8
Self-referral to hospital, 3.2
Senior nursing staff, 4.3.5
Sensitivity of test, 1.7.2
Sexually transmitted disease, 2.5.30
Side effects of medication, 2.5.4; 6.2.5.2
Size of waiting list, 3.4; 3.5
Skin disease, 2.2.2.4
Skinfold thickness, measurement of, 1.7.4; 2.2.2.2;
    2.5.26
Smoking habits, 1.7.3; 1.7.6; 2.2.1.2; 2.2.2.2; 2.5.3;
    2.5.31
Smoking, schoolboy, 2.5.31
Social Science Research Council, 1.10.3; 1.10.5
Social security data, 2.4; 6.2.5.2
Social services, use of health and personal, 2.2.1.2
Social Workers, Association of Psychiatric, 5.3.3
Society of County Treasurers, 4.1.1; 4.1.5; 4.3.2; 5.3
Society of Medical Officers of Health, 4.2.1; 4.3.3
Sources of official data, 1.10.2
Sources of social statistics, 1.10.2
South Wales, population studies in, 2.2.2.2
Southwark, Bermondsey and, 2.2.2.3
Specialist group on management services and statis-
    tics, 7.3

Specialist in community medicine, 1.4.4
Specialists Association, Hospital Consultants and, 4.2.5
Specificity of test, 1.7.2
Speech therapists, professions supplementary to medicine and, 4.4
Spina bifida, 6.2.5.2
Sputum cytology, 5.5.1
SSRC survey archive, 1.10.5
Standing Maternity and Midwifery Advisory Committee, 4.3.6
State Enrolled Nurses, 4.3.4
State Registered Nurses, 4.3.4
Statistics, Specialist Group on Management Services and, 7.3
Sterilization, 5.1.2.5
Stillbirth, 2.5.10.1; 2.5.10.3
Stroke, acute, 2.1.2
Student doctors, 4.2.7
Student nurses, 4.3.8
Study design, 1.7.1
STYCAR hearing test, 2.5.10.1
STYCAR vision test, 2.5.10.1
Subnormal children, educationally, 2.5.10.5; 2.5.24
Subnormality, mental, 2.5.23; 2.5.24; 5.6.5
Sudden death in infancy, 2.5.10.3
Suicide, 2.2.2.2; 2.5.3; 2.5.23
Survey control unit, CSO, 1.10.4
Survey of sickness, 1.7.3; 2.2.1.1; 2.2.1.2
Survival data, 6.2.5.1
Symptoms index, health, 6.2.5.3
Symptoms of respiratory disease, 1.7.2; 1.7.3; 2.2.2.2
Systolic blood pressure, 2.2.2.2

Teaching hospitals, 1.4.3
Technical manpower, professional and, 4.4
Technical Whitby Council, Professional and, 4.4
Terminal care, 2.5.32
Thalidomide, 6.2.5.2
The Medical Directory, 4.2; 4.2.1; 4.2.8; 5.1.2.7
The Medical Register, 4.2; 4.2.1
Thyroid drugs, 5.1.2.8
Time on waiting list, 3.3; 3.4; 5.4.3.2; 7.2.1.2
Time spent in hospital, 5.6.2
Tobacco consumption, 2.2.1.2
Traffic and Road Research Laboratory, 2.5.2
Tranquillizers, 5.1.2.8
Transportation systems, patient, 5.1.2.6
Treatment, evaluation of, 6.2.4.1
Treatment room, health centre, 5.4.2
Tuberculosis, 1.7.6; 2.3.1; 2.5.33
Tuberculosis dispensaries, 5.4.3.3
Tuberculosis visitors, 4.3.3; 5.3
Tuberculosis dispensaries, 5.4.3.3
Tuberculosis visitors, 4.3.3; 5.3

Ulcer, duodenal, 2.2.2.4
Unemployment of married women doctors, 4.2.5
Urinary disease, 2.2.2.2; 2.5.20
Use of accident and emergency services, 5.4.1
Use of acute beds, 5.6.2; 6.2.4.1
Use of beds, 2.3.3
Use of community health services, 5.3.1
Use of dental services, 5.2.1
Use of general practitioner services, 5.1.1
Use of health and personal social services, 2.2.1.2
Use of hearing aids, 6.2.3
Use of in-patient services, 5.6.1
Use of out-patient services, 5.4.1
Utilization, WHO International Collaborative Study of Medical Care, 5.1.1

Vaccination, 5.1.2
Validity of data, 1.7.2; 1.7.3; 1.7.9; 2.1.1
Varicose veins, 2.2.2.2
Venepuncture, 2.2.2.2
Vision test, STYCAR, 2.5.10.1
Visiting hours, 6.2.5.3
Vitamin D intake, 2.5.25

Waiting list, size of, 3.4; 3.5
Waiting list, time on, 3.3; 3.4; 5.4.3.2; 7.2.1.2
Waiting lists, 4.1.2
Waiting time at out-patient department, 3.3; 5.4.3; 5.4.3.2
Waiting time at surgery, 3.1; 5.1.2.3
Weight of children, 2.5.26
Welfare milk, 2.5.25
Well-being, indicator of, 6.2.5.2
Whitby Council, Professional and Technical, 4.4
WHO angina questionnaire, 2.2.2.4
WHO International Collaborative Study of Medical Care Utilization, 5.1.1
Women doctors' careers, 4.2.5; 4.2.8
Women's Federation, Medical, 4.2.8
Work study projects, 1.3
Working Party on Collaboration between NHS and Local Government, 7.3
Working time, general practitioner, 5.1.2.2
Workload, dentists', 5.2.2
Workload, general practitioner, 5.1.2
World Health Organization, 2.1

X-ray data, 2.2.2.2
X-ray departments, 5.5.1
X-rays, interpretation of, 1.7.5

Young chronic sick, 2.5.21.1